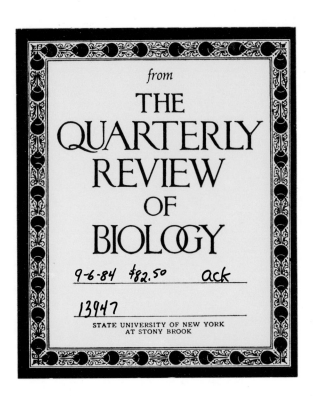

from

THE
QUARTERLY
REVIEW
OF
BIOLOGY

9-6-84 $82.50   ack

13947

STATE UNIVERSITY OF NEW YORK
AT STONY BROOK

CENTRAL NERVOUS SYSTEM PHARMACOLOGY

ANALGESICS: NEUROCHEMICAL, BEHAVIORAL, AND
CLINICAL PERSPECTIVES

Central Nervous System Pharmacology

Editor-in-Chief: S. J. Enna, Ph.D.

Antidepressants: Neurochemical, Behavioral, and Clinical Perspectives
S. J. Enna, Jeffrey B. Malick, and Elliott Richelson, editors, 1981.

Anxiolytics: Neurochemical, Behavioral, and Clinical Perspectives
Jeffrey P. Malick, S. J. Enna, and Henry I. Yamamura, editors, 1983.

Neuroleptics: Neurochemical, Behavioral, and Clinical Perspectives
Joseph T. Coyle and S. J. Enna, editors, 1983.

Stimulants: Neurochemical, Behavioral, and Clinical Perspectives
Ian Creese, editor, 1983.

Analgesics: Neurochemical, Behavioral, and Clinical Perspectives
Michael J. Kuhar and Gavril W. Pasternak, editor, 1984.

Hallucinogens: Neurochemical, Behavioral, and Clinical Perspectives
Barry L. Jacobs, editor, 1984.

Central Nervous System Pharmacology

Analgesics: Neurochemical, Behavioral, and Clinical Perspectives

Volume Editors

Michael J. Kuhar, Ph.D.
*Professor of Neuroscience, Pharmacology
and Psychiatry
Johns Hopkins University School
of Medicine
Baltimore, Maryland*

**Gavril W. Pasternak,
M.D., Ph.D.**
*Associate Professor of Neurology
and Pharmacology
Memorial Sloan-Kettering Cancer Center
and Cornell University Medical College
New York, New York*

Raven Press ■ New York

Raven Press, 1140 Avenue of the Americas, New York, New York 10036

Made in the United States of America

Library of Congress Cataloging in Publication Data

Main entry under title:
Analgesics: neurochemical, behavioral, and clinical
   perspectives.

   (Central nervous system pharmacology series;)
   Includes bibliographical references and index.
   1. Analgesics. I. Kuhar, Michael J. II. Pasternak,
Gavril, W. III. Series. [DNLM: 1. Analgesics. QV 95
A5315]
RM319.A518   1984
      615'.783   84-3437
ISBN 0-89004-793-6

Preface

Pain remains one of the most difficult and widespread problems in medicine, a problem which confronts virtually all physicians regardless of their particular sub-specialty. Both the clinical assessment and management of pain is difficult. It requires a knowledge of mechanisms of pain and an understanding of the drugs used in its treatment, as well as a commitment to the patient. Opiates have remained the mainstay of pain management for hundreds and probably thousands of years. However, their use has a price which includes tolerance, physical dependence, respiratory depression, constipation, and sedation. In the 10 years since the demonstration of opiate receptors and the subsequent discovery of the vast family of opioid peptides, our knowledge of opioid actions has expanded greatly. In addition to opioid-related drugs, some nonopioid compounds have been found which are analgesic. Recent years have also seen the development of a number of novel peripherally-acting drugs. While most of these agents have ceiling effects which appear to limit their use in very severe pain, the absence of tolerance and physical dependence makes them quite important clinically. We have made a special effort to have all of this new information included in this volume. We have attempted to bring together both the basic mechanisms and clinical use of both opiate and nonopiate analgesics to help scientists and clinicians in their understanding of the actions of these agents and hopefully, to provide information which could be used in new drug development. We have also included material on the evaluation of these agents in man and animals so that the properties of potentially new and useful drugs can be compared with those in existence.

This book will be of interest to a wide range of basic and clinical scientists studying analgesics. The book includes practical information which would be helpful both in the development of new analgesics, as well as in the testing and comparison of various analgesics.

Gavril Pasternak, M.D., Ph.D.
Michael J. Kuhar, Ph.D.

Acknowledgments

The editors are grateful to the authors for their individual contributions, to Dr. Ray Houde, to Dr. Sam Enna for his helpful suggestions, to Darlene Weimer, and especially Mary Flutka for editorial assistance.

Contents

Contributors

Eugene R. Baizman, Ph.D.
Senior Research Biologist
Department of Pharmacology
Sterling-Winthrop Research Institute
Columbia Turnpike
Rensselaer, New York 12144

Allan I. Basbaum, Ph.D.
Associate Professor
Department of Anatomy
University of California, San Francisco
San Francisco, California 94143

Kay Brune, M.D.
Professor of Pharmacology
Institute of Pharmacology and Toxicology
University of Erlangen-Nürnberg
Universitatsstrasse 22
D-8520 Erlangen, West Germany

Kathleen M. Foley, M.D.
Associate Attending Neurologist
Department of Neurology
Memorial Sloan-Kettering Cancer Center
1275 York Avenue
New York, New York 10021

Robert C. A. Frederickson, M.D., Ph.D.
Research Associate
Lilly Research Laboratories
Eli Lilly and Company
307 E. McCarty Street
Indianapolis, Indiana 46285

Robert R. Goodman, M.D., Ph.D.
Resident in Neurosurgery
Department of Surgery
Columbia-Presbyterian Medical Center
W. 168th Street
New York, New York 10032

Dean R. Haubrich, Ph.D.
Section Head, Neuropsychopharmacology
Department of Pharmacology
Sterling-Winthrop Research Institute
Columbia Turnpike
Rensselaer, New York 12144

Charles E. Inturrisi, Ph.D.
Professor
Department of Pharmacology
Cornell University Medical College
New York, New York 10021

Thomas G. Kantor, M.D.
Professor of Clinical Medicine
New York University Medical Center
Department of Medicine
550 First Avenue
New York, New York 10016

Riní Lanz, Ph.D.
Post-Doctoral Fellow
Institute of Pharmacology and Toxicology
University of Erlangen-Nürnberg
Universitatsstrasse 22
D-8520 Erlangen, West Germany

Louis Lasagna, M.D.
Professor
Department of Pharmacology
University of Rochester
School of Medicine and Dentistry
Rochester, New York 14642

William F. Michne, Ph.D.
Section Head
Medicinal Chemistry Department
Sterling-Winthrop Research Institute
Rensselaer, New York 12144

Barry A. Morgan, Ph.D.
Group Leader
Medicinal Chemistry Department
Sterling-Winthrop Research Institute
Columbia Turnpike
Rensselaer, New York 12144

Gavril W. Pasternak, M.D., Ph.D.
Associate Professor of Neurology and
*   Pharmacology*
Department of Neurology
Memorial Sloan-Kettering Cancer Center
*   and Cornell University Medical*
*   College*
1275 York Avenue
New York, New York 10021

Jeffrey K. Saelens, Ph.D.
Departmental Director
Department of Pharmacology
Sterling-Winthrop Research Institute
Columbia Turnpike
Rensselaer, New York 12144

Stanley L. Wallenstein, M.S.
Assistant Member
Sloan-Kettering Institute for Cancer
*   Research*
New York, New York 10021

E. Leong Way, Ph.D.
Professor
Department of Pharmacology
University of California, San Francisco
San Francisco, California 94143

Paul L. Wood
Neuroscience Research
CIBA-GEIGY
Summit, New Jersey 07901

Analgesics: Neurochemical, Behavioral, and Clinical Perspectives, edited by M. Kuhar and G. Pasternak. Raven Press, New York © 1984.

Historical Overview

Louis Lasagna

Department of Pharmacology, University of Rochester, School of Medicine and Dentistry, Rochester, New York 14642

There were two key forces in the evolution of analgesic testing in the United States—the Committee on Drug Addiction and Narcotics and Henry K. Beecher.

In 1929, the National Academy of Sciences (NAS)/National Research Council (NRC) set up a program to discover a nonaddicting substitute for morphine (11). At first the program was funded by grants from the Rockefeller Foundation and the Bureau of Social Hygiene in New York City. Later, funds were donated by a number of pharmaceutical companies and distributed by the NAS/NRC Committee on Drug Addiction and Narcotics, which was later to evolve into the now free-standing Committee on Problems of Drug Dependence.

This program was important for several reasons. First, it provided an identifiable motivating force and research support umbrella. Second, it was able not only to achieve a "marriage" between investigators (both in industry and academia) and drugs deserving investigation, but to arrange for the addiction liability testing of promising drugs both at the primate facility at the University of Michigan and at the clinical testing facility at the Addiction Research Center in Lexington, Kentucky. Third, the program supported methodologic research, which was badly needed at that time. Such research had never had a high priority at the National Institutes of Health, so that NAS/NRC support was crucial for the evaluation of the testing methods (both animal and human) which have now become routine. Finally, the NAS/NRC program provided for annual meetings that brought together everyone who was actively toiling in the analgesic vineyard, with up-to-date presentations of research in progress, in a lively atmosphere of free exchange and criticism that was as pleasant as it was instructive. Many of us still recall those old days with nostalgia. The only drawback to these meetings was the nonarchival nature of the proceedings of the Committee. For those who were present at the meetings and were recipients of the reports, there was no great problem. Much of the information presented orally or in writing at these meetings, however, only appeared as published minutes, and was therefore lost to the world at large.

The second key force was Henry K. Beecher, Henry Isaiah Dorr Professor of Research in Anesthesia and Head of the Anesthesia Laboratory of the Harvard Medical School at the Massachusetts General Hospital (MGH) in Boston, Massachusetts. Beecher, having received an M.S. in Chemistry at Kansas University,

I

took his medical training at the Harvard Medical School. His scientific and personal home then became Boston. Having started out as a surgical housestaff officer, Beecher became a protégé of Dr. Edward D. Churchill, Professor of Surgery at Harvard and Head of the Surgical Service at MGH. Beecher then spent an academic leave in the laboratory of August Krogh at the University of Copenhagen. Krogh, who had won the Nobel Prize in Physiology and Medicine in 1920 for his work on the regulation of capillary blood supply in muscle, combined research interests in respiration and circulation, an ideal background for the future anesthesiologist. On Beecher's return to Boston, he was made Chief of Anesthesia at MGH.

Although such figures as Crawford Long, Horace Wells, and W. T. G. Morton deserve great credit, Beecher probably ranks as the most colorful and innovative scientist in American anesthesiology. Certainly he was without peer in 20th century anesthesiology.

As a surgeon, Beecher had ample opportunity to appreciate the need of patients to be free of pain not only during surgery, but also afterward. During World War II, he was involved in the planning of medical services for United States troops in Italy. He was impressed by the instances of opiate poisoning resulting from the use of Syrettes by corpsmen on the battlefield, and by the difference between wounded servicemen and injured civilians in their requests for pain relievers.

These Syrettes contained 30 mg of morphine, a large individual dose by any standard. The injured GIs were often in a condition of shock or near shock. Hence, subcutaneous or intramuscular morphine was often not well absorbed. In the face of inadequate pain relief, repeated doses of morphine were administered to these men. Then, as the patients reached facilities where parenteral fluids or plasma were available, their circulatory status improved, and the large doses of morphine were suddenly absorbed from what had inadvertently become "depot" injections. As a result, classical opiate poisoning resulted, with impaired consciousness, depressed respiration, and pinpoint pupils (1). These poisonings were at times fatal.

Beecher's observation, that wounded GIs were less likely to complain of pain than civilians suffering from injury of similar severity, made him curious about the possible role of psychological factors in the modification of pain (4,6). He hypothesized that for a civilian, injury was almost invariably disastrous, whereas for a soldier, injury was possibly a blessing, because it could mean a departure (temporary or permanent) from the battlefield, where death was ever a serious possibility. In fact, an examination of the data in Beecher's paper leaves one in doubt about the fact; the soldiers did indeed want a narcotic less often, but most seemed to have received a prior dose (usually large) of morphine, whose effects may still have been manifested at the time of the interview. Nevertheless, the Beecher hypothesis was typical of the man in its imagination and drama, and predictive of much to come.

Although Beecher ultimately became quite interested in the psychophysics of pain, he did not, to my knowledge, have much contact with colleagues at Harvard University, such as S. S. Stevens, editor of the *Handbook of Experimental Psychol-*

ogy, who had analogous interests in the quantification of the intensity of sound and light.

What did become a focus of Beecher's thinking was his conviction that experimental pain in humans (as opposed to animals) was not particularly useful for evaluating analgesics. In theory, the ability to control irrelevant variables should make the laboratory a splendid venue for such purposes. Certainly there was no dearth of stimuli and techniques suggested and applied by different investigators: thermal (both hot and cold), mechanical, chemical, ischemic, etc. Tourniquets were applied to extremities to induce pain, biliary trees were distended by hydrostatic distension through indwelling T-tubes, electric shocks were applied, and hypertonic saline was injected into muscles.

At one point, Beecher himself was co-author of a paper that described the successful use of the Hardy-Woolf-Goodell technique (shining radiant heat at a blackened spot on the forehead) to quantify the analgesic power of nitrous oxide (7). Hardy and his colleagues were prolific researchers, and argued that individuals varied remarkably little in their threshold for pain (10), an idea that was later rejected by Beecher, at least in so far as it pertained to clinical situations.

However, when Beecher tried to repeat the early success of his own colleagues in subsequent studies, utilizing double-blind controls, he was no longer able to detect reproducibly the effectiveness of clinically useful doses of morphine. He began to suspect that the Hardy-Woolf-Goodell team, who seemed often to serve as their own experimental subjects, had been misled by their failure to use appropriately stringent controls.

It is perhaps worth recounting that Beecher did not deny the utility of animal testing in the laboratory. He believed that for animals, "stress" was present in experimental pain, whereas this was not true, or the stress was significantly less, for human subjects. He was aware that many drugs had been successfully picked for human trial by rodent testing, although it was obvious that conventional tests in animals failed to pick up salicylates with any ease. Later on, with the failure of the standard tests to anticipate the analgesic potency of nalorphine, it became clear that new tests were also needed at the animal level.

In C. A. Strong, Beecher found just the theoretician he wanted (19). In 1895, Strong had published his notion that pain had two components—sensation and reaction. Beecher reasoned that in clinical pain, reaction was more important than sensation in determining the amount of distress. Thus, the psychological reverberation set in motion by central perception of noxious stimuli could vary significantly from person to person. This construct not only fit in with the obviously great difference between the postoperative course of different people after a standard operation, but with the effect of placebos and the data of Beecher referred to above.

Parenthetically, late in his career, Beecher and his psychologist colleague Gene Smith successfully employed ischemic tourniquet pain to evaluate analgesics of various kinds. Beecher seemingly had no difficulty accepting these results from his own laboratory, despite years of blistering attacks on the uselessness of experimental pain in humans (12).

Beecher was impressed with the evolving methodology for controlled trials, including the need for blinding of both observer and patient, the use of placebos, and the statistical analysis of data. (To help in this last regard, Beecher added, as a part-time staff member, the distinguished statistician Fred Mosteller of Harvard University.) One ingredient that he was less concerned with was randomization. For most, if not all, of his analgesic testing career, simple alternation of treatments was used. It is of interest that the results of his experiments were invariably validated in replications by other investigators, despite this lack of strictly randomized allocation of patients to the treatments under study.

Harry Gold of Cornell, an early pioneer in control trial methodology and a student of the placebo response, was highly esteemed by Beecher, who ultimately became very much interested in what he dubbed "the powerful placebo (5)."

Many collaborators worked closely and sequentially with Beecher over several decades, each one contributing to the development of analgesimetry. The list included, among others, Jane E. Denton, Arthur Keats, J. M. Von Felsinger, Louis Lasagna, and Joachim S. Gravenstein.

The early years were not without error. In the first work with Denton, for example, Beecher was convinced that 8 mg of morphine was the maximum dose needed for any patient in pain (8). In retrospect, this was owing to the inclusion in these early studies of patients with operations now recognized as generating little pain on average, and responding well to modest doses of drugs. Later, such patients were not included in analgesic trials. There was also an exaggerated emphasis on the importance of the crossover technique. Beecher argued that since pain was such a personal and internal phenomenon, the only way to accurately and fairly compare two treatments was to give them successively to the same patient. The trouble with this approach is that postoperative pain is waning with time, so the challenge to the second treatment is not necessarily equal to the challenge to the first. Today, parallel studies (i.e., noncrossover) are usually favored over crossover by most investigators and drug companies.

Beecher's use of 24 hr coverage by interviewers may or may not have been a mistake. It certainly introduced a new variable, i.e., different interviewers for the same patient. It did allow studies to be completed more expeditiously. Today, for logistic purposes only, most investigators employ one technician and do not collect data during the night hours.

A serious deficiency was the absence of informed consent procedures, especially paradoxical in view of Beecher's later diatribes against other investigators for similar ethical lapses (2). (He never publicly admitted his own sins.) Patients were not asked whether they wished to participate in Beecher's experiments, whether an old drug was being used, a new one, or placebos. Such a strategy made the studies easier and quicker to perform, but I do not believe that this was the reason for selecting this approach. Rather, I believe it was owing to a simple failure of imagination and to the spirit of the times. Most investigators in those years did not seem to consider seriously the possibility that patients might want to know (or should know) that they were a part of an experiment. Beecher did, to be sure, argue with justification that patients in his studies were often better off than patients who were not. Not only were the experimental subjects interviewed hourly as to their discomfort, but they ended up requiring, on average, fewer doses of drugs than did other patients. (Since patients on the private service were never used for these studies, Beecher quipped that he now knew why rich patients had poor appetites, and that although the rich shouldn't have better care than the poor, they shouldn't have worse.)

Beecher's preoccupation with crossover studies probably helps to explain why he never considered the possibility that patients should be allocated to treatments on the basis of their initial pain level, i.e., the treatments should have equal exposure to patients with severe pain, moderate pain, etc. Today, many people believe that stratified randomization improves the power of analgesic studies.

At first, Beecher's laboratory relied on questions such as "Is your pain more or less than half gone?" Later, his associates adopted the use of ordinal scales for various levels of pain severity (0 for none, 1 for mild, 2 for moderate, 3 for severe, etc.). Statistical analysis of such data assumed that the intervals between pain levels were of equal importance, despite some evidence of the contrary (15).

Beecher and his colleagues, while at an early stage using set criteria for deciding whether a given dose was "effective" or not (using speed of effect, duration, etc.), never asked patients for a global assessment of the medication. This may have been forced by Beecher's technique of alternating treatments, because such exposure would make it impossible for patients to make judgments, especially because they were even unaware that different drugs were being administered. Today, investigators often add global assessments, with the patient being asked to describe an analgesic as "excellent," "good," "fair," or "poor." The single dose parallel design makes this eminently feasible. There is no attempt made usually to get the patient to explain the basis of the evaluation, and at least in theory, such judgments consider both desired and undesired effects. But displaying the distribution of these responses for a drug (or several drugs) not only allows readers to come to clinical judgments more readily than from any display of pain intensity difference scores, but allows both the sponsor and physicians to predict how patients will accept a drug if marketed.

Beecher and his colleagues made many important contributions to science. By helping to set human analgesimetry on a sound basis, the clinical evaluation of analgesics was made more reliable. Dependable potency ratios are an indispensable requirement, for example, to a valid comparison of the side action liability of drugs.

Furthermore, the general evolution of standard methods for pain studies in man, in which Beecher's laboratory played such a key role, established the fact that type of pain was less important for evaluating general analgesics then was the use of valid techniques. Thus, it is now acknowledged that cancer pain, postoperative pain, dental pain, and postpartum pain, when studied by similar techniques, come up with very similar potency ratios for any two given drugs. (Rheumatoid arthritis is an obvious exception.)

Beecher's group also developed methods for quantifying the adverse effects of analgesics. These included techniques for assessing respiratory depression, as well as subjective side effects. Although these studies were almost always conducted on healthy volunteers rather than patients, they were useful for estimating relative side action liability.

All of these studies provided invaluable feedback to industrial and academic chemists in the search for better analgesics. Empiric studies led to considerable modification of older theories about potent analgesics. The intact basic morphine molecule was shown not to be necessary for activity, as much simpler structures provided analgesics that were more effective, milligram for milligram, than morphine itself.

Old drugs as well as new drugs were studied by the newer techniques, placing clinical use on a much more scientific basis than it had been.

The placebo phenomenon was repeatedly emphasized by Beecher and his group. Lasagna et al., for example, initiated research on the psychological characteristics of placebo reactors (17). Unfortunately, some erroneous concepts evolved. To begin with, the term "placebo reactor" should probably never have been coined. Placebo reactivity is probably like honesty or suggestibility—people differ in their likelihood for responding to placebos in general, but specific events and circumstances also affect this likelihood. Also, Beecher popularized the notion that placebo rates were invariably close to 35%. This came out of a published analysis, by him, of drug trials in many different types of situations (5). In fact, placebo "success rates" are highly variable (and were even in Beecher's paper), depending both on the disease or symptom under study and the definition of response. (If one were foolish enough to study the ability of a placebo to prevent death after the common cold, it would have a 100% success rate.)

In addition, none of Beecher's work seemed to appreciate the two components of the placebo response. A patient may improve or deteriorate for psychological reasons, but "spontaneous" change can also occur. Most people assume that what happens after a placebo is given to a patient is exclusively a reflection of psychological causes, but sometimes it is entirely nonpsychological. The relative contributions of the two components can, unfortunately, only be appreciated by using a "no treatment" control as well as a placebo control (13).

Beecher's work, and that of others in the field, reminded everyone of the variability in response both to painful stimuli and to drugs, with the obvious lesson that flexibility is necessary for optimal clinical care.

One of the most interesting contributions of the new methodology was the accidental finding by Lasagna and Beecher that nalorphine was an analgesic (16). Animal experiments gave no hint of this possibility. The realization came from clinical trials that were initiated by a desire to discover a mixture of morphine and nalorphine that would be free of at least some of the undesired effects of morphine. As a control, nalorphine was administered by itself to postoperative patients, and seemed to have analgesic activity. As higher doses of nalorphine were employed, it became obvious that this was indeed the case. Other groups soon corroborated these surprising findings. Nalorphine's psychotomimetic properties precluded its marketing as a nonaddicting substitute for morphine, but subsequent research allowed the marketing first of pentazocine and then of other narcotic antagonist-analgesics.

Another lesson of nalorphine was the inadequacy of older animal tests for detecting the considerable analgesic activity of nonmorphine-like drugs. The subsequent introduction of inhibition of phenylquinone-induced "writhing" in rodents has, at least partially, corrected this deficiency. (It is of interest that the new nonsteroidal anti-inflammatory analgesics would have been completely missed in animals had only older analgesic tests been in place. Yet at least one of these newer analgesics seems to be as effective by mouth as morphine is by injection.)

In retrospect, clinical trials also provided evidence of the existence of enkephalins, long before the recent activity in that field. In our first nalorphine experiments, Beecher and I had noticed that several patients, instead of reporting pain relief after nalorphine, complained of severe pain "all over." I did not understand this, but knew it was both unusual and important. Our submitted paper contained the case reports, but the editor, in his wisdom, insisted on the deletion of these "anecdotes." Some years later, a repeat of this experience was seen in a clinical trial evaluating the analgesic potential of naloxone (14). Two milligrams of naloxone seemed to have some analgesic effect. Five milligrams, however, was less effective than two milligrams, and at eight milligrams, all 3 patients who received the dose complained so bitterly that the study was promptly terminated. Today I would explain this finding as evidence of mobilization of endogenous opioids in patients subjected to operative stress. When such mobilization is significant, narcotic antagonists can block the body's attempt to relieve pain through its own resources, with the result that pain is actually increased.

Perhaps even more important than all of the above, however, was the opening up of the entire field of subjective responses. Before the 1950s, science had a general scorn for subjective responses. Any data that were "in somebody's head" were ipso facto suspect as capricious and unquantifiable. Beecher and his associates changed that for all time, and showed that humans could be used to bioassay analgesics with acceptable precision.

Analgesia was followed by euphoria, dysphoria, "mental clouding," "hangover," and hallucinations as topics that deserved to enter the tent of science. Cough (9) and pruritus (18) were also studied by Gravenstein et al. and Morris et al., with less success, but the general point had been made and was never to be lost. Hypnotics were successfully studied using subjective responses long before the application of the EEG in human drug trials (13). The psychotropic drugs have obviously also benefitted from the principles elaborated initially in the field of pain studies.

I can close in no better way than to quote Beecher, from his book entitled *Management of Subjective Responses:*

"Quantitative work with pain is possible and rewarding. Experience in this area has already served as a prototype to guide work with other subjective responses. Quantitative study of the psychological effects of drugs is an urgent need; such work is properly a part of pharmacology. The possibility of accurate quantitative work in this field has been demonstrated; but even so, accomplishments to date constitute no more than a beginning in what promises to be a great development in pharmacology. Successful pursuit of studies in this field is basic to the sound growth of the behavioral sciences (3)."

REFERENCES

1. Beecher, H. K. (1944): Delayed morphine poisoning in battle casualties. *J.A.M.A.*, 124:1193–1194.
2. Beecher, H. K. (1966): Ethics and clinical research. *N. Engl. J. Med.*, 274:1354–1360.
3. Beecher, H. K. (1959): Measurement of subjective responses. In: *Quantitative Effects of Drugs*, pp. 189–190. Oxford University Press, New York.
4. Beecher, H. K. (1956): Relationship of significance of wound to the pain experienced. *J.A.M.A.*, 161:1609–1613.
5. Beecher, H. K. (1955): The powerful placebo. *J.A.M.A.*, 159:1602–1606.
6. Beecher, H. K. (1946): Pain in men wounded in battle. *Ann. Surg.*, 123:96–105.
7. Chapman, W. P., Arrowood, J. G., and Beecher, H. K. (1943): The analgesic effects of low concentrations of nitrous oxide compared in man with morphine sulphate. *J. Clin. Invest.*, 22:871–875.
8. Denton, J. E., and Beecher, H. K. (1949): I. Methods in the clinical evaluation of new analgesics. *New Analgesics*, 141:1051–1057.
9. Gravenstein, V. S., Denloo, R. A., and Beecher, H. K. (1954): Effect of antitussive agents on experimental and pathological cough in men. *J. Appl. Physiol.*, 7:119–139.
10. Hardy, J. D., Wolff, H. G., and Goodell, H. (1952): *Pain Sensations and Reactions.* Williams and Wilkins, Baltimore.
11. Isbell, H. The search for a nonaddicting analgesic: Has it been worth it? *Clin. Pharmacol. Ther.*, 22:377–384.
12. Keats, A. S., Beecher, H. K., and Mosteller, F. C. (1950): Measurement of pathological pain in distinction to experimental pain. *J. Appl. Physiol.*, 1:35–44.
13. Lasagna, L. A comparison of hypnotic agents. *J. Pharmacol. Exp. Ther.*, 111:9–20.
14. Lasagna, L. (1965): Drug interaction in the field of analgesic drugs. *Proc. R. Soc. Med.*, 58:978–983.
15. Lasagna, L. (1960): The clinical measurement of pain. *Am. N.Y. Acad. Sci.*, 86:28–37.
16. Lasagna, L., and Beecher, H. K. (1954): The analgesic effectiveness of nalorphine and nalorphine-morphine combinations. *J. Pharmacol. Exp. Ther.*, 112:356–363.
17. Lasagna, L., Mosteller, F., von Felsinger, J. M., and Beecher, H. K. (1954): A study of the placebo response. *Am. J. Med.*, 16:770–779.
18. Morris, S. G., Smith, G. M., and Beecher, H. K. (1958): Comparison of the anti-pruritic effect of morphine and papaverine in experimental and pathological itch in man. *J. Pharmacol. Exp. Ther.*, 123:220–223.
19. Strong, C. A. (1895): The psychology of pain. *Psychol. Rev.*, 2:329–347.

Analgesics: Neurochemical, Behavioral, and Clinical Perspectives, edited by M. Kuhar and G. Pasternak. Raven Press, New York © 1984.

Endogenous Opioids and Related Derivatives

Robert C. A. Frederickson

Lilly Research Laboratories, Eli Lilly and Company, Indianapolis, Indiana 46285

THE ENDOGENOUS OPIOIDS—TERMINOLOGY AND CANDIDATES

The story of the endogenous opioids has grown very complex, indeed, since the first reports of such activity in brain and CSF by Hughes (131) and by Terenius and Wahlstrom (279). The first identified endogenous opioids were the pentapeptides, methionine (Met)- and leucine (Leu)-enkephalin (132). It was surprising at that time to find that there were two such substances, but the widespread studies stimulated by these first reports have made it clear that there are even more numerous opioid peptides of many different sizes in the brain, and also in various peripheral sites and body fluids. The physiological roles of these many related peptides, i.e., whether they serve as hormones, neurotransmitters, precursors or metabolites, or whether they may be artifacts of some sort, remain substantially uncertain even at this time. These circumstances provide some problems with terminology.

The term endogenous opioid refers to any material occurring in the brain or other organs which has pharmacological properties similar to those of the opiate (derived from opium) substance morphine. Endogenous opioids are for the most part peptides, although there are reports of a nonpeptide endogenous opioid (92,141). The term endorphin, coined from *end*ogenous m*orphin*e by Eric Simon, is synonymous with endogenous opioid, and is used also to designate the whole class of such compounds. Since these materials are structurally very different from morphine, and may in many ways be different also pharmacologically, it might be more appropriate although less elegant, to designate them as endogenous opioids or endopioids. It would be premature, however, to begin changing the terminology before the significance and functions of the various materials are established, and therefore I will continue using the term endorphin to refer to the general class of endogenous opioids. The enkephalins are thus a subclass of the group of endorphins as are other identified opioid peptides such as beta-endorphin, alpha-endorphin, gamma-endorphin, and dynorphin. A list of the various specific endorphins which have been reported to date is given in Table 1.

Our understanding of the significance and possible function of the various endorphins is greatest for beta-endorphin and the enkephalins. This review, therefore, will concentrate mainly on these specific endorphins. Many of the others may be

TABLE 1. *Endogenous opioids[a]*

Characterized opioids	Amino acid sequence[b]
β-LPH (61-91) β-Endorphin (C fragment)	Tyr[61]-Gly-Gly-Phe-Met-Thr-Ser-[67]...-Thr[76]-Leu[77]...-Tyr[87]-Lys-Lys-Gly-Glu[91]-OH
β-LPH (61-87) δ-Endorphin (C' fragment)	Tyr[61]-Gly-Gly-Phe-Met-Thr-Ser-[67]...-Thr[76]-Leu[77]...-Tyr[87]-OH
β-LPH (61-77) γ-Endorphin	Tyr[61]-Gly-Gly-Phe-Met-Thr-Ser-[67]...-Thr[76]-Leu[77]-OH
β-LPH (61-76) α-Endorphin	Tyr[61]-Gly-Gly-Phe-Met-Thr-Ser-[67]...-Thr[76]-OH
β-LPH (62-77) des-Tyr-γ-endorphin[c]	Gly[62]-Gly-Phe-Met-Thr-Ser-[67]...-Thr[76]-Leu-OH
β-LPH (62-76) des-Tyr-α-endorphin[c]	Gly[62]-Gly-Phe-Met-Thr-Ser-[67]...-Thr[76]-OH
β-LPH (61-65) Met-enkephalin	Tyr-Gly-Gly-Phe-Met-OH
Dynorphin	Tyr-Gly-Gly-Phe-Leu-Arg-Arg-Ile-Arg-Pro-Lys-Leu-Lys-Trp-Asp-Asn-Gln-OH
Leu-enkephalin	Tyr-Gly-Gly-Phe-Leu-OH
β-Casomorphin	Tyr-Pro-Phe-Pro-Gly-Pro-ILeu-OH
Morphiceptin	Tyr-Pro-Phe-Pro-NH$_2$
Dermorphin	Tyr-D-Ala-Phe-Gly-Tyr-Pro-Ser-NH$_2$
Kyotorphin	Tyr-Arg-OH
Uncharacterized opioids	
Humoral (H) endorphin	
Anodynin	
Endorphin fractions I and II	
Nonpeptide morphine-like factor	

[a]For specific reference to each of these materials, see ref. 76.
[b]The missing sequences represented by ellipses are Glu[68]-Lys-Ser-Gln-Thr-Pro-Leu-Val[75]- and Phe[78]-Lys-Asn-Ala-Ile-Lys-Asn-Ala-[86].
[c]These are not truly opioids, because loss of the N-terminal tyrosine eliminates opioid activity.

hormones or transmitters in their own right, or they may be precursors, metabolites, or even artifacts; they will receive very brief treatment throughout the following sections only where it seems appropriate, and where time, space, and available information permit.

PHYSIOLOGY OF SELECTED OPIOID PEPTIDES

Methodology

In order to investigate the presence, distribution, synthesis, release, and degradation of materials such as the opioid peptides, a means of measuring these substances is necessary. There are many different assay systems available to detect and quantitate the opioid peptides. These include the guinea pig ileum bioassay, the mouse vas deferens bioassay, the radioreceptor assay, and the radioimmunoassay with its immunocytochemical extensions. The ileum and vas deferens preparations measure biological activity, which reflects both affinity and efficacy at the receptor. But these assays do not readily distinguish the different opioid structures. The radioreceptor assay measures only affinity for an opioid binding site; it provides no information on efficacy, and therefore, cannot readily differentiate agonists and antagonists, nor distinguish the different opioid structures other than into broad classes. The radioimmunoassay recognizes structural features, not biological activity, and is, therefore, capable of distinguishing different opioid peptides on a structural but not a pharmacological basis.

The immunocytochemical techniques are very powerful and their extensive use over the last few years in the study of the opioid peptides has shed much light on the distribution and possible functions of the latter. These techniques do have limitations, however, and much care must be taken in interpreting the resulting data. The various antisera available have different degrees of cross reactivity with other peptides than their intended antigen. For example, many of the determinations of beta-endorphin have used an antibody that recognizes beta-lipotropic hormone as well, with equimolar sensitivity.

The development of more sensitive and more specific antisera, the simultaneous use of several antisera with different relative sensitivities, and chromatographic separation before assay have allowed careful, accurate quantitation of the different opioid components. The chromatographic techniques, of course, cannot be used with the immunocytochemical approach, and in most cases it is probably more appropriate to refer to the identified materials as enkephalin-like immunoreactivity or beta-endorphin-like immunoreactivity rather than as enkephalin or beta-endorphin, respectively. The combined use of various of the assay techniques described above, however, has provided a reasonably consistent picture of the distribution of the opioid peptides.

Distribution

Beta-Endorphin

High concentrations of beta-endorphin are found in the pituitary, with the greatest amounts being found in the anterior and intermediate lobes (71,176,238,239). The amounts in the intermediate lobe exceed those in the anterior lobe (25,176,320). The major immunoreactive peptides in both lobes of the rat pituitary have been found to be C′-fragment (beta-LPH 61-87) and N-acetyl C′-fragment (264,320). These are both inactive, or only weakly active as opiates, indicating that in the rat, the circulating endorphins released from the pituitary probably have little morphinomimetic activity.

The same four immunoreactive peptides observed in the pituitary have also been observed in the rat brain, namely beta-endorphin or C-fragment, (N-acetyl) beta-endorphin, beta-endorphin 61-87 or C′-fragment, and (N-acetyl) C′-fragment (264,320). The highest concentrations of beta-endorphin have been found in the hypothalamus, including the preoptic nucleus, paraventricular nucleus, and median eminence. High levels are also found in the paraventricular thalamus, periaqueductal gray, zona compacta of the substantia nigra, medial amygdaloid nucleus, zona incerta, and locus coeruleus. In the hippocampus and midbrain, the C′-fragment is present in greater amounts than beta-endorphin, but in hypothalamus, beta-endorphin is the major opioid peptide (320). The pituitary is a potential source for beta-endorphin found in the brain, but several studies have clearly demonstrated that the brain and pituitary beta-endorphin stores have separate origins (26,299). Hypophysectomy or adrenalectomy produce no change in the brain levels of beta-endorphin (149,238,239). Therefore, brain cells most likely synthesize their own supplies of beta-endorphin.

Beta-endorphin cell bodies in the brain are localized to the arcuate nucleus of the hypothalamus. Radioimmunoassay, immunocytochemistry, and *in vitro* biosynthetic studies with this tissue have demonstrated that beta-endorphin is present in and can be synthesized by neurons in this basal hypothalamic region (26,177,238). Fibers from this hypothalamic region, containing beta-endorphin, innervate the median eminence and project through the anterior hypothalamus to the dorsal midline thalamus (26,148). Additional fibers have been shown to innervate the amygdala, preoptic area, ventral medial nuclei, and periventricular nucleus as well as the periaqueductal gray, reticular formation, and stria terminalis (238). Destruction of the hypothalamic nuclei by sodium glutamate-induced lesions resulted in a significant decrease in immunoreactive beta-endorphin in these other brain regions (151). Treatment of rats, furthermore, with colchicine, an inhibitor of axonal transport, followed by immunocytochemistry, showed a significant increase in staining of the cell bodies in the arcuate nucleus. These data support the view that the hypothalamic neurons are the source of brain β-endorphin. The distribution and levels of beta-endorphin in the brain are illustrated in Table 2 and Fig. 1.

Beta-endorphin has been extracted also from human placenta (175,211). A high molecular weight glycoprotein similar to pro-opiomelanocortin, the precursor isolated from pituitary, is thought to be the source of this peptide. Processing of this precursor resembles the pathway demonstrated in the intermediate lobe of the pituitary; alpha-MSH and beta-endorphin are the major products rather than ACTH and beta-lipotropic hormone (LPH) which predominate in the anterior pituitary. Studies of immunoreactivity have also detected beta-endorphin-like material in the pancreas, gastrointestinal tract, thyroid gland, and mast cells (29,55,140). Plasma and CSF levels of beta-endorphin, and the factors that regulate these levels will be discussed in detail in a later section.

The Enkephalins

Numerous and extensive studies have been undertaken, utilizing the various methodologies discussed above such as radioreceptor assay, bioassay, radioimmunoassay, and immunocytochemistry, on the distribution of the enkephalins in brain and elsewhere. Many of these studies (26,62,238,299) have made it clear that the enkephalins and beta-endorphin have distinctly different distributions throughout the brain and pituitary. The distribution of the enkephalins is illustrated in Table 2 and Fig. 1.

In the pituitary, the highest concentrations of beta-endorphin and acetylated beta-endorphin occur in the anterior and intermediate lobes (238,320), whereas

TABLE 2. *Distribution of opioid peptides in the brain and pituitary gland*

	β-Endorphin, ng/mg tissue		Enkephalin, mU-Enk/mg tissue	
Pituitary				
Whole	269 ± 20	(11)	72 ± 4	(6)
Adenohypophysis	128 ± 9	(3)	3.7 ± 0.7	(3)
Neurohypophysis and pars intermedia	1,500 ± 600	(3)	740 ± 47	(3)
Pineal	4.8 ± 0.8	(10)	19 ± 2	(7)
	ng/gram tissue		U-enkephalin/ gram tissue	
Brain				
Whole	108 ± 8	(10)	25 ± 2	(6)
Hypothalamus	490 ± 30	(5)	120 ± 7	(6)
Septum	234 ± 34	(3)	85 ± 7	(6)
Midbrain	207 ± 15	(5)	32 ± 1	(6)
Medulla and pons	179 ± 5	(5)	30 ± 4	(6)
Striatum	None	(5)	112 ± 11	(6)
Hippocampus	None	(5)	13 ± 1	(6)
Cortex	None	(5)	15 ± 2	(6)
Cerebellum	None	(5)	5 ± 1	(6)

Rat brains were dissected as outlined by Glowinski and Iversen (93a). Data are means ± SEM; numbers of animals are shown in parentheses. One unit of immunoreactive enkephalin corresponds to 1 ng of Leu[5]-enkephalin or 30 ng of Met[5]-enkephalin. (From ref. 238.)

enkephalin appears to occur in the highest concentration in the posterior lobe (239,320), although there has been some controversy on this latter point. In the brain, although beta-endorphin cell bodies occur only in the arcuate nucleus, and terminals are distributed in a midline periventricular fashion as discussed above, the enkephalin cell bodies and terminals are more broadly distributed (68,242). Cell bodies containing enkephalin-like immunoreactivity have been found in the caudate nucleus, nucleus interstitialis stria terminalis, central nucleus of the amygdala, periventricular and supraoptic nuclei, perifornical region of the hypothalamus, interpeduncular nucleus, nucleus cochlearus dorsalis, nucleus vestibularis medialis, nucleus vestibularis spinalis, the central gray and reticular formation, nucleus tractus solitarius, nucleus tractus spinalis nervi trigemini, Golgi type II cells of the cerebellum, olfactory bulb, olfactory tubercle, the lateral preoptic nucleus, suprachiasmatic nucleus, periventricular nucleus of the hypothalamus, lateral amygdaloid nucleus, cortical amygdaloid nucleus, basal amygdaloid nucleus, medial amygdaloid nucleus, hippocampus, neocortex, cingulate cortex, posterior mammillary nucleus, medial nucleus of the optic tract, brachium of the inferior colliculus, ventral tegmental nucleus, nucleus reticularis lateralis, and laminae II, III, and VII of the cervical spinal cord.

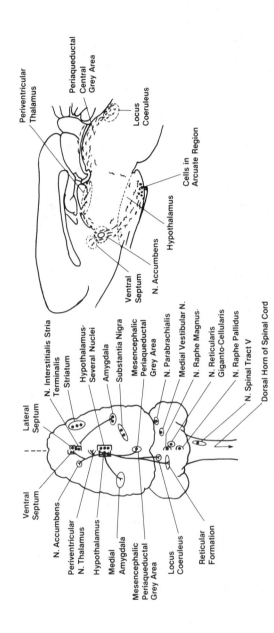

FIG. 1. A, comparative distribution of beta endorphin neuronal systems and enkephalin neuronal systems in the brain. The Met- and Leu-enkephalin neuronal systems are depicted on the right. These show mainly cell bodies because they are comprised for the most part of local interneuronal short-fiber systems. The amygdala-stria terminalis pathway is discussed in section 3.4 of the text. The beta-endorphin system is shown on the left and consists of a single hypothalamic cell group providing long fiber paths innervating regions distributed along the midline periventricular-periaqueductal system. **B**, a cross-sectional view of the beta-endorphin/beta-LPH/ACTH system originating in the arcuate region of the basal hypothalamus. (From Barchas, ref. 15a, and Watson and Barchas, ref. 300a.)

Neuronal processes containing enkephalin-like immunoreactivity have been observed in the lateral septum, central nucleus of the amygdala, area CA2 of the hippocampus, parts of the cortex, corpus striatum, bed nucleus of the stria terminalis, parts of the hypothalamus including the median eminence, parts of the thalamus and subthalamus, the interpeduncular nucleus, reticular formation, periaqueductal gray, parabrachial nucleus, locus coeruleus, raphe nuclei, cochlear nucleus, nucleus tractus solitarius, nucleus tractus spinalis nervi trigemini, motor nuclei of certain cranial nerves, nucleus commissuralis, and substantia gelatinosa. As was found with beta-endorphin, hypophysectomy does not significantly alter brain levels of the enkephalins (145,305,307). With a few exceptions, the general distribution of enkephalin parallels that of the opioid receptors as measured by tritiated diprenorphine binding (152).

The ratio of Met-enkephalin to Leu-enkephalin is not constant from one brain region to another, but Met-enkephalin levels are generally greater than the levels of Leu-enkephalin (169). A major question is whether Met-enkephalin and Leu-enkephalin share common neurons and common precursors. Larsson et al. (156) investigated this question. They prepared a Met-enkephalin antiserum that did not cross react with Leu-enkephalin by selectively absorbing cross reacting antibodies in crude anti-Met-enkephalin antiserum. They used Leu-enkephalin antiserum to localize Leu-enkephalin in acid permanganate-treated tissues in which Met-enkephalin immunoreactivity was destroyed. They observed separate populations of Met-enkephalin neurons and Leu-enkephalin neurons in the caudate nucleus, putamen, globus pallidus, and guinea pig ileum, and concluded that the two enkephalins often occur in separate neurons. This evidence for independent production of the two enkephalins in separate systems appears to be in conflict, however, with other evidence suggesting a large common precursor which will be discussed in a later section.

The enkephalins are also found in substantial amounts in tissues other than the brain and pituitary. Endocrine cells in the gastrointestinal mucosa, containing enkephalin, were first reported by Polak et al. (224). In addition to endocrine cells, enkephalin-containing neurons have been found throughout the gastrointestinal tract in man, mouse, chicken, rat, guinea pig, rabbit, cat, monkey, and pig (13). Enkephalin-containing fibers were found in the highest density in the myenteric plexus and circular muscle layers of the rat and guinea pig, virtually along the entire length of the tract (137,257). Immunoreactive neuronal perikarya were observed in the myenteric plexus of both species, with greater numbers being found in the guinea pig. The enkephalins are also present in the substantia gelatinosa of the spinal cord (138,152), neurons of the mesenteric ganglia (138), and the pancreas (29). Large amounts of enkephalins have also been identified in the adrenal medulla (254,255). Enkephalin-like immunoreactivity is found in gland cells of the adrenal medulla, and also in nerve terminals which appear to be terminals of the splanchnic nerve, because they disappear on sectioning of this nerve (179,254,255).

Synthesis, Release, and Degradation

Beta-Endorphin

A large precursor protein, or glycoprotein of 31 kd (31 kd precursor, pro-opiomelanocortin), has been identified (116) as the source of corticotropin (ACTH), beta-LPH, beta-endorphin, alpha-MSH, gamma-LPH, and corticotropin-like intermediate lobe peptide (CLIP) (Fig. 2). The identification of precursor-product relationships was made primarily through radiolabeling studies in mouse pituitary ACTH-producing tumor cells (AtT-20) and through cell-free biosynthesis directed by mRNA prepared from bovine pituitary or AtT-20 cells (184,202,231). The nucleotide sequence of the complimentary DNA which codes for the precursor has been determined in bovine (203,204), human (39), and rat (58) tissues. This has made it possible to determine the complete amino acid sequence of pro-opiomelanocortin (203).

ACTH and beta-LPH are the primary products in the anterior pituitary, whereas in the intermediate lobe, beta-endorphin and alpha-MSH are predominant (25,176, 183). Zakarian and Smyth (320) were able to identify four fragments from the anterior and intermediate pituitary lobes which are recognized by beta-endorphin antibodies: beta-endorphin (C-fragment), N-acetyl-beta-endorphin, beta-endorphin 61-87 (C'-fragment) and N-acetyl-beta-endorphin 61-87. In the anterior pituitary, the ratio of C-fragment to C'-fragment is 1:4, whereas in the intermediate lobe, the ratio is about 1:15. The amount of actual beta-endorphin in the intermediate lobe is about 17 to 18 times the amount in the anterior lobe.

Biosynthesis of beta-endorphin has also been demonstrated in the arcuate nucleus (177,322). The details of the synthetic process have been worked out primarily in studies with pituitary tissue, but it is presumed that the same process occurs in the basal hypothalamus. For reviews of this work, see Herbert (116), Miller (194), Beaumont and Hughes (19), and Imura and Nakai (133).

The release of opioid peptides from the pituitary has been investigated with mouse, rat, and human tissue or cultured primary or tumor cell lines (11,91,183, 227,260,291). These studies have demonstrated a coordinate regulation of release

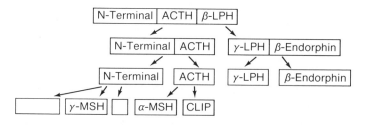

FIG. 2. Schematic representation of generation of beta-endorphin, ACTH, and other peptides from pro-opiomelanocortin. The single large precursor (31K) is the source of beta-LPH, gamma-LPH, beta-endorphin, corticotropin (ACTH), gamma-MSH, alpha-MSH, and CLIP. (Modified from ref. 116).

of ACTH, beta-LPH, and beta-endorphin from the anterior pituitary, with the relative composition of the opioid peptides in the released material being about 70% beta-LPH and 30% beta-endorphin. This release is calcium-dependent and is stimulated by high K^+, adrenal steroids, lysine-vasopressin, and hypothalamic extracts. Cortisone and dexamethasone inhibit stimulated release (11,91,227,288), and hydrocortisone was reported to inhibit basal release as well (91). Vale et al. (288) have recently purified a 41 amino acid peptide from ovine hypothalamic extracts, which stimulates the simultaneous release of ACTH, beta-LPH, and beta-endorphin from primary cultures of rat anterior pituitary. No autoinhibition of release has been reported.

Beta-endorphin was reported to constitute about 97% of the release from the intermediate lobe (291) and this release appears to be regulated in a different fashion than release from the anterior pituitary. Hypothalamic extract and lysine-vasopressin had no effect on release from this lobe, whereas dopamine inhibited release and this could be blocked by a dopamine antagonist, domperidone (291). Isoprenalin, a beta-adrenergic agonist, furthermore, caused a three to fourfold stimulation of beta-endorphin release from the intermediate lobe, and this could be blocked by propranolol, a beta-adrenergic blocker.

In the brain, beta-endorphin concentrations were not affected by steroid hormones or stress (239), but chronic exposure to opiates has been reported to lower beta-endorphin both in the pituitary and brain (125). Factors affecting the release of beta-LPH and beta-endorphin as reflected in blood and CSF levels will be discussed in more detail later in this chapter.

Removal of tyrosine from the N-terminal of beta-endorphin results in loss of activity at opioid receptors and loss of analgesic potency. Fragments of beta-endorphin shortened at the C-terminal, such as alpha-endorphin (beta-LPH 61-76) or gamma endorphin (beta-LPH 61-77), have reduced opioid activity (e.g., 173). Graf et al. (102) have demonstrated that cathepsin D, a soluble lysosomal enzyme, is capable of hydrolyzing beta-endorphin at the Leu^{77}-Phe^{78} site, yielding gamma-endorphin. Suhar and Marks (273) have shown that cathepsin B is capable of hydrolyzing beta-LPH to a peptide similar in size to beta-LPH 1-77, but whose identity remains to be clearly established. It has been suggested, however, that the acidic pH optimum of these enzymes, as well as their subcellular localization in lysosomes, makes them unlikely candidates for the processing of *in vivo* stores of beta-endorphin and beta-LPH (33). Austin et al. (15) have reported, however, that gamma-endorphin and alpha-endorphin can be formed from beta-endorphin by rat brain membranes. Burbach et al. (32,33), furthermore, have described an enzyme with spcificity for the Leu^{77}-Phe^{78} site, which is tightly associated with synaptic plasma membranes. This enzyme has a neutral pH optimum and is not sensitive to pepstatin, a cathepsin D inhibitor.

Removal of the N-terminal tyrosine from alpha-endorphin and gamma-endorphin produces des-Tyr-alpha-endorphin and des-Tyr-gamma-endorphin, nonopioid peptides with reportedly potent neuroleptic effects (54,142). Hersh et al. (118) have purified a soluble amino-peptidase from rat brain, which has a high affinity for

Met-enkephalin, but which will also release tyrosine from alpha-, gamma-, and beta-endorphin. Under their conditions, the rate of release of tyrosine was greatest with Met-enkephalin. Alpha- and gamma-endorphin also gave high rates, but beta-endorphin, known to be relatively resistant to aminopeptidase, was a poor substrate.

The presence of beta-endorphin 61-87, N-acetyl-beta-endorphin 61-87, and N-acetyl-beta-endorphin, as well as beta-endorphin itself in the pituitary, has been discussed above. The regulation of the relative amounts of the endorphins, and their des-Tyr and acetylated derivatives, and the mechanisms of production and inactivation of these peptides have only begun to be examined. The clarification of the biological significance of these various peptides awaits resolution.

The Enkephalins

The recognition that the N-terminal sequence of beta-endorphin consists of the Met-enkephalin sequence, and the apparent greater potency of beta-endorphin compared to Met-enkephalin, led to the suggestion of precursor-products or hormone-metabolite relationships between these two peptides. The prevailing evidence, however, does not support such relationships between these two peptides, but rather, that they are independent entities serving separate functions.

No physiological processing of beta-endorphin to enkephalin has been demonstrated, although enzymes capable of releasing Met-enkephalin from beta-endorphin have been reported (143,146). Beta-endorphin and Met-enkephalin have a markedly different distribution in the brain and pituitary, and their levels in the brain increase at different rates during development (238). Immunohistofluorescence studies have demonstrated that the enkephalins and beta-endorphin are present in different and separate neuronal systems (26,299).

Large peptides containing the Leu-enkephalin sequence have also been demonstrated, such as alpha-neoendorphin (139) and dynorphin (94,95). These larger peptides are reported to be more potent than Leu-enkephalin, however, in studies *in vitro* with mouse vas deferens and guinea pig ileum preparations, and, thus, it has been suggested that they may be neurotransmitters or hormones in their own right rather than precursors. The data are not yet adequate to establish the various roles of these peptides, but immunocytochemical studies now indicate that the dynorphin neuronal system is separate from the Met- and Leu-enkephalin neuronal systems (300). Immunocytochemical evidence has been recently reported for concomitant storage of alpha-neoendorphin and dynorphin in rat hypothalamic neurons suggesting origin from a common precursor molecule (301). Further immunocytochemical studies and investigation of the release and action of these large peptides will be important to help resolve their roles. It is possible that, analogous to the differential processing of the pro-opiomelanocortin molecule in the anterior and intermediate pituitary lobes, processing of a common precursor may vary between regions.

Another pertinent question is whether Met- and Leu-enkephalin share common neurons and/or common precursors or represent different neuronal systems as mentioned earlier. Larsson et al. (156) observed separate populations of Met-enkephalin-containing neurons and Leu-enkephalin-containing neurons in the caudate nucleus, putamen, globus pallidus, and ileum of the guinea pig. None of the cells contained both enkephalins. These observations suggested that the varying amounts of enkephalin found throughout the brain are owing to independent synthetic pathways. Evidence for this is also derived from studies that demonstrated labeling of the enkephalins *in vitro* using cultured adrenal medulla cells. Wilson et al. (309) observed a preferential increase in the relative amount of labeling of enkephalins compared to other opioid peptides after exposure of these cultured cells to reserpine, and this was attributed to an increase in biosynthesis. They observed, furthermore, preferential increases in Met-enkephalin over Leu-enkephalin and suggested that the regulation of synthesis, processing, degradation, storage, and secretion of these two enkephalins may be independent of each other.

This concept of independent biosynthesis is, however, in conflict with the evidence suggesting a large common precursor. The adrenal medulla has been identified as a tissue rich in enkephalin (254,255). This tissue has been exploited by Rossier and colleagues to identify potential precursors of Met- and Leu-enkephalin, and to demonstrate the biosynthesis of enkephalin from radiolabeled amino acids (240). Large peptide fragments containing multiple copies of met-enkephalin and single copies of Leu-enkephalin have been isolated from this tissue (165). This observation may explain the ratio, in adrenal medulla and various brain regions, of Met- to Leu-enkephalin which ranges from 4 to 1 to 7 to 1. The apparently different concepts of a common macroprecursor and independent enkephalinergic system could be compatible if, for example, the designation of a neuron as Met-enkephalinergic or Leu-enkephalinergic lies simply in the differential processing of such a common precursor.

The 50,000 dalton precursor has not yet been purified to homogeneity and sequenced (236), but two groups have cloned DNA sequences complementary to the bovine mRNA coding for this protein. Nucleotide sequence analysis of this cloned cDNA has revealed the whole amino acid sequence of the bovine adrenal precursor. Gubler et al. (108) refer to this precursor as proenkephalin and Noda et al. (209) refer to the same material as preproenkephalin. There is only one amino acid difference, at position 44 of the material of Noda et al., between the two published sequences, but Gubler et al. did not present the first 21 amino acids of the complete structure presented by Noda et al. The structure of this enkephalin precursor is shown in Fig. 3. This protein is composed of 263 amino acids and has a calculated molecular weight of 29,786. It contains four copies of Met-enkephalin and one copy each of Leu-enkephalin, Met-enkephalin-Arg[6]-Phe[7], and Met-enkephalin-Arg[6]-Gly[7]-Leu[8]. These sequences are each bound by paired basic residues, except at the carboxyl terminus, implying that they can be formed by proteolytic processing of the precursor molecule.

A biosynthetic pathway for Met-enkephalin was previously proposed involving first a trypsin-like cleavage to produce arginine- and lysine-extended Met-enkephalins, followed by carboxypeptidase-B-like cleavage to yield free Met-enkephalin

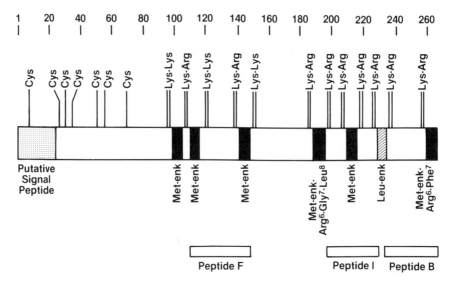

FIG. 3. Schematic representation of the structure of bovine preproenkephalin. The sequences of Met-enkephalin, Met-enkephalin-Arg^6-Phe^7, and Met-enkephalin-Arg^6-Gly^7-Leu^8 are indicated by *closed boxes*, the sequence of Leu-enkephalin by a *shaded box*, and the putative signal peptide by a *stippled box*. All the paired basic amino acid residues and cysteine residues are shown. Amino acid numbers are given above. The known peptide structures, peptide F (residues 104–137), peptide I (residues 192–230), and peptide B (residues 233–263), are displayed underneath by *open bars*. (From ref. 208, with permission.)

(127,269). Bovine chromaffin granules were reported to contain an enzyme and a precursor which generate Met-enkephalin *in vitro* (284). More recently, a trypsin-like enzyme, which appears to be a serine protease, has been purified from bovine adrenal chromaffin granules. It is able to generate Met-enkephalin directly from endogenous substrates (170). It remains to be established whether this enzyme operates *in vivo* to generate Met-enkephalin. Fricker and Snyder (83), furthermore, have purified and characterized a specific carboxypeptidase, dubbed enkephalin convertase, which converts Arg^6- and Lys^6-enkephalin precursors into enkephalin.

It has been suggested that these large precursors isolated from chromaffin granules in the adrenal medulla may also be present in the brain (130,164,268). Indeed, hexapeptides and heptapeptides containing the Met- and Leu-enkephalin sequences have been purified from the brain, but the larger peptides containing the Met-enkephalin and Leu-enkephalin sequences have not yet been identified there. Of course, alpha-neoendorphin and dynorphin, as already mentioned, have been demonstrated in the brain but it is not yet clear what relationship they have to Leu-enkephalin or to the large precursor peptides. There is no sequence in the adrenal precursor corresponding to α-neo-endorphin or dynorphin.

The release of enkephalins has been demonstrated from several brain regions. Both Met- and Leu-enkephalin were released by high potassium in a calcium-dependent manner from perfused slices of rat globus pallidus (18,134,168). Substantial degradation of the enkephalins occurred in these studies even though bacitracin was used in the perfusion medium. Release of enkephalins from the globus pallidus *in vivo* has been demonstrated by Glowinski (93). Using a push-pull cannula, he demonstrated a release of Met-enkephalin of 20 to 30 pg/15 min. A 20–30-fold increase of release was observed in the presence of 60 mM potassium. Veratridine produced similar increases in release.

A potassium-stimulated calcium-dependent release of enkephalins has also been demonstrated from slices of corpus striatum (114,168,217,230,251). In these studies, the ratio of Met- to Leu-enkephalin released was 3 or 4 to 1, which compares well with the ratios reported for levels in intact tissue. Richter et al. (230) passed perfusate from the striatal tissue directly over columns of Amberlite AXD-2 and did not need to include enzyme inhibitors such as bacitracin to detect released Met- and Leu-enkephalin. The high potassium stimulated release was transient in nature and a total of only 2 to 3% of the tissue stores could be released (168,217,230). Basal release rates of 0.1 to 0.2% of tissue stores per minute were reported and stimulated release rates reached 0.6 to 0.8% of tissue stores per minute (168). Veratridine (50 μM) was observed to increase release of both enkephalins in parallel (114,168). Richter et al. (230) were unable to demonstrate any effect of either morphine or naloxone on release stimulated by 50 mM potassium. Sawynok et al. (251), conversely, were able to demonstrate an inhibitory effect of both morphine and naloxone on the release of Met-enkephalin evoked by lower concentrations of potassium (30 mM). In agreement with Richter et al., this effect was not observed at higher potassium levels (47 mM). The inhibitory effect of morphine could be caused by action on an enkephalin autoreceptor, but the effect of the antagonist, naloxone, is puzzling unless naloxone is perceived as an agonist at this receptor. This point needs further investigation.

The effects of several γ-aminobutyric acid (GABA) receptor agonists and antagonists have been examined on Met-enkephalin release. Osborne and Herz (216) reported that both GABA and muscimol decreased potassium-evoked release of Met-enkephalin. Sawynok and Labella (249), conversely, reported that GABA and baclofen, but not muscimol, potentiated the potassium-evoked release of Met-enkephalin from rat striatal slices. Picrotoxin, but not bicuculline, blocked this stimulatory effect of GABA on Met-enkephalin release. The stimulatory effects of GABA and baclofen on enkephalin release were observed only at an intermediate potassium concentration (30 mM). Further investigations will be necessary to clarify these apparent discrepancies and to elucidate the role of GABA receptors in the regulation of enkephalin release.

Patey et al. (220) observed that incubation of striatal slices with thiorphan, a potent inhibitor of enkephalinase A (*see* section on analgesic activity of peptidase inhibitors), resulted in a 100% increase in the potassium-stimulated release of Met-enkephalin. Other inhibitors, puromycin (0.1 μM) and captopril (0.1 mM), which inhibit aminopeptidase and angiotensin converting enzyme, respectively, did not enhance the recovery of Met-enkephalin. The authors suggest from these data that it is enkephalinase at the release site rather than other enzymes, such as aminopeptidases, which is responsible for the inactivation of enkephalin. Sullivan et al. (274), however, reported that degradation of enkephalins in brain homogenates was inhibited at a concentration of puromycin of 0.1 mM. It is possible that the concentration of puromycin of 0.1 μM, used by Patey et al. (220), was insufficient, or that loosely bound aminopeptidase activity may have been washed out during preincubations. Alternatively, the brain homogenate may expose aminopeptidases which do not function synaptically. Investigation of the effects of higher concentrations of puromycin and/or bacitracin and/or other better aminopeptidase inhibitors on release from slices might help determine whether aminopeptidase contributes to the metabolism.

The following characteristics are necessary to distinguish enzymes which might degrade enkephalins in a physiologically relevant manner: high affinity for the enkephalins, narrow substrate specifity, a regional distribution which parallels the distribution of enkephalin stores and opiate receptors, and a subcellular distribution which is compatible with the actions of enkephalins at the synaptic site. Among the enzymes which can digest enkephalins are aminopeptidases, di-peptidyl carboxypeptidases (enkephalinase and angiotensin converting enzyme), and carboxypeptidase A.

At least five aminopeptidases within the brain have been described (16,112,117, 253,282,283,294,295). Another aminopeptidase from plasma has also been characterized (46). These are all soluble enzymes and the five isolated from brain tissue are metalloenzymes which can be inhibited by chelating agents such as o-phenanthroline and EDTA. These enzymes all have a high affinity for the enkephalins, but their relative substrate specificities differ, and estimations of molecular weight also indicate that they are not identical enzymes. Those from rat and human brain have neutral pH optima, ruling out lysosomal origin. The distributions of the separate aminopeptidases have not been examined, but the distribution of total undifferentiated aminopeptidase activity does not parallel that of the opioid receptor. Immunohistochemical mapping of the separate enzymes would help in evaluating the extent of their participation in enkephalin metabolism in vivo. Puromycin is an effective inhibitor of aminopeptidase in the brain and ileum homogenates, and potentiates the inhibition of guinea pig ileum contractions produced by Met-enkephalin (275,293). Bacitracin, a less potent aminopeptidase inhibitor, has been reported to produce a dose-dependent naloxone-reversible analgesia in mice tested in the tail flick assay, when the drug is administered by the intracerebroventricular route (261).

The digestion of the enkephalins by a dipeptidylcarboxypeptidase (called enkephalinase A) was first reported by Malfroy et al. (185) and Sullivan et al. (274). The possible identity of this enzyme with angiotensin converting enzyme (ACE) became the subject of investigation. Although these two enzymes have properties in common (22,276), and captopril, an ACE inhibitor, was reported to potentiate met-enkephalin analgesia (270), several distinguishing features have been reproducibly observed. Differential inhibition of these enzymes can be obtained using thiorphan and captopril (233). Thiorphan is more potent against enkephalinase, whereas captopril is a more potent inhibitor of ACE. Enkephalinase is inhibited or unaffected by chloride ions, whereas ACE is activated in the presence of chloride ions (98,277). The distribution of ACE in the brain does not parallel that of enkephalins or opioid receptors as does that of enkephalinase, and furthermore, these enzymes are chromatographically separable (99,100,277). Gorenstein and Snyder (98–100) have described two enkephalinases; enkephalinase B is a dipeptidylaminopeptidase which cleaves the Gly^2, Gly^3 bond, whereas enkephalinase A is the dipeptidylcarboxypeptidase which cleaves the Gly^3, Phe^4 bond of enkephalin. Studies of subcellular distribution (52) and regional distribution (186) have demonstrated a close association between enkephalinase A and nerve endings and opiate receptors. Enkephalinase B has not been well characterized, and more information on the specificity and properties of this enzyme is needed before its importance can be evaluated. Carboxypeptidase A is a lysosomal enzyme which cleaves the c-terminal amino acid from enkephalin (53). The amino acid, D-phenylaline, is a weak inhibitor of carboxypeptidase A (111). Carenzi et al. (37) have reported that this compound potentiated the inhibition by Met-enkephalin of guinea pig longitudinal muscle contractions and also potentiated the analgesic response to Met-enkephalin in the rat hot plate jump assay. It seems unlikely, however, because of its lysosomal origin, that this enzyme plays a significant role in the physiological disposition of enkephalin.

It is not yet clear to what extent aminopeptidase and enkephalinase A contribute to the physiological degradation of the enkephalins. Each may function in different neuronal pathways. Further immunocytochemical localization of the separate enzymes, in correlation with opiate receptor distribution, will help answer these questions. Such data, followed by a study of the effect of specific enzyme inhibition on the actions of enkephalins administered microiontophoretically onto neurons in specified brain areas, should significantly advance our understanding of synaptic regulation of the enkephalins. The enzymes which can inactivate the enkephalins and their probable roles are summarized in Fig. 4.

EVIDENCE FOR PHYSIOLOGICAL FUNCTION OF ENDOGENOUS OPIOID PEPTIDES

Levels of Opioid Peptides in Blood and CSF

There have been numerous reports over the last 5 years of efforts to identify and quantitate the opioid peptides in body fluids. These have demonstrated substantial differences in apparent plasma levels and also in CSF levels, as measured in different laboratories. These differences were most likely attributable to differences in methodology as discussed previously. Levels have been measured in unextracted plasma, in extracted plasma, and after chromatographic separation.

Unidentified Endorphins

Terenius and colleagues (280,281) developed one of the first procedures for measuring opioid peptides in CSF. This consisted of a chromatographic separation

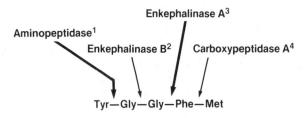

FIG. 4. Enzymes that have been shown to degrade enkephalins. The two most important are shown with bold arrows. **1:** Aminopeptidase, five or six different species identified; these are potent inactivators of enkephalins (including exogenously administered), but their role in synaptic inactivation of endogenous materials is uncertain. **2:** Enkephalinase B, this is a dipeptidylam-inopeptidase which has been only minimally characterized; there is no evidence for a role in synaptic inactivation. **3:** Enkephalinase A, this is a dipeptidylcarboxypeptidase which best meets the criteria for providing physiologically relevant synaptic inactivation of the enkephalins. **4:** Carboxypeptidase A, there is no evidence for a physiological role in the inactivation of the enkephalins.

(Sephadex G10) followed by a radioreceptor assay with dihydromorphine as the labeled ligand. They observed two major opioid components in CSF, which they referred to as fraction 1 and fraction 2. The respective basal levels of these fractions were 1.4 ± 0.4 and 5.2 ± 1.8 pmoles enkephalin equivalents per ml CSF. The active components in both fractions were peptide-like, but the main active component for fraction 1 did not coelute with the enkephalins or beta-endorphin, nor react with antiserum to these known opioid peptides. The enkephalins coeluted with fraction 2, but the major component from this fraction was different from the enkephalins because it was not recognized by antiserum to Met-enkephalin or beta-endorphin. Patients with chronic pain syndromes of an organic, but not those considered of psychogenic, nature were found to have significantly lower levels of fraction 1 than controls, and these levels were increased after successful electroacupuncture analgesia (12,263). There was, however, no correlation between duration or severity of pain and the fraction 1 levels. In another study, investigators (144) observed lower CSF fraction 1 levels in pain sensitive patients, compared with pain insensitive patients, classified on the basis of pain threshold to electrical stimulation applied to the fingers. They concluded that endorphins are physiological factors which can contribute to pain threshold and tolerance.

A factor was found in human plasma by Ho et al. (120), which was active on the guinea pig ileum, displaced Met-enkephalin from opiate receptors, and cross reacted with beta-endorphin antiserum, but which eluted from a Biogel P-2 column between beta-endorphin and Met-enkephalin. Sarne et al. (243–245) observed a similar material, which they called humoral endorphin, in blood and CSF of humans and rats. Humoral endorphin was active on the guinea pig ileum but cross reacted with Leu-enkephalin antibody only after treatment with trichloroacetic acid. The concentration of this substance in CSF ranged from 4 to 8 ng/ml. Its molecular weight was determined by chromatography to be 1,000 to 1,400 daltons, similar to fraction 1 of Terenius and colleagues (280,281), and to the material reported by Ho et al. (120).

Naber et al. (199), using a radioreceptor assay, measured opioid activity in human plasma and monkey CSF at 2-hr intervals during a 24-hr period. Human plasma levels ranged from 0.7 to 4.4 pmoles enkephalin equivalents per ml, whereas the monkey CSF levels ranged from 2.1 to 11.1 pmoles enkephalin equivalents per ml. This opioid activity showed a significant variation over time in both plasma and CSF, suggesting a diurnal rhythm with higher levels in the morning when pain sensitivity in man is lowest. This demonstrates a phase shift with respect to the diurnal rhythm reported for a nocturnal rodent (78,303).

A nonpeptide opiate-like material has also been found in rodent brain and human CSF and urine. Gintzler et al. and Spector and colleagues (92,266) utilized antibodies generated to morphine to detect this material which also has affinity for the opiate receptors in the NG108-15 hybrid cell line. The material has a MW less than 1,000, but has not been further characterized. Its physiological significance is still unclear.

Met-Enkephalin

Reports of the extremely rapid degradation of Met-enkephalin in blood and brain (110) suggested that it would not be found intact in body fluids such as plasma and CSF. Wahlstrom et al. (296), however, reported that their fraction 2 co-chromatographed with authentic enkephalins and that they ocassionally found a small portion of this material to be immunoreactive with enkephalin antiserum. Akil et al. (8), furthermore, reported an enkephalin-like material in CSF taken from the third ventricle of pain patients, which was observed to increase after stimulation of periventricular brain sites to produce analgesia. The material was measured by radioreceptor assay (0.69 ± 0.2 pmoles/ml) and by mouse vas deferens bioassay (2.15 ± 0.8 pmoles/ml). Higher base-line levels (3.12 to 3.25 pmoles/ml) were observed by these investigators in lumbar CSF from normal control subjects (9). This material was chromatographically similar to fraction 2 of Wahlstrom et al. (296), and also immunogenically similar to Met-enkephalin, but was not conclusively identified as such. Furui et al. (84) found, similarly, that levels of a Met-enkephalin-like material determined by radioreceptor assay were higher in spinal CSF than in ventricular CSF. They reported a mean level, in samples obtained from normal subjects by lumbar puncture, of 2.6 ± 1.0 pmoles/ml. Anselmi et al. (14) reported levels of a Met-enkephalin-like material in CSF measured by a radioreceptor assay, of approximately 25 pmoles/ml. These levels were decreased after migraine and cluster headache attacks. Again, this material was not conclusively identified as Met-enkephalin.

Clement-Jones et al. (42,44) developed a highly specific assay for Met-enkephalin, in which the sample was prepared by extraction with high performance liquid chromatography and oxidation before assay with antiserum to Met-enkephalin sulfoxide. It did not cross react with beta-LPH, beta-endorphin, or Leu-enkephalin. They measured mean control levels of Met-enkephalin of 13.3 pg/ml in CSF and 69.3 pg/ml in plasma. They observed somewhat reduced levels in heroin addicts of 4.5 pg/ml in CSF and 40.4 pg/ml in plasma. After successful treatment of withdrawal symptoms, with electroacupuncture, plasma levels of Met-enkephalin were unchanged, whereas CSF levels were increased. Beta-endorphin levels were increased in the addict, but they remained unchanged in both plasma and CSF after the electroacupuncture treatment. Clement-Jones et al. suggested that Met-enkephalin release may be involved in the physiological basis of effective electroacupuncture treatment of withdrawal symptoms. They reported subsequently (45) that in recurrent pain patients, CSF enkephalin levels (7.3 ± 0.8 pg/ml) were not different from those in pain-free control subjects (<4.6 pg/ml), nor were these levels increased after electroacupuncture to relieve pain.

Using this highly specific radioimmunoassay these investigators (43,44) confirmed the presence of Met-enkephalin in human plasma as the intact pentapeptide, but observed levels much lower than those reported previously by others. They reported a range in plasma (20 normal subjects) of 14 to 140 pg/ml and in CSF of 5 to 29 pg/ml. Their data suggested that the Met-enkephalin-like immunoreactivity in plasma is independent of circulating ACTH, beta-LPH, and beta-endorphin, and is possibly secreted by the adrenal medulla. Concentrations were twice as high in adrenal effluent (116 pg/ml) as in other venous samples of central or peripheral origin. In confirmation of this, Hexum et al. (119) observed more Met-enkephalin-like peptide in plasma from the left adrenal lumbar vein of the dog than in plasma from the jugular and femoral veins or from the femoral artery. They found, furthermore, that splanchnic nerve stimulation resulted in an increase in Met-enkephalin-like material in lumbar vein plasma. Base-line plasma and CSF levels of Met-enkephalin and factors which increase or decrease these levels are summarized in Table 3.

TABLE 3. *Factors that influence Met-enkephalin levels in blood and CSF[a]*

	Increase	Decrease	No change
Human CSF Third ventricle[b]	Stimulation in periventricular region to produce analgesia		
Lumbar[c]	Electroacupuncture for opiate withdrawal	Migraine attack Cluster headache Heroin addiction	Recurrent pain Electroacupuncture for analgesia
Human plasma[d]		Heroin addiction	Electroacupuncture for analgesia
Dog plasma[e]	Splanchnic nerve stimulation		

[a]Reported levels are in the range, [b]0.7–2.2 pmoles/ml, [c]<0.01–25 pmoles/ml, [d]0.02–0.2 pmoles/ml, [e]0.16 pmoles/ml. (See ref. 76 for more details.)

Shanks et al. (259) used the highly specific radioimmunoassay for Met-enkephalin discussed above to study the 24-hr profile of Met-enkephalin in man. In this study, they found basal levels in six subjects of 57 ± 19.9 pg/ml, but no regular rhythm in plasma levels of Met-enkephalin was discernible during the 24-hr period. This is in contrast to uncharacterized opioid activity, and to beta-LPH and beta-endorphin, for which there do seem to be circadian rhythms with highest levels in the early morning hours and lowest levels in the late evening (198,199,259).

Beta-Endorphin and Beta-LPH

Basal levels of beta-endorphin-like immunoreactivity (beta-ELI) in rat plasma ranging from 250 to 1,500 pg/ml have been reported (10,109,124). These assays did not distinguish between beta-endorphin and beta-LPH. The proportions of each peptide contributing to the measured levels are somewhat uncertain. Hollt et al. (124) were unable to detect beta-endorphin in unextracted plasma from nonstressed rats.

Krieger et al. (150) reported the first determination of human plasma levels of beta-LPH using a specific antiserum. They measured normal plasma beta-LPH levels of 47.9 ± 5.7 pg/ml, and a ratio of ACTH to beta-LPH of about 4.6 to 1 on a molar basis. They subsequently claimed, however, that beta-endorphin is not detectable in plasma from normal human subjects (278). The detection limit in these assays was 8.5 pg/ml. Subsequent to these studies, however, several laboratories managed to measure beta-endorphin in normal human plasma. Nakao et al. (205) used nonspecific antiserum, but separated beta-endorphin and beta-LPH with gel exclusion chromatography, and observed levels of plasma beta-endorphin and beta-LPH in normal male volunteers of 5.8 ± 1.1 and 111.2 ± 17.4 pg/ml, respectively. Wardlaw and Frantz (297) used a talc extraction procedure and separation on Sephadex G50. They reported mean basal plasma beta-endorphin and beta-LPH concentrations in five normal subjects of 21 ± 7.3 and 114 ± 50 pg/ml, respectively. The molar ratio of beta-LPH to beta-endorphin in these studies was 2.2. The mean beta-ELI was 33 ± 1.5 pg/ml. Akil et al. (10) reported levels of beta-ELI in plasma of five normal human males of 41 pg/ml. Hollt et al. (126) separated beta-endorphin and beta-LPH in plasma of four normal humans on Sephadex G50 and measured levels of 16 ± 2.4 and 48 ± 19 pg/ml, respectively. Ghazarossian et al. (88) separated beta-endorphin and beta-LPH on Biogel P-60 and measured levels of 24.1 and 129 pg/ml, respectively. Yamaguchi et al. (319) submitted plasma extracts to immunoaffinity chromatography to provide simultaneous determinations of beta-LPH, gamma-lipotropin, and beta-endorphin which were 61 ± 8, 25.5 ± 2.9, and $<7.8 \pm 0.7$ pg/ml, respectively. Weidemann et al. (302) used a sensitive and highly specific antiserum (5 to 6% molar cross reactivity with beta-LPH) to measure beta-endorphin in 'raw' plasma of 14 normal subjects without extraction or separation, and observed levels ranging from less than 5 to 45 pg/ml.

Increases in plasma beta-ELI ranging from 150 to 600% after stress or physical trauma in rats have been reported (109,193,237). The immunoreactive material was reported to consist of about 70% beta-endorphin and 30% beta-LPH, and the increase in plasma levels coincided with a decrease in levels in the anterior and intermediate lobes of the pituitary.

Beta-endorphin is elevated in plasma from heroin addicts but does not change during electroacupuncture which suppresses the clinical features of withdrawal (42). Beta-ELI in plasma from schizophrenic patients appears not to differ from levels in normal controls (235). Plasma beta-endorphin increases dramatically during labor and delivery and levels are significantly reduced 1 day postpartum (49,69). Levels do not increase until cervical dilatation is greater than 4 cm and are highest during delivery (96). Levels are also high in cord blood. Csontos et al. (49) reported no arteriovenous difference in neonatal plasma, whereas Wardlaw et al. (298) reported beta-ELI to be higher in the artery than in the vein. The latter group observed, furthermore, a significant negative correlation between umbilical arterial pH and PO_2 and beta-ELI levels, and concluded that hypoxia and secondary acidosis may be major stimuli to the release of beta-endorphin and beta-LPH. They observed beta-ELI in umbilical cord plasma of 45 term human fetuses to be significantly higher (91 ± 16 pg/ml) than the normal adult level (30.7 ± 2.7 pg/ml). Chromatographic analysis indicated the mean beta-endorphin and beta-LPH concentrations to be 57 ± 12.8 and 455 ± 101 pg/ml, respectively. Fetal beta-endorphin appears to be of fetal rather than maternal origin (49,96). Fletcher et al. (69) observed no correlation between plasma beta-ELI during labor and delivery and pain scores. Human plasma, however, contains high levels of opioid peptides other than enkephalins, beta-endorphin, or beta-LPH, including several which are dynorphin-like (28).

Strenuous physical exercise has also been shown to cause a marked increase in plasma beta-endorphin, concomitant with an increase in plasma ACTH (47,70). Any relevance of these findings to runners high is very unlikely, however, because the increased levels are still too low by at least three orders of magnitude to produce any effects in the central nervous system. Levels in CSF might be expected to have a better correlation to such effects.

Acute morphine treatment has been reported to cause an increase in plasma beta-ELI in the rat (125) and the dog (159). Naloxone was reported to have little direct effect in the rat (125), but surprisingly produced an even larger increase in plasma beta-ELI than did morphine in the dog (159). Chronic treatment with morphine caused a decrease in basal plasma levels of beta-ELI in the rat, but did not prevent the poststress increase, which was at least as great as in naive rats (193). Anesthesia induction is reported to have no effect, but surgical stress increases human plasma beta-ELI and these levels are reduced after postoperative morphine (59).

Plasma levels of beta-endorphin and beta-LPH may be dramatically increased, concomitant with ACTH, in patients with endocrine diseases such as Addison's disease, Cushing's disease, or Nelson's syndrome (126,150,201,272,297). Levels of these peptides are also increased after adrenalectomy or treatment with insulin or the synthetic glucocorticoid metyrapone, and are decreased after hypophysectomy or treatment with the synthetic glucocorticoid dexamethasone. Base-line plasma and CSF levels of beta-endorphin and factors which increase or decrease these levels are summarized in Table 4.

There is a significant correlation between levels of beta-ELI and levels of ACTH-ELI in CSF, suggesting a common regulatory mechanism in the brain as in the pituitary, but there is no correlation between beta-ELI levels in CSF and the levels in plasma. Beta-endorphin levels in CSF tend to be higher than the levels in plasma. Indeed, separate beta-endorphin-producing systems in the pituitary and brain have been described (26,299,322), and a better correlation with centrally-mediated phenomena, such as analgesia, might be expected with endorphin levels in CSF than with plasma levels. Akil et al. (7) examined levels of beta-ELI in CSF (third ventricle) before and after electrical stimulation of a periventricular medial thalamic site which produced relief of chronic intractable pain. Levels increased from less than 85 pg/ml before stimulation to $1,636 \pm 382$ pg/ml at 0 to 5 min after stimulation, and the levels were still substantially increased at 20 min. Hosobuchi et al. (129) reported increases of beta-endorphin in CSF after stimulation of the periaqueductal gray matter to give relief to patients with pain of peripheral origin. Levels increased from 193.3 ± 12 pg/ml to 763.3 ± 345.3 pg/ml immediately after a 15-min period of stimulation, and were still elevated 30 min after cessation of stimulation. Levels were not similarly increased after nonanalgesic stimulation of the

TABLE 4. *Factors that influence beta-endorphin levels in blood and CSF[a]*

	Increase	Decrease	No change
Human CSF[a]	Stimulation of PAG for pain relief Stimulation of periventricular medial thalamus for pain relief Electroacupuncture for pain relief Heroin addiction	Cushing's disease	Stimulation of posterior limb of internal capsule Electroacupuncture to relieve withdrawal Nelson's syndrome Glucocorticoids Schizophrenia Acromegaly
Human plasma[b]	Surgical stress Exercise stress Heroin addiction Labor/delivery Adisson's disease Cushing's disease Nelson's syndrome Morphine	Dexamethasone	Anesthesia
Rodent plasma[c]	Noxious stress Morphine Naloxone Vasopressin Chronic metyrapone Adrenalectomy Insulin	Chronic morphine Hypophysectomy Dexamethasone	

[a]Reported levels are in the range: [a]5.3–155 fmoles/ml, [b]0.74–13.2 fmoles/ml, [d]75–441 fmoles/ml. (See ref. 76 for more details.)

posterior limb of the internal capsule in patients suffering deafferentation dysesthesia.

Clement-Jones et al. (42) reported elevated levels of CSF beta-endorphin in heroin addicts, but observed no changes in these levels after auricular electroacupuncture which suppressed withdrawal phenomena. Beta-endorphin levels in the lumbar CSF of patients with recurrent pain was not different from levels in pain-free control subjects, but did show a significant increase after 30 min of low frequency acupuncture which relieved the pain. There was, however, no obvious correlation between the original severity of the pain, or the degree or duration of pain relief, and the basal or elevated levels of beta-endorphin in CSF. CSF levels of beta-ELI were not different from controls in patients with schizophrenia or acromegaly (206,207).

Analgesic Activity of Peptidase Inhibitors

Several enzymes, including aminopeptidases, carboxypeptidases, and dipeptidylcarboxypeptidases, have been reported to degrade enkephalins. If endogenous enkephalins indeed play a physiological role to modulate pain perception, then inhibition of the enzymes that inactivate this released enkephalin might be expected to produce an analgesic effect. Demonstration of such analgesia could be taken as evidence for the proposed role for the enkephalins.

Bacitracin, an aminopeptidase inhibitor, was reported to produce a dose-dependent and naloxone-reversible analgesia in mice tested in the tail flick assay, when administered by the intracerebroventricular route (261). Another aminopeptidase inhibitor, d-leucine, has been reported to potentiate stress-induced analgesia in the rodent (37). D-phenylalanine, a weak inhibitor of carboxypeptidase A, was reported to potentiate the analgesic response to Met-enkephalin in the rat hot-plate jump assay, and also stress-induced analgesia in rats (37). The role of these particular enzymes in the synaptic inactivation of the enkephalins is, however, presently unknown.

As discussed above, the dipeptidyl carboxypeptidase, enkephalinase A, is the enzyme most likely to have a physiological role in inactivating enkephalins at the synapses. The most potent ($K_I = 4.2$ nM for enkephalin) and selective inhibitor of enkephalinase A reported to date is thiorphan, 3-mercapto-2-propionylglycine (233). In the mouse tail withdrawal and mouse hot-plate tests, thiorphan administered either intracerebroventricularly or intravenously significantly potentiated the analgesic effect of D-Ala^2-Met^5-enkephalin or D-Ala^2-Met^5-enkephalin amide (76,233). In the jump response of the hot plate assay, thiorphan even produced a small but significant antinociceptive effect when administered alone intracerebroventricularly (Fig. 5). This antinociceptive effect could be antagonized by naloxone and was more readily elicited in the afternoon hours (Fig. 5), when it has been reported that enkephalinergic systems may be more active and when naloxone's hyperalgesic effect is most readily demonstrable (78).

Captopril (SQ14225), an angiotensin converting enzyme inhibitor, which is a less potent inhibitor of enkephalinase ($K_I = 10$ μM, 233) than is thiorphan, has also

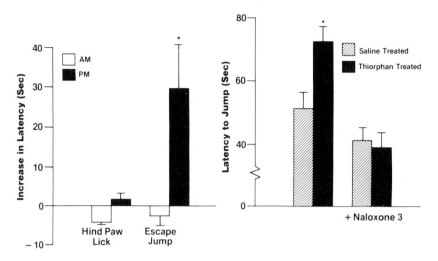

FIG. 5. The *left* graph shows that analgesic activity of thiorphan depends on the time of day. The changes in latency (compared to saline-treated controls) to the hind paw lick and escape jump responses in the mouse hot-plate (55°C) test for analgesia at 30 min after 30 μg intracerebroventricular thiorphan were measured. Thiorphan had no effect on the hind paw lick response in either the a.m. or the p.m. but did increase the latency to the jump response in the p.m. when enkephalinergic systems may be most active (78,303–306). The *right* graph shows antagonism of thiorphan analgesia by naloxone. The latencies to the jump response at 30 min after either saline (10 μl) or thiorphan (30 μg/10 μl) intracerebroventricularly were measured. Naloxone administered at 3 mg/kg, subcutaneously, 15 min before testing, completely antagonized the analgesic activity of thiorphan.

been evaluated for analgesic activity. Buckett (31) reported that captopril at 100 mg/kg intraperitoneally did not influence stimulation-produced analgesia nor show direct analgesic properties. Carenzi et al. (37), to the contrary, reported that captopril given intracerebroventricularly produced dose-related naloxone-reversible analgesia in the hot plate assay. Stine et al. (270) found that captopril administered intracerebroventricularly was analgesic in the tail flick assay and also potentiated the analgesia owing to Met-enkephalin. The analgesic activity of these agents appears weak and variable, but further studies with combinations of these inhibitors, may prove interesting.

Actions of the Opioid Antagonist Naloxone

Antagonism of Exogenous Opioid Peptide-Induced Analgesia

Analgesia has been widely demonstrated after intracerebral or intraventricular administration of the natural enkephalins, but this activity is weak and short-lived owing to the enzymatic lability of these peptides (21,34,78,79,317). Beta-endorphin is more potent and produces analgesia of much longer duration than do the natural enkephalins after intracerebroventricular administration (64,72,178,221) because of its greater resistance to enzymatic degradation (57,187,195). Very slight modifications of the enkephalin structure, to provide analogs with increased enzymatic stability, have been made (*see* more detailed discussion later in this chapter), and these analogs produce analgesia of a much greater degree and a longer duration than do the natural enkephalins after intracerebroventricular administration (72, 101,223,317). Indeed, such peptide analogs have been synthesized which are at least 100 times more potent than morphine given intracerebroventricularly. They produce analgesia even after systemic administration (82,232). These will be discussed further in a later section. The analgesic activity of the opioid peptides and analogs, furthermore, can be blocked by naloxone (e.g., Fig. 6), demonstrating that they produce analgesia by their action on opioid receptors. The interpretation of such results, of course, is that the exogenous peptides produce analgesia by their action on receptors for endogenous opioid peptides. Would action of these endogenous ligands on these receptors also produce analgesia? This question is discussed in following sections of this chapter.

Hyperalgesic Activity—Antagonism of Endogenous Opioids

If an endogenous opioid modulates the perception of pain in such a manner as to reduce the averseness of this pain, then treatment with an antagonist such as naloxone, by blocking the action of the endogenous opioid, should have the opposite effect, i.e., produce hyperalgesia. This concept sounds simple enough, but caution must be taken when attempting to apply this approach and to interpret the results. Naloxone may, for example, produce some of its effects by direct actions other

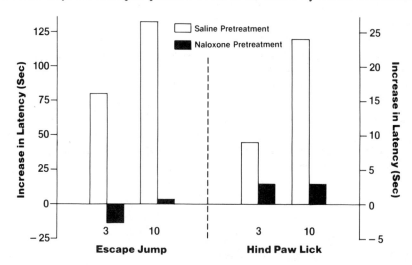

FIG. 6. Naloxone antagonism of metkephamid analgesia. The increases in latency to the escape jump and hind paw lick responses in the mouse hot-plate test caused by metkephamid (3 and 10 mg/kg, subcutaneously) compared to saline. Either saline or naloxone (1 mg/kg, subcutaneously) was injected immediately before metkephamid and the latencies were measured 15 min later. The pretreatment with naloxone completely blocked the increases in latency to both responses produced by metkephamid at both doses.

than blockade of opioid receptors. This concern has been discussed in some detail by Sawynok et al. (250). The subtlety of the effects of blocking endogenous opioid systems is emphasized by the conflicting reports on the effects of the narcotic antagonist, naloxone, in various pain models. This indicates the importance, in attempting to study the results of interfering with the activity of endogenous opioid systems, of measuring the appropriate parameters under the appropriate conditions to expect them to be active. The status of this work has been previously reviewed in some detail (73,76).

Jacob et al. (135) were the first to report a hyperalgesic effect of naloxone in rodents. Frederickson et al. (78,79), also using the mouse hot-plate test, reported similar results and both groups claimed the effect to be specific to the jump response, the hind paw lick response being rather insensitive to naloxone. This has been explained on the basis of a selective action of the endogenous opioids on tolerance to pain as opposed to the threshold for perception of pain (79). This hyperalgesic effect of naloxone in the rodent has been confirmed in several other test systems (23,104,147).

The initial studies in man used *experimental* pain models to measure pain *threshold* in *unselected* subjects, and failed to demonstrate a hyperalgesic effect of naloxone (63,105,106). The effect of naloxone in the absence of exogenous opioids, however, appears to be dependent on many factors such as dose, test system, parameter measured, and the nature of the subjects and their environment. Levine et al. (161) thought that clinical pain might be a more appropriate model than experimental pain to study the actions of endorphins and naloxone. They tested this idea successfully in patients undergoing oral surgery. They concluded that the prolonged duration and stress associated with clinical pain make it particularly effective for activating the endogenous analgesic systems.

Buchsbaum et al. (30) divided subjects into pain sensitive and pain insensitive groups, and found the pain insensitive subjects to perceive electrical shock as more painful after naloxone administration, whereas pain sensitive subjects perceived them as less painful, i.e., experienced an analgesic effect. Levine et al. (162) divided subjects into placebo responders and placebo nonresponders, and observed a biphasic effect in the placebo responders. This group experienced analgesia at low doses of naloxone (0.4 and 2 mg) and hyperalgesia at higher doses (7.5 and 10 mg). These results are qualitatively similar to earlier reports of Lasagna (157). Placebo nonresponders had a final mean pain rating identical to that of placebo responders who received the high dose of naloxone. Investigators have interpreted this as evidence that endorphin release mediates placebo analgesia (160).

Stress-induced analgesia, which can be antagonized by naloxone, has been reported in both the rodent (182) and man (308). It seems, however, that both opioid and nonopioid mechanisms of analgesia can be activated by stress (163). Naloxone-reversible analgesia has been produced by high-intensity low-frequency transcutaneous electrical stimulation (TENS; 40,262), and it is likely that both opioid and nonopioid mechanisms may be activated depending on the nature of the stimulation, just as reported for stress-induced analgesia (163). In rodents, naloxone-reversible analgesia could be elicited with peripheral electrical stimulation at various frequencies, and the degree of analgesia appeared to be directly dependent on pulse widths and frequency (312). Acupuncture or electrical stimulation in appropriate brain areas can produce analgesia which can be antagonized by naloxone (3,6,41,189). These observations all certainly support the concept that endogenous opioid systems can be activated to modulate nociceptive processes.

Almay et al. (12) reported that CSF endorphins in chronic pain patients with pain of organic origin were lower than in healthy volunteers. Lindblom and Tegner (171), however, reported no significant effect of naloxone (0.8 mg) on levels of spontaneous pain or on heat pain thresholds in 10 chronic pain patients. It is possible that sensitivity to pain in such patients is already maximum. Abram et al. (2) reported the failure of naloxone to reverse analgesia produced by low-intensity high-frequency TENS in patients with chronic pain. They concluded that this sort of stimulation, unlike high-intensity low-frequency stimulation, which does produce naloxone-reversible analgesia as discussed above, provides analgesia not associated with release of endogenous opioids. The doses of naloxone used in these studies, however, were in the lower range (0.4 to 1.2 mg), reported by Levine et al. (162) to produce analgesia rather than hyperalgesia. Higher doses of naloxone (>7.5 mg) will have to be tried in this paradigm to clarify whether or not endorphins play a role in this phenomenon.

Another factor, which can contribute to contradictory results in these studies, is the existence of a diurnal rhythm in sensitivity to pain. Such a rhythm was demonstrated in the latency to jump response in the mouse hot-plate test for analgesia (78). Such a rhythm has been reported in man also (226), but man, not being nocturnal as is the rodent, demonstrates a reverse cycle. Thus, for man, the greatest tolerance to pain occurs in the morning hours and diminishes in the afternoon and evening hours. Frederickson et al. (78) observed a diurnal variation also in the hyperalgesic activity of naloxone, which coincided with the variation in sensitivity to painful stimuli. Naloxone was most effective during the times of highest control latencies, i.e., the times of highest tolerance to pain. The small and variable effects of naloxone during the morning hours, when the basal latencies were already at a minimum, may explain some of the discrepancies between different studies of the hyperalgesic action of naloxone. Such a rhythm in naloxone hyperalgesia, paralleling the rhythm in basal responsiveness to pain, has been confirmed in various other test systems and species, including man (51,234). It has been suggested that the diurnal rhythm follows food intake patterns, rather than a circadian rhythm (190), but more recent work supports a circadian rhythm cued to a photo-period (155).

These rhythms in pain responsiveness and the effects of naloxone could be most readily explained by a diurnal rhythm in the levels of endogenous opioid activity. Indeed, a diurnal rhythm in the brain levels of Met-enkephalin has been observed in rodents (303,305,306). Basal Met-enkephalin levels were not observed to vary diurnally, but when animals were exposed to noxious stimuli before sacrifice, levels increased in the afternoon only, when mice are most tolerant to pain (303). It was mentioned previously in this chapter that pituitary-derived blood-borne opioid peptides are not likely to have any direct influence on centrally-mediated opioid actions such as analgesia. Indeed, hypophysectomy was found to have no effect on the diurnal rhythm in pain tolerance, naloxone hyperalgesia, or brain Met-enkephalin levels (305). The diurnal increase in brain Met-enkephalin levels in response to noxious stress was found to be restricted to the striatal region, more specifically to the globus pallidus as determined by the punch technique (Fig. 7). The significance of this unexpected localization is not yet known.

A circadian rhtyhm in rat brain opioid receptors has also been demonstrated (200). The differences observed throughout the 24-hr period were not because of changes in affinity, but rather to changes in the number of binding sites. This rhythm in binding sites closely parallelled the rhythm reported earlier in tolerance to pain (78). Thus, the ability of rodents to tolerate noxious stress in the late afternoon and evening, appears to be provided by both an increase in ability to produce opioid peptides in response to the stress, and also an increased number of receptors for these peptides.

Endogenous Opioids as Neurotransmitters, Neuromodulators, or Neurohormones

The enkephalins have been shown to meet many of the criteria for neurotransmitters, and this has been the subject of several previous reviews (60,72,265). The distribution, synthesis, release, and metabolism of the opioid peptides have been reviewed in previous sections of this chapter. The functional aspect of neurotrans-

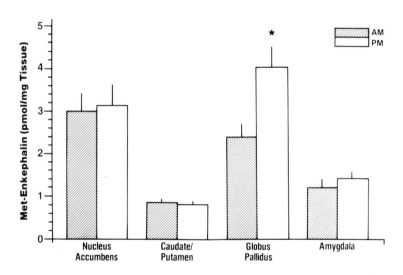

FIG. 7. Levels of Met-enkephalin (measured by radioimmunoassay) in specific striatal nuclei in the a.m. and in the p.m. after exposure to noxious stimuli. *, difference is significant at the $p < 0.01$ level (306).

mitter action is the effect on neuronal activity after activation of neuronal receptors, and this has been studied by electrophysiological techniques. The enkephalins inhibit neuronal firing in many brain areas containing opioid receptors, such as the caudate nucleus, hippocampus, hypothalamus, thalamus, periaqueductal gray region, and frontal cortex. These electrophysiological actions have also been reviewed in previous articles (60,72,210). Although the actual enkephalinergic pathways are for the most part unknown, there are several areas for which the neuronal circuitry has been proposed.

There is evidence for an inhibitory enkephalinergic pathway from the amygdala to the bed nucleus of the stria terminalis (BST). High levels of Met-enkephalin occur in the BST (107), and an enkephalin-containing pathway from the central nucleus of the amygdala to the BST has been demonstrated immunohistochemically (286). Sawada and Yamamoto (248) reported that an enkephalin analog (Dalamid) suppressed spontaneous and glutamate-evoked spike discharges, and also field potentials and spike discharges elicited by stimulation of the stria terminalis in thin sections of BST from the guinea pig brain. These actions of Dalamid were blocked by naloxone. Stimulation of the lateral division of the stria terminalis, furthermore, produced a late inhibitory action on neurons in the BST, which could be antagonized by naloxone in a portion of the neurons tested.

Opioids have been reported to excite hippocampal pyramidal cells, in contrast to their inhibitory actions on most other neurons in the brain. This has been attributed to a disinhibition rather than a direct excitation, i.e., to result from inhibition of GABAergic inhibitory interneurons (321). This has been confirmed with *in vitro* hippocampus slices (61,158,208) and cultured hippocampal pyramidal cells (86). Thus, an endogenous opioid, possibly Met-enkephalin, is released from its nerve terminals to act on postsynaptic receptors on GABAergic cell bodies, which provide tonic inhibition to the pyramidal cells unless shut down by the endogenous opioid. A similar mechanism was earlier postulated for the actions of opioids in the periaqueductal gray matter (74,75). Nicoll et al. (208) have reported such an action in other neuronal circuits such as the postsynaptic inhibition of olfactory bulb mitral cells, and presynaptic inhibition of spinal primary afferents. They suggest that this type of inhibition may be an important general mechanism of opioid action in the CNS, and that local GABA-containing inhibitory interneurons may be primary targets of Met-enkephalin containing fiber systems.

The relative lack of susceptibility of beta-endorphin to enzymatic degradation, its resultant long duration of action, and the strategic location of beta-endorphinergic cell bodies and terminals for release into the ventricular system, all implicate a neurohormonal role for this peptide. Nevertheless, a neurotransmitter role as well cannot be discounted. The enkephalins may also function as neurohormones in the peripheral circulation since the adrenal glands secrete large amounts of various enkephalin-like peptides into the blood (48,119), but the target tissues are not well known at this time.

Coexistence of Opioid Peptides and Other Neurotransmitters

Almost 50 years ago, Dale (50) propounded his "principle" that neurons release the same transmitter at all their terminals. This has been extrapolated to suggest that only one particular neurotransmitter is associated with any one particular neuron. It has recently been pointed out (122), however, that Dale's concept emphasized, rather, that if one knows the neurotransmitter in the peripheral branch of a sensory neuron, then this reveals the nature of the transmission process at a central synapse of the same neuron. This does not preclude the possible existence of more than one transmitter substance in a given terminal, but only requires that the situation be the same at all the terminals for a given neuron.

Indeed, examples suggesting the coexistence of different transmitters in the same neuron have been reported (122,123). It has been cautioned, however, that the evidence is mainly morphological and the classical transmitter criteria have not yet been satisfied for two substances within the same neuron. The immunohistochemical technique is the main approach used to demonstrate the coincidence of neurotransmitters. These studies may be conducted in a single section of tissue if the appropriate and compatible processing techniques are available, or, alternatively, in consecutive or serial sections. There are of course many limitations to this technique, as discussed in an earlier section. A major concern is the identity and integrity of the immunoreactive antigens. Supportive biochemical and chromatographic analyses may be used to further characterize them.

An enkephalin-like peptide has been observed in some of the principle ganglion cells of the rat superior cervical ganglion and in the guinea pig prevertebral ganglia (256). Enkephalin-like, but not beta-endorphin-like, immunoreactive material has been also observed in adrenal gland cells in the rat, guinea pig, cat, cow, monkey, and human (179,181,254,255). This peptide was present in both epinephrine- and norepinephrine-containing cells. This immunoreactive material increased after sectioning of the splanchnic nerve such that it could be demonstrated in almost all gland cells. These immunohistochemical data are in accord with biochemical data (radioimmunoassay, bioassay) demonstrating the presence of both Met-enkephalin and Leu-enkephalin, and various larger precursors in chromaffin cells of the adrenal medulla and in sympathetic ganglia (48,56,166). Figure 8 shows immunofluorescence micrographs demonstrating the coexistence of Met-enkephalin-like immunoreactivity, and dopamine beta-hydroxylase in adrenal medullary gland cells of the cat, and enkephalin-positive fibers in the guinea pig adrenal medulla, which disappeared after denervation.

Enkephalin-like, but not beta-endorphin-like, peptides have also been demonstrated in dopamine-containing neurons (glomus cells) in the carotid body of the cat, dog, and monkey (180,181). Evidence has been obtained for the coexistence in neurons in the central nervous system of serotonin and substance P (24,38,121), but not yet for opioid peptides and other transmitter candidates.

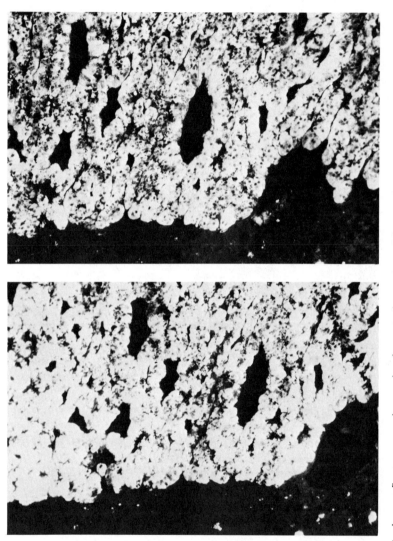

FIGS. 8 A and B. Immunofluorescence micrographs of consecutive sections of the cat adrenal gland after incubation with **(A)** Met-enkephalin antiserum, **(B)** dopamine β-hydroxylase antiserum. In this section all medullary gland cells contain enkephalin-like immunoreactivity **(A)** as well as dopamine β-hydroxylase **(B)**. No immunofluorescence was observed after treatment with Met-enkephalin control serum or with beta-endorphin antiserum.

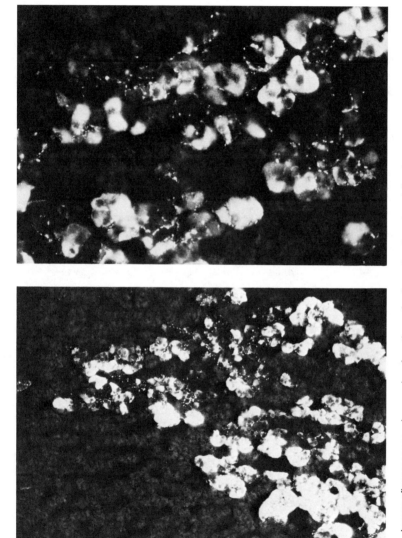

FIGS. 8 C and D. Immunofluorescence micrographs of sections of guinea pig adrenal medulla after incubation with Met-enkephalin antiserum. Note the Met-enkephalin positive fibers. These disappear after denervation (from ref. 254, with permission).

Such coexistence of putative neurotransmitters in neurons has led to the suggestion that one may function as a neurotransmitter and the other as a neuromodulator. Costa et al. (48) presumed the peptide to be the likely neuromodulator and attempted to examine this phenomenon by using as a model system, the synapse between splanchnic nerves and chromaffin cells of the adrenal medulla. These cells are innervated by splanchnic cholinergic neurons which apparently contain multiple forms of an enkephalin-like peptide in addition to acetylcholine (153,154). They reported that the opioid peptides appear to modulate, via an allosteric action, the number of cholinergic receptors available to regulate catecholamine secretion from the chromaffin cells. Thus, in this system, acetylcholine would appear to act as the primary transmitter, while the enkephalins act as modulators.

Electrophysiological evidence has been presented to show that in some systems in the brain the roles may be reversed. Catecholamines, for example, may act as modulators to augment the responsiveness of cerebral cortical neurons to enkephalins (219). Cortical neurons have not yet been reported, however, in which catecholamines coexist with enkephalins. Of course, there are other possibilities for the functions of coexisting peptides and biogenic amines. One may have a transmitter function, for example, and the other a trophic or metabolic function. Alternatively, one may activate receptors on the postsynaptic cell, while the other acts on autoreceptors to regulate their release from the presynaptic terminals.

Sites and Mechanisms of Analgesic Actions of the Endogenous Opioids

The probable sites in the central nervous system where the endogenous opioids function to modulate nociception have been mapped by using the stereotactic techniques of electrostimulation and microinjection of exogenous opioids (167,189, 222,228,229,246,247,278,313,315). The major sites involved include the PA-periventricular gray, nucleus reticularis giganto-cellularis, medial thalamus, mesencephalic reticular formation, lateral hypothalamus, raphe nuclei, and spinal cord.

Microinjection of opioids into the periaqueductal gray (PAG) or electrical stimulation of this area both produced analgesia which could be at least partially antagonized by naloxone (3,6,128,136,189,285,315). That both opioids and electrical stimulation in the PAG produce analgesia is surprising because the opioids are generally inhibitory on single neurons in the PAG (74,75,79,115,310). An increase in multiunit activity results, however, when opioids are injected into the PAG (287). This puzzle would be explained if the opioids had a disinhibitory action in the PAG. This has been previously postulated (74,75,189). Indeed, evidence for such a disinhibitory action of opioids has been obtained in the hippocampus (321) as previously discussed.

There is both anatomical (1,87,241) and electrophysiological (258) evidence for a direct connection from PAG to nucleus raphe magnus (NRM). Stimulation in the PAG (66), systemic morphine (212), or microinjection of morphine into the PAG (20) all excite neurons in the NRM. Stimulation of the PAG or NRM, furthermore, inhibits spinothalamic neurons (89,167,214) and produces analgesia (214,215).

Selective destruction of the dorsolateral funiculus of the spinal cord, containing the descending axons of the NRM projecting to the dorsal horn of the spinal cord, blocked the inhibition of spinothalamic neurons (67), and also the analgesia elicited by PAG stimulation (17). There is evidence that this raphe spinal system mediating opioid- and stimulation-produced analgesia from the PAG has a major serotonergic component (4,5,113,196,314,316).

A proposed scheme of the mechanism of action of opioid-induced analgesia in the PAG is presented in Fig. 9. This is not likely an endogenous analgesic system, but rather, a trans-synaptic feed back circuitry meant to regulate the spinothalamic pain transmission neuronal circuitry. It might produce analgesia during a period of continuous activity, such as during electrical stimulation of the PAG, or after introduction of an opioid, which is resistant to enzymatic degradation. But, the released endogenous enkephalins would be rapidly inactivated by the synaptic

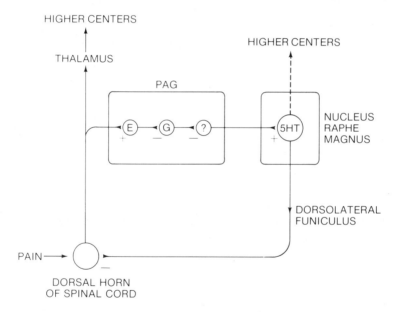

FIG. 9. Simplified schematic of proposed circuitry for the action of opioid-, stimulation-, and stress-induced analgesia via the periaqueductal gray matter (PAG). This scheme involves an enkephalinergic interneuron in the PAG which inhibits a tonically active GABAergic inhibitory interneuron. The enkephalinergic neuron would be driven by pain stimuli or by electrical stimulation in the PAG. This would result in disinhibition of the output neuron (?, neurotransmitter unknown), which would activate a descending spinal "gating" system via the nucleus raphe magnus. Administration of an opioid into the PAG would produce disinhibition of the output neuron by action on the opioid receptors on the GABAergic interneuron. Electrical stimulation in the PAG, besides providing naloxone-reversible analgesia by releasing enkephalins, would provide analgesia insensitive to naloxone by directly activating the output neuron. The descending system from raphe to dorsal horn appears to be at least partly serotonergic. The normal function of this system is not likely to provide analgesia, but rather to provide feedback regulation of the spinothalamic pain transmission system. + = excitatory synapse; − = inhibitory synapse; E = enkephalin; G = GABA; 5HT = 5-hydroxytryptamine (serotonin). (From ref. 76, with permission.)

enkephalinases. Some forms of stress- or stimulation-produced analgesia have long durations which outlast the stimulus. Such analgesia may result from the release of beta-endorphin into the CSF. Via the CSF, this beta-endorphin might find its way to enkephalin receptors in the PAG, and activate the gating mechanism for prolonged periods of time, because it is only slowly inactivated by the synaptic enzymes. Alternatively, such analgesia may be mediated via other neuronal systems and/or by nonopioid mechanisms as well.

Evidence has been reported that the PAG system need not be intact for analgesia induced by systemic morphine (225). This is not surprising because there are brain sites other than the PAG through which morphine may induce analgesia (189,192, 213,246,247,292,313,315).

SUMMARY AND COMMENTS

Endogenous opioids, particularly beta-endorphin and the enkephalins, have been demonstrated to occur in specific brain regions in association with opioid receptors. The mechanisms of their synthesis and degradation are being studied. These endogenous opioids have been detected in both plasma and CSF in animals and in man. Factors that regulate the levels in these body fluids have been discussed. A diurnal rhythm has been observed in the levels of some of these materials in both body fluids. Higher levels occur in human plasma in the early morning hours, which correlates with the lower sensitivity to pain reported during this time period. Important questions remain concerning the sources and functions of the various endogenous opioid peptides in plasma and CSF. It seems clear, however, that levels in plasma and levels in CSF derive from different sources and reflect different roles, although there may be some feed back regulation between the two systems. Blood levels of beta-endorphin appear to originate from the pituitary, whereas CSF levels derive from the periventricular system in the brain. The levels in the CSF may reflect function in the modulation of pain, but it is unlikely that plasma levels reflect any such role. Levels in the two body fluids appear to be under separate controls, and vary differently in different conditions. It is unlikely that there is any substantial transport of beta-endorphin or beta-LPH from plasma to CSF. The source of Met-enkephalin in plasma appears to be the adrenal glands, and unlike beta-endorphin levels in plasma, the Met-enkephalin levels do not appear to vary according to a diurnal rhythm. Cell bodies and nerve terminals synthesizing and releasing enkephalins are distributed throughout the brain. Different large precursors, pro-opiomelanocortin and preproenkephalin, respectively, have been described for beta-endorphin and the enkephalins.

Evidence about whether endogenous opioids function to modulate nociceptive processes has been reviewed. CSF levels of beta-endorphin are increased after brain stimulation to produce pain relief or after acupuncture for the same purpose. The levels are also increased in heroin addiction. Levels of Met-enkephalin in human CSF appear to be reduced during migraine attacks and cluster headaches, and also in heroin addicts, but not in patients suffering from recurrent pain. These levels may be increased in human CSF after stimulation of the periventricular region to produce analgesia, and after electroacupuncture for relief of withdrawal symptoms in heroin addicts. Met-enkephalin levels in CSF were not reported to be changed, however, in patients with recurrent pain, nor were they increased after electroacupuncture to relieve this pain. Some caution must be advised, however, in interpreting such negative findings for Met-enkephalin. The CSF levels of this peptide may not be an adequate reflection of levels at the site of action in the brain, owing to the enzymatic lability of this material.

Evidence has also derived from investigations of the ability of enzyme inhibitors to potentiate, and of antagonists such as naloxone to block, analgesia induced by acupuncture, brain stimulation or exposure to stress, and from the ability of naloxone to produce hyperalgesia in the normal condition. Further evidence derives from the ability of the natural peptides, and analogs, administered exogenously, to produce analgesia that can be antagonised by naloxone.

At the present time, there is positive evidence that endogenous opioids function in some manner to modulate nociception. The tonic activity of these systems, however, is apparently very low, and many factors appear to influence their likelihood of becoming activated. Another confounding factor is the diurnal rhythm in the levels of the endogenous opioids and the receptors upon which they act. Further complications arise from the existence of both opioid and nonopioid mechanisms of analgesia. These factors have probably contributed to some of the negative results reported. A possible mechanism for the modulation of nociceptive processes by the endogenous opioids has been proposed, and will be used in subsequent sections to provide a rationale for developing new analgesic interventions.

ANALGESIC PHARMACOLOGY OF OPIOID PEPTIDES AND THEIR DERIVATIVES

Rationale for Development of Opioid Peptides as Analgesics

The endogenous opioids themselves have no apparent clinical utility as analgesics. The enkephalins are too rapidly degraded enzymatically, and the more enzymatically stable beta-endorphin does not appear to cross the blood brain barrier readily enough. There are, however, approaches that may be used to overcome these problems and to develop agents with therapeutic potential. The basic mechanistic model upon which these approaches are based is shown in Fig. 10.

An attractive possibility is the development of specific inhibitors of the enzyme or enzymes that inactivate enkephalins at their synapses. A carboxydipeptidase discussed earlier, enkephalinase A, may be such an enzyme (185,186). An effective inhibitor of this enzyme, thiorphan (3-mercapto-2-benzylpropionyl glycine) has been prepared (233), but does not appear likely to have clinical utility. Its systemic bioavailability may not be adequate, and, furthermore, although it is very effective at potentiating the analgesic activity of exogenously administered opioid peptides, it appears to exert rather limited analgesic activity on its own. This relative lack

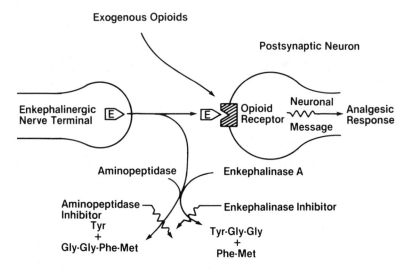

FIG. 10. Neuronal model for mechanisms for producing analgesia by compounds interacting with enkephalinergic systems. The natural enkephalins are not analgesics themselves, but rather neurotransmitters sending brief neuronal messages as discussed in Fig. 9. The message is brief because the enkephalins are rapidly inactivated by the enzymes as shown. Beta-endorphin, reaching these receptors as a circulating neurohormone, on the other hand, might be able to provide a sustained enough message to be perceived as analgesia since it is less susceptible than the shorter enkephalins to these degradative enzymes. One approach to developing analgesics based on the enkephalins is to modify the structure to provide protection from these enzymes, so that when they are applied exogenously, they produce analgesia as discussed above for beta-endorphin. Another approach would be to develop inhibitors of the degradative enzymes so that the activity of the natural enkephalins would be prolonged sufficiently to provide an analgesic effect. These approaches are discussed further in the text.

of apparent direct activity may be explained by a very low basal activity of the enkephalinergic systems. Of course, if clinical pain were to activate such systems, compounds of this nature might have very desirable clinical utility not detected by standard analgesic model systems.

An intact and active endogenous opioid system would not be required, however, for the production of analgesic activity by enkephalin analogs which are resistant to enzymatic degradation. The challenge in this approach is to develop analogs with receptor selectivity and sufficient bioavailabiilty to achieve adequate concentration at the desired receptors in the brain. The emerging multiple receptor concept raises the possibility that it may yet be possible to develop the elusive analgesic structure devoid of physical dependence, or respiratory depression, or other unwanted side effects. There are also other advantages to be provided by these new structures. These will be discussed in a later section. Since high activity resides in the enkephalin-like pentapeptide and tetrapeptide sequences, the preparation of analogs of these or even smaller fragments is more economically feasible than analogs of the much larger beta-endorphin. Indeed, many hundreds of such enkephalin analogs have been synthesized, and considerable structure activity data have already been reported (72,174,197). We will briefly discuss some of the more basic aspects of this structure activity information in the next section.

Structure Activity Relationships of Opioid Peptides and Derivatives

Many factors may confound the interpretation of structure activity studies, and this is particularly so for peptides and their derivatives. Many of the factors that influence the outcome of structure activity relationship (SAR) studies are illustrated in Fig. 11. An example of how the unique enzymatic degradability of the opioid peptides can lead to errors is provided, for example, by the conclusion reached earlier concerning the minimum sequence of the peptide for opioid activity. The essential lack of activity of the tetrapeptide structure (Tyr-Gly-Gly-Phe) in either the mouse hot-plate test for analgesia or even on the mouse vas deferens preparation *in vitro* suggested that the pentapeptide sequence must be the shortest chain length with significant activity (72). Subsequent studies with derivatives of the tetrapeptide more resistant to enzymatic degradation, however, demonstrated high activity in the tetrapeptide sequence (Table 5; 191,290). The structure activity relationships of the opioid peptides, the enkephalins in particular, have been discussed in detail elsewhere (72,174,196,197).

Because the natural enkephalins are too labile to have therapeutic utility, a research challenge to be met in exploring such potential utility has been to provide structural modification, which would infer enzymatic protection without destroying affinity and efficacy at the desired receptors. A number of analogs of Met-enkephalin have been prepared toward these ends, and two, metkephamid and FK33

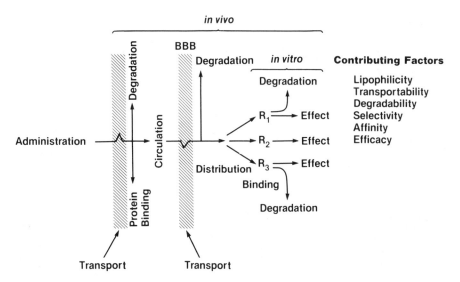

FIG. 11. Factors that can influence the outcome of SAR studies. These factors can distort possible correlations between structure and activity, particularly in *in vivo* studies, if they are not properly accounted for. This can lead to erroneous conclusions.

TABLE 5. *Relative opioid activities of several tetrapeptide analogs of enkephalin*

| | Molar potency ratios[a] | | |
| | Mouse Hot-plate | | |
Compound	MVD	ICV	SC
Morphine	1.0	1.0	1.0
Tyr-Gly-Gly-Phe-Met-OH	20.0	<0.003	0
Tyr-Gly-Gly-Phe-OH	<0.2	<0.003	0
Tyr-D-Ala-Gly-Phe-NH$_2$	0.8	25.0	0.7
Tyr-D-Ala-Gly-N(Me)Phe-NH$_2$	10.0	200.0	4.0

[a]The molar potency ratios relative to morphine were calculated from the molar IC$_{50}$ values on mouse vas deferens (MVD) preparation and from ED$_{50}$ values on the jump response in the mouse hot-plate test for analgesia after intracerebroventricular (ICV) or subcutaneous (SC) administration.

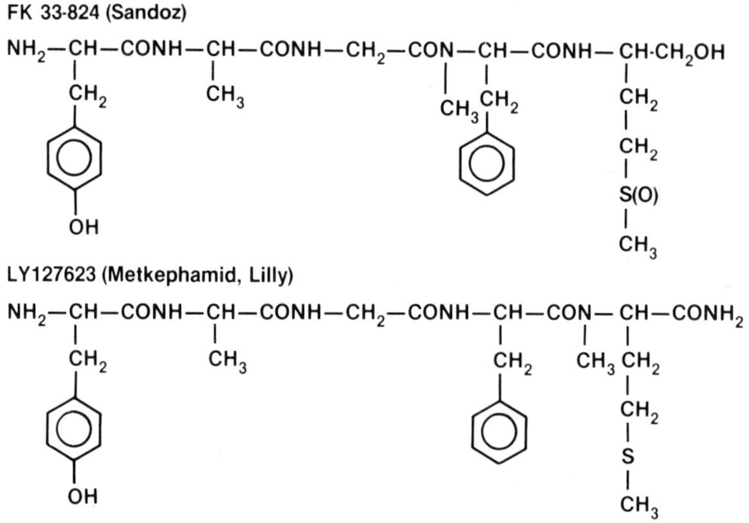

FK 33-824 (Sandoz)

LY127623 (Metkephamid, Lilly)

FIG. 12. Structures of the two Met-enkephalin analogues: FK33 824 (Tyr-D-Ala-Gly-N(Me)Phe-Met(S-O)-carbinol, Sandoz) and metkephamid (Tyr-D-Ala-Gly-Phe-N(Me) Met-amide, LY 127623). These are both systemically active analgesics.

824 (Fig. 12), have progressed to the clinic. These will be discussed in some detail in the next sections.

μ-Receptors vs. δ-Receptors in Analgesia

The discovery of the opioid peptides has provided an explanation for the proposed multiple opioid receptors—i.e., that there are probably multiple opioid ligands serving multiple functions. The μ, κ, and σ receptors were proposed earlier by Martin and colleagues (90,188) on the basis of differential pharmacological activity of various analgesic agents in the spinal dog preparation. Several others, including the δ-receptors, have been proposed since the discovery of the endogenous opioid peptides. Several lines of evidence support the existence of separate μ- and δ-receptors (82,97). The opioid receptors will be discussed in detail in the following chapter, but I would like to discuss in this section the roles of δ versus μ receptors in mediating analgesic activity and physical dependence.

The prevalent opinion has been that the μ-receptor rather than the δ-receptor mediates analgesia. Goodman et al. (97) reported a differential distribution of μ- and δ-receptor binding in brain, and suggested that the areas of concentration of μ-receptors appeared to correlate better with the probable mediation of analgesic activity. Gacel et al. (85) attempted to differentiate the μ versus δ involvement in analgesia by making comparative studies of enkephalin analogs selective for peripheral μ or δ receptors, as defined by potencies on guinea pig ileum (GPI) or mouse vas deferens (MVD), respectively. They concluded that the dissociation between antinociceptive properties in mice and potencies on the mouse vas deferens unambiguously reflected preferential implication of μ-receptors in analgesia. There are problems with this conclusion, however. The two δ-selective ligands used had unmodified amino acids at the c-terminal, and thus little protection from carboxypeptidase or enkephalinase activity, whereas the μ-selective agents were modified at the c-terminal. The authors provided no data concerning the relative enzymatic lability of the peptide analogs compared. They attempted to 'circumvent' possible differences in pharmacokinetic properties by using intracerebroventricular injection, but this is not totally adequate because the brain possesses potent enkephalin c-terminal inactivating activity. Dose-response curves, furthermore, were not generated, but only single doses were evaluated.

Pasternak et al. (218) have used an irreversible antagonist, naloxazone, to define a high affinity μ-receptor (μ_1), and lower affinity μ (μ_2)- and δ-receptors. They were able to antagonize analgesia with this agent, and concluded that analgesia was mediated by the high affinity μ_1-receptor, but it is not clear that the doses of naloxazone used *in vivo* were not able to block the lower affinity δ- and μ_2-receptors also. I will now discuss some new data from cross tolerance and naloxazone antagonism studies, which suggest that δ-receptors as well as μ-receptors can mediate analgesia.

Cross-tolerance between metkephamid and morphine was assessed in the mouse writhing test for analgesia (80). The mice were treated chronically with either saline or morphine on a 5-day schedule with four doses per day. Sixteen to twenty hr after the last injection of morphine, dose-response curves were generated to morphine and met-kephamid. The dose-response curve for morphine was shifted to the right in the morphine-treated animals resulting in a 3.5-fold increase in the ED_{50} value for morphine. A similar shift to the right in the dose-response curve was not observed for metkephamid in the morphine-tolerant mice. Only at the higher end of the dose-response curve was there some reduction in the analgesic

activity of metkephamid in the morphine-tolerant mice. These results were interpreted to indicate that a δ-receptor-mediated mechanism contributes to the analgesia
produced by metkephamid, although a μ-mechanism appears to become more
prominent at the higher doses.

Yaksh and colleagues (318) have reported similar findings of a relative lack of
tolerance to metkephamid in morphine-tolerant animals, using both the shock
titration model with the monkey, and the hot-plate model with the rat. Figure 13
provides an example of the data generated in the monkey. Tolerance to morphine
and beta-endorphin, but not D-Ala²-D-Leu⁵-enkephalin (DADL) or metkephamid
occurred after chronic treatment of the animal with morphine. These results suggest
analgesic activity of DADL and metkephamid at a spinal δ-receptor. In these studies,
tolerance to morphine in animals treated chronically with metkephamid was more
readily produced than tolerance to metkephamid in animals treated chronically

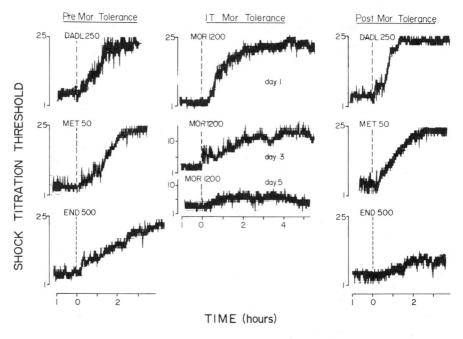

FIG. 13. Shock titration threshold records for a rhesus monkey after the intrathecal administration of D-Ala²-D-Leu⁵-enkephalin (DADL, 250 μg), metkephamid (MET, 50 μg) or beta-endorphin (END, 500 μg). The drugs were tested at 7-day intervals. The first panel shows the responses
before the development of tolerance to morphine. The *middle panel* shows the development of
tolerance to intrathecal morphine. Morphine (MOR, 1,200 μg) was administered daily for 5 days.
The records from days 1, 3, and 5 are shown. The *last panel* shows the results during the post-
morphine tolerance phase. The animals received DADL (250 μg) followed by 2 days of morphine
(1,200 μg), then metkephamid (50 μg) followed by 2 days of morphine (1,200 μg) and finally
beta-endorphin (500 μg). Injections were made at the times indicated by the *vertical dashed lines*.
The ordinate represents the shock titration threshold steps and the abscissa represents the time
in hours after the intrathecal administration of the opioid agonist. Cross-tolerance occurred to
END but not to DADL or MET. (From ref. 318, with permission.)

with morphine. This is not surprising since metkephamid is a better ligand for the μ-receptor than morphine is for the δ-receptor.

It might seem fair to question whether the non-μ-receptor-activated analgesia produced by metkephamid may be κ-rather than δ-mediated analgesia, but this is not likely since metkephamid has negligible activity at the κ-receptor (311). One might question, in fact, whether analgesia previously attributed to the activation of κ-receptors may not have been mediated rather by δ-receptors. This question has not yet been fully explored, but evidence has been recently obtained that non-μ-receptor-mediated spinal analgesia correlates better with δ-than with κ activity (173).

Further support for the concept that metkephamid produces analgesia by action on δ-receptors was provided by studies with naloxazone (80). It was possible to determine a dose of this irreversible antagonist, which, given 20 hr earlier, would selectively antagonize morphine-induced analgesia without affecting analgesia produced by metkephamid. The importance of careful dose-ranging in cross-tolerance or antagonism studies to distinguish receptor types must be emphasized; as of yet, we have no pharmacological tools with absolute specificity for the μ- or δ-receptor.

A word of caution or admonition must be given at this point. Considerable effort has been devoted to demonstrating that tolerance, cross-tolerance, and dependence as well as analgesia can be produced by the opioid peptides. The general conclusions reached from most of these studies has been that the μ- and not the δ-receptor mediates analgesia, and that the natural peptides and their derivatives offer no promise of reduced tolerance or physical dependence. Unfortunately, the approach in such studies has been to attempt to swamp the receptors by either perfusing the brain directly or in other ways pushing the dose until tolerance or dependence is demonstrated. This approach will wash out any chance of distinguishing different receptor mechanisms, which should be an object of such studies. The presence of multiple receptors and the lack of absolutely specific ligands demand a more refined approach to dissect the differing mechanisms.

Consider the work discussed above with metkephamid and morphine. By using the appropriate treatment regimen, it was possible to produce selective tolerance to morphine, presumably a μ-receptor phenomenon. By increasing the chronic dosage of morphine, however, the δ-receptor will be affected also, and tolerance will be seen to metkephamid as well. Indeed, cross-tolerance to morphine in chronic metkephamid-treated animals is more readily demonstrated than the reverse, because metkephamid is a better μ-agonist than morphine is a δ-agonist. Similarly, by using a high enough dose of naloxazone, which presumably inactivates both receptor types, it was possible to antagonize the analgesia induced by both morphine and metkephamid. By lowering the dose of naloxazone, however, it proved possible to selectively antagonize morphine-induced analgesia, presumably by selective antagonism of the μ-receptor at the lower doses of naloxazone. Such approaches, with full dose-response considerations, are critical and essential to obtaining meaningful information from this kind of study.

None of the above considerations suggest that analgesia is a δ-mediated rather than a μ-mediated phenomenon, but rather that analgesia can be produced by activation of δ- as well as μ-receptor activation. It is not yet clear whether δ-receptor activation alone is sufficient to produce analgesia or whether δ-mediated analgesia requires activation of μ-receptors as well. Indeed, Vaught et al. (289) have suggested a receptor model proposing coupling between μ- and δ-receptors, such that δ-receptor activation facilitates analgesia produced by μ-receptor activation. It remains to be established whether this is the case or whether δ-activation alone is sufficient to induce analgesia.

Preclinical Pharmacology of FK33 824 and Metkephamid (LY127623)

The work with these two enkephalin analogs confirmed the important concept that appropriate modification of the natural enkephalin structure can produce systemically active analgesic agents. The preclinical pharmacology of FK33 824 has been reported by Roemer et al. (232) and that of metkephamid by Frederickson et al. (77,80,81,82).

These compounds competed with labeled opioid ligands for binding in brain homogenate and produced potent naloxone-reversible depression of the electrically-induced twitch of both mouse vas deferens and guinea pig ileum. The IC_{50}s for these effects were in the nanomolar range. pA_2 values (252) for naloxone versus metkephamid, normorphine, and Met-enkephalin on the mouse vas deferens preparation were determined to be 7.60, 8.32, and 7.54, respectively. These data suggested that metkephamid and Met-enkephalin shared a similar receptor, the δ-receptor, differing from the μ-receptor used by normorphine. This was corroborated by the GPI/MVD ratios which were about 4.1 for metkephamid and 0.25 for morphine, suggesting a 16-fold greater δ-selectivity for metkephamid over morphine. This contrasted with the ratios for competing with ^{3}H-N$_x$ versus ^{3}H-DADL which were 0.6 and 0.1, respectively, for metkephamid and morphine. These latter data indicated that, although metkephamid had a sixfold greater preference for the δ-receptor than did morphine, it still had a slight absolute preference for the μ-receptor. This difference between the binding ratios and the ratios on the isolated muscle preparations has been interpreted to suggest that metkephamid may have considerably greater efficacy than morphine at the δ-receptor (80).

The cross-tolerance and naloxazone antagonism data discussed in the previous section clearly demonstrated that metkephamid could produce analgesia utilizing a different receptor, presumably the δ-receptor, than does morphine. In *in vivo* tests for analgesia, when given by the intraventricular route, metkephamid and FK33 824 were greater than 100-fold more potent than morphine. They were also analgesic by systemic routes of administration, being anywhere from ⅓ to 10 times as potent as morphine, depending on the test system and the route of administration.

Roemer et al. (232) reported that naloxone precipitated a marked withdrawal syndrome in monkeys self-administering FK33 824. In contrast, Frederickson et al. (82) reported that chronic treatment of rats with metkephamid produced little more physical dependence than did saline, unlike other drugs similarly tested such as morphine, meperidine, and pentazocine. Metkephamid, similarly, produced little locomotor activity or naloxone-precipitated withdrawal jumping in mice compared to morphine (80). Metkephamid was also reported to have a much lesser depressant effect on respiration in a rodent model than did morphine.

The ability of metkephamid to cross the placental barrier was assessed by measuring maternal and fetal serum levels in rats and sheep at various times after intramuscular injection of metkephamid (80). In the rat, the fetal:maternal ratio of metkephamid in blood at 1 hr after injection was about 1:60 compared to 1:1.8 for meperidine. In sheep, the fetal:maternal ratio for metkephamid was less than 1:200 compared to 1:1 reported for meperidine. This indicates a remarkable advantage for metkephamid over meperidine for use in obstetric analgesia.

Based on the preclinical pharmacological profile of these peptide analogs, it was considered justified to submit them to clinical testing. The clinical results to date will be discussed in the following section.

Clinical Studies

Safety

The first report of the effects of a modified opioid peptide in man was that of Graffenried et al. (103) who examined FK33 824 in normal male volunteers. After 0.1 to 1.2 mg intramuscular, all subjects experienced a 'feeling of heaviness in all the muscles of the body, often combined with a feeling of oppression on the chest or tightness in the throat which induced a certain amount of anxiety.' Other symptoms noted were a marked increase in bowel sounds, redness of face, injection of the conjunctivae, chemosis, whole body flush, rhinitis vasomotorica, and a flare reaction after intradermal injection. Plasma prolactin and growth hormone were increased. Expected morphine-like effects such as changes in emotional behavior or mental alertness, formication, and nausea were not observed, and the unexpected signs observed were not blocked by opioid, histamine, serotonin, or cholinergic antagonists. The lack of blockade with nalorphine suggested that the effects were not mediated by opioid receptors, but a subsequent report (271) claimed that the hormonal effects and other side effects could be blocked by the more pure opioid antagonist naloxone.

Metkephamid was administered to normal male volunteers in single intramuscular doses ranging from 0.5 to 150 mg (81). No clinically relevant effects were seen by routine clinical chemistry, electrolytes, urinalysis, hemograms, EKGs, blood pressure, or heart rate. At doses greater than 12.5 mg, subjects reported a mild retro-orbital burning which progressed to nasal congestion and dry mouth. A heavy sensation in the extremities, emotional detachment, and conjunctival injection were also reported, but no flushing or changes in bowel sounds were noted, and a flare formation did not occur after intradermal administration. Serum prolactin was increased, but no change in serum growth hormone was observed after 75 mg.

Thus, there are differences even between these enkephalin analogs as well as between enkephalin analogs and morphine.

Efficacy

As mentioned in the previous section, metkephamid and FK33 824 are both systemically active analgesics in standard animal model systems (82,232). FK33 824 was reported to have analgesic activity against experimental pain in man (267). A single intramuscular dose of 1 mg produced a significant increase in tolerance to electrically-evoked pain, but caused no change in the threshold to pain. Neither 0.5 nor 1.0 mg of FW 34-569, an [N-Me]Tyr^1 analog of FK33 824, influenced the pain threshold in human volunteers subjected to a hot-plate analgesimeter but both doses stimulated growth hormone and prolactin release and inhibited the release of cortisol and LH (172).

Metkephamid is presently undergoing clinical tests in postoperative pain, and these tests are demonstrating it to be efficacious as an analgesic. In one study, metkephamid at 70 or 140 mg was compared with 100 mg meperidine and placebo in 60 hospitalized women with severe postepisiotomy pain (27). Two separate trials were run using single intramuscular doses in parallel, randomized double-blind designs. Metkephamid, at 140 mg, produced the most effective analgesia followed by 100 mg meperidine, 70 mg metkephamid and placebo. The effect of 140 mg of metkephamid had a duration of about 6 hr.

In another study, the analgesic efficacy of 70 mg metkephamid was compared with that of 100 mg meperidine and placebo in the treatment of postoperative pain (35,36). This was a double-blind randomized controlled clinical trial of single intramuscular doses in 30 postsurgical patients. All measures indicated that the analgesic activity of 70 mg metkephamid was significantly greater than placebo, and not less than that of 100 mg meperidine. The duration of activity was about 4 hr, and up to the 4-hr point, 70 mg metkephamid appeared more efficacious than did 100 mg meperidine (Fig. 14). The frequency of remedication with metkephamid was also less than with meperidine or placebo.

There was a higher incidence of side effects with metkephamid than with the other treatments in these studies, but these effects were not distressing to the patients. The spectrum of these side effects were transient and suggested that the pharmacological properties of metkephamid are different from those of standard narcotic analgesics. It was suggested that this might be owing to greater utilization of the δ-rather than the μ-receptor, which is preferred by the standard analgesics.

Final Summary and Future Possibilities

The natural opioids appear to have little clinical utility because of enzymatic instability and poor passage of the blood-brain-barrier. Methods for overcoming this limitation include the development of specific enzyme inhibitors or structurally stabilized analogs of the natural peptides. The utility of enkephalinase inhibitors

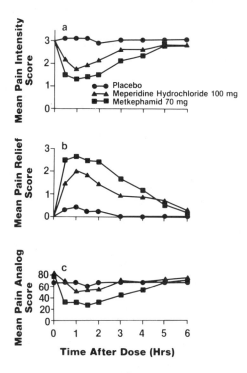

FIG. 14. Time-effect curves of analgesic activity of metkephamid (70 mg) compared to placebo and meperidine (100 mg). Thirty postoperative patients experiencing 'alot' of pain received one intramuscular dose of the allotted treatment in a double-blind randomized manner at time 0. The patients were interviewed at the time of medication and at ½, 1, 1½, 2, 3, 4, 5, and 6 hr after medication. Pain was assessed subjectively at each interview by (1) a reported pain score on an ordinal scale of 0 (no pain) to 4 ("terrible" pain), (2) a reported score for pain relief compared to premedication pain level on an ordinal scale of 0 (no relief) to 4 (complete relief), and (3) an analog scale of pain consisting of a 20-cm line marked 0 ("no pain") at one end and 100 ("worst pain I have ever felt") at the other end. From these observations, the mean pain intensity scores, mean pain relief scores, and mean pain analog scores were calculated for each observation time and plotted as shown. The placebo generally had no effect on pain. By contrast, metkephamid and meperidine had begun to reduce pain by ½ hr, with peak analgesic effect usually at 1 hr; the analgesic effect was considerably diminished by 4 hr. Up to the 4-hr point, metkephamid (70 mg) appeared more effective than meperidine (100 mg). (From ref. 36, with permission).

appears to be limited by the low basal activity of enkephalinergic systems, but there may be a unique potential here if clinical pain activates these systems.

More headway has been made to date, however, with the latter approach. An intact and active endogenous system is not required for analgesic activity of analogs modified structurally to provide protection from enzymatic degradation. Hundreds, possibly thousands, of analogs have been synthesized, many of which have analgesic activity. Two of these, FK33 824 and metkephamid (LY127623), have been tested for analgesic efficacy in man. FK33 824 is apparently no longer being pursued as an analgesic agent, but metkephamid is still being tested in the clinic for its analgesic properties. The analgesic efficacy of this slightly modified Met-enkephalin structure has been demonstrated in several clinical settings with 70 to 140 mg being roughly equivalent to 100 mg meperidine. Several potential advantages for this compound as a new analgesic are becoming apparent. Such a compound represents a unique analgesic structure closely related to a natural substance. It is potent on both μ and δ receptors *in vitro*, but *in vivo* it appears to have analgesic activity via a receptor, presumably the δ-receptor, not utilized by existing analgesic agents. It presents a different side effect spectrum with the likelihood of reduced physical dependence and respiratory depression, although the latter phenomena have not yet been demonstrated in man. Even more exciting is the finding in rats and sheep of a markedly reduced passage of the placental barrier by metkephamid compared to meperidine. If this is true also for the human, metkephamid will provide a significant therapeutic advance and a real advantage for use in labor and delivery as well as other obstetric and gynecologic uses.

Further advances will come from the development and study of more selective analogs and antagonists, which should help elucidate the role of the various different receptor types.

REFERENCES

1. Abols, I. A., and Basbaum, A. L. (1979): Afferent input to the medullary reticular formation and raphe magnus of the cat: An HRP study. *Anat. Rec.*, 93:467.
2. Abram, S. E., Reynolds, A. C., and Cusick, J. F. (1981): Failure of naloxone to reverse analgesia from transcutaneous electrical stimulation in patients with chronic pain. *Anesth. Analg.*, 60:81–84.
3. Adams, J. E. (1976): Naloxone reversal of analgesia produced by brain stimulation in the human. *Pain*, 2:161–166.
4. Akil, H., and Liebeskind, J. C. (1975): Monoaminergic mechanisms of stimulation-produced analgesia. *Brain Res.*, 94:279–296.
5. Akil, H., and Mayer, D. J. (1972): Antagonism of stimulation-produced analgesia by p-CPA, a serotonin synthesis inhibitor. *Brain Res.*, 44:692–697.
6. Akil, H., Mayer, D. J., and Liebeskind, J. C. (1976): Antagonism of stimulation-produced analgesia by naloxone, a narcotic antagonist. *Science*, 191:961–962.
7. Akil, H., Richardson, D. E., Barchas, J. D., and Li, C. H. (1978): Appearance of β-endorphin-like immunoreactivity in human ventricular cerebrospinal fluid upon analgesic electrical stimulation. *Proc. Natl. Acad. Sci. U.S.A.*, 75:5170–5172.
8. Akil, H., Richardson, D. E., Hughes, J., and Barchas, J. D. (1978): Enkephalin-like material elevated in ventricular cerebrospinal fluid of pain patients after analgesic focal stimulation. *Science*, 201:463–465.
9. Akil, H., Watson, S. J., Sullivan, S., and Barchas, J. D. (1978): Enkephalin-like material in normal human CSF: Measurement and levels. *Life Sci.*, 23:121–126.
10. Akil, H., Watson, S. J., Barchas, J. D., and Li, C. H. (1979): β-Endorphin immunoreactivity in rat and human blood: Radioimmunoassay, comparative levels and physiological alterations. *Life Sci.*, 24:1659–1666.
11. Allen, R. G., Herbert, E., Hinman, M., Shibuya, H., and Pert, C. B. (1978): Coordinate control of corticotropin, β-lipotropin, and β-endorphin release in mouse pituitary cell cultures. *Proc. Natl. Acad. Sci.*, 75:4972–4976.
12. Almay, B. G. L., Johansson, F., Von Knorring, L., Terenius, L., and Wahlstrom, A. (1978): Endorphins in chronic pain. I. Differences in CSF endorphin levels between organic and psychogenic pain syndromes. *Pain*, 5:153–162.
13. Alumets, J., Hakanson, R., Sundler, F., and Chang, K.-J. (1978): Leu-enkephalin-like material in nerves and enterochromaffin cells in the gut. *Histochemistry*, 56:187–196.
14. Anselmi, B., Baldi, E., Cassacci, F., and Salmon, S. (1980): Endogenous opioids in cerebrospinal fluid and blood in idiopathic headache sufferers. *Headache*, 20:294–299.

15. Austin, B. M., Smyth, D. G., and Snell, C. R. (1977): γ-Endorphin, α-endorphin and met-enkephalin are formed extracellularly from lipotropin C-fragment. *Nature*, 269:619–621.
15a. Barchas et al. (1980): Behavioral neurochemistry: Neuroregulators and behavioral states. *Science*, 200:964–973.
16. Barclay, R. K., and Phillipps, M. A. (1980): Inhibition of enkephalin-degrading aminopeptidase activity. *Biochem. Biophys. Res. Commun.*, 96:1732–1738.
17. Basbaum, A. I., Marley, N., and O'Keefe, J. (1975): Effects of spinal cord lesions on the analgesic properties of electrical brain stimulation. In: *Proc. First World Congress on Pain*, p. 268.
18. Bayon, A., Rossier, J., Mauss, A., Bloom, F. E., Iversen, L. L., Ling, N., and Guillemin, R. (1978): In vitro release of [5-methionine]enkephalin and [5-leucine]-enkephalin from the rat globus pallidus. *Proc. Natl. Acad. Sci.*, 75:3503–3506.
19. Beaumont, A., and Hughes, J. (1979): Biology of opioid peptides. *Ann. Rev. Pharmacol. Toxicol.*, 19:247–267.
20. Behbehani, M. M., and Pomeroy, S. L. (1978): Effect of morphine injected in periaqueductal gray on the activity of single units in nucleus raphe magnus of the rat. *Brain Res.*, 149:266–269.
21. Belluzzi, J. D., Grant, N., Garsky, V., Sarantakes, D., Wise, C. D., and Stein, L. (1976): Analgesia induced *in vivo* by central administration of enkephalin in rat. *Nature*, 260:625–626.
22. Benuck, M., and Marks, N. (1979): Co-identity of brain angiotensin converting enzyme with a membrane bound dipeptidyl-carboxypeptidase inactivating met-enkephalin. *Biochem. Biophys. Res. Commun.*, 88:215–221.
23. Berntson, G. G., and Walker, J. M. (1977): Effect of opiate receptor blockade on pain sensitivity in the rat. *Brain Res. Bull.*, 2:157–159.
24. Bjorklund, A., Emson, P. C., Gilbert, R. T. F., and Skagerberg, G. (1979): Further evidence for the possible coexistence of 5-hydroxytryptamine and substance P in medullary raphe neurons of rat brain. *Br. J. Pharmacol.*, 66:112–113.
25. Bloom, F. E., Battenberg, E., Rossier, J., Ling, N., Leppaluoto, J., Vargo, T. M., and Guillemin, R. (1977): Endorphins are located in the intermediate and anterior lobes of the pituitary glands, not in neurohypophysis. *Life Sci.*, 20:43–48.
26. Bloom, F. E., Battenberg, E., Rossier, J., Ling, N., and Guillemin, R. (1978): Neurons containing β-endorphin in rat brain exist separately from those containing enkephalin: Immunocytochemical studies. *Proc. Natl. Acad. Sci. U.S.A.*, 75:1591–1595.
27. Bloomfield, S. S., Barden, T. P., and Mitchell, J. (1982): Metkephamid and merperidine analgesia in postepisiotomy pain. *Clin. Pharmacol. Ther.*, 31:205.
28. Boarder, M. R., Erdelyi, E., and Barchas, J. D. (1982): Opioid peptides in human plasma: Evidence for multiple forms. *J. Clin. Endocrin. Metabol.*, 54:715–720.
29. Bruni, J. F., Watkins, W. B., and Yen, S. S. C. (1979): β-endorphin in the human pancreas. *J. Clin. Endocrinol. Metab.*, 49:649–651.
30. Buchsbaum, M. S., Davis, G. C., and Bunney, Jr., W. E. (1977): Naloxone alters pain perception and somatosensory evoked potentials in normal subjects. *Nature*, 270:620–622.
31. Buckett, W. R. (1979): The actions of enkephalins are not modified by the kininase-II inhibitor captopril. *Eur. J. Pharmacol.*, 57:267–271.
32. Burbach, J. P. H., Loeber, J. G., Verhoef, J., and de Kloet, E. R. (1980): β-Endorphin biotransformation in brain: Formation of γ-endorphin by a synaptosomal plasma membrane associated endopeptidase distinct from cathepsin D. *Biochem. Biophys. Res. Commun.*, 92:725–732.
33. Burbach, J. P. H., Loeber, J. G., Verhoef, J., Wiegant, V. M., de Kloet, E. R., and de Wied, D. (1980): Selective conversion of β-endorphin into peptides related to γ- and α-endorphin. *Nature*, 283:96–97.
34. Buscher, H. H., Hill, R. C., Romer, D., Cardinaux, F., Closse, A., Hauser, D., and Pless, Jr., D. (1976): Evidence for analgesic activity of enkephalin in the mouse. *Nature*, 261:423–424.
35. Calimlim, J. F., Wardell, W., Sriwatanakul, K., and Lasagna, L. (1982): Analgesic efficacy of a single intramuscular dose of LY127623. *Clin. Pharmacol. Ther.*, 31:208–209.
36. Calimlim, J. F., Wardell, W. M., Sriwatanakul, K., Lasagna, L., and Cox, C. (1982): Analgesic efficacy of parenteral metkephamid acetate in treatment of post-operative pain. *Lancet*, 1:1374–1375.
37. Carenzi, A., Biacini, F., Frigeni, V., and Della Bella, D. (1980): On the enzymatic degradation of enkephalins: Pharmacological implications. In: *Advances in Biochemical Psychopharmacology, Vol. 22*, edited by E. Costa and M. Trabucchi, pp. 237–246. Raven Press, New York.

38. Chan-Palay, V., Jonsson, G., and Palay, S. L. (1978): Serotonin and substance P coexist in neurons of the rat's central nervous system. *Proc. Natl. Acad. Sci. U.S.A.*, 75:1582–1586.
39. Chang, A. C. Y., Cochet, M., and Cohen, S. N. (1980): Structural organization of human genomic DNA encoding pro-opiomelanocortin peptide. *Proc. Natl. Acad. Sci. U.S.A.*, 77:4890–4894.
40. Chapman, R. N., and Benedetti, C. (1977): Analgesia following transcutaneous electrical stimulation and its partial reversal by a narcotic antagonist. *Life Sci.*, 21:1645–1648.
41. Chiang, C. Y., Chang, C. T., Chu, H. L., and Yang, L. F. (1973): Peripheral afferent pathway for acupuncture analgesia. *Sci. Sin.*, 16:210–217.
42. Clement-Jones, V., McLoughlin, L., Lowry, P. J., Besser, G. M., Rees, L. H., and Wen, H. L. (1979): Acupuncture in heroin addicts: Changes in met-enkephalin and β-endorphin in blood and cerebrospinal fluid. *Lancet*, 2:380–383.
43. Clement-Jones, V., Lowry, P. J., Rees, L. H., and Besser, G. M. (1980): Met-enkephalin circulates in human plasma. *Nature*, 283:295–297.
44. Clement-Jones, V., Lowry, P. J., Rees, L. H., and Besser, G. M. (1980): Development of a specific extracted radioimmunoassay for methionine enkephalin in human plasma and cerebrospinal fluid. *J. Endocrinol.*, 86:231–243.
45. Clement-Jones, V., McLoughlin, L., Tomlin, S., Besser, G. M., Rees, L. H., and Wen, H. L. (1980): Increased β-endorphin but not met-enkephalin levels in human cerebrospinal fluid after acupuncture for recurrent pain. *Lancet*, II:946–948.
46. Coletti-Previero, M.-A., Mattras, H., Descomps, H., and Previero, A. (1981): Purification and substrate characterization of a human enkephalin-degrading aminopeptidase. *Biochem. Biophys. Acta*, 657:122–127.
47. Colt, E., Wardlaw, S., and Frantz, A. (1981): The effect of running on plasma β-endorphin. *Life Sci.*, 28:1637–1640.
48. Costa, E., Guidotti, A., Hanbauer, I., Hexum, T., Saiani, L., Stine, S. and Yang, H.-Y. T (1981): Regulation of acetylcholine receptors by endogenous cotransmitters: Studies of adrenal medulla. *Fed. Proc.*, 40:160–165.
49. Csontos, K., Rust, M., Hollt, V., Mahr, W., Kromer, W., and Teschemacher, H. J. (1979): Elevated plasma β-endorphin levels in pregnant women and their neonates. *Life Sci.*, 25:835–844.
50. Dale, H. H. (1935): Pharmacology and nerve endings. *Proc. R. Soc. Med.*, 28:319–332.
51. Davis, G. C., Buchsbaum, M. S., and Bunney, Jr., W. E. (1978): Naloxone decreases diurnal variation in pain sensitivity and somatosensory evoked potentials. *Life Sci.*, 23:1449–1460.
52. De La Baume, S., Patey, G., and Schwarz, J.-C. (1981): Subcellular distribution of enkephalin-dipeptidyl carboxypeptidase (enkephalinase) in rat brain. *Neuroscience*, 6:315–321.
53. Della Bella, D., Carenzi, A., Frigeni, V., and Santini, V. (1979): Effect of carboxypeptidase inhibition on the in vivo and in vitro pharmacological properties of morphine and enkephalins. *Neuropharmacology*, 18:719–721.
54. DeWied, D., Kovacs, G. L., Bahus, B., Van Ree, J. M., and Greven, H. M. (1978): Neuroleptic activity of the neuropeptide β-LPH$_{62-77}$ (Des-Tyr^1) γ-endorphin: (DT$_\gamma$E). *Eur. J. Pharmacol.*, 49:427–436.
55. Di Augustine, R. P., Lazarus, L. H., Jahnke, G., Kahn, M. N., Erisman, M. D., and Linnoila, R. I. (1980): Corticotropin/β-endorphin immunoreactivity in rat mast cells: Peptide or protease. *Life Sci.*, 27:2663–2668.
56. DiGiulio, A. M., Yang, H.-Y. T., Lutold, B., Fratta, W., Hong, J., and Costa, E. (1978): Characterization of enkephalin-like material extracted from sympathetic ganglia. *Neuropharmacology*, 17:989–992.
57. Doneen, B. A., Chung, D., Yamashiro, D., Law, P. Y., Loh, H. H., and Li, C. H. (1977): β-Endorphin: Structure-activity relationships in the guinea pig ileum and opiate receptor binding assay. *Biochem. Biophys. Res. Commun.*, 74:656–662.
58. Drouin, J., and Goodman, H. M. (1980): Most of the coding region of rat ACTH β-LPH precursor gene lacks intervening sequences. *Nature*, 288:610–612.
59. Dubois, M., Pickar, D., Cohen, M. R., Roth, Y. F., Macnamara, T., and Bunney, W. E., Jr. (1981): Surgical stress in humans is accompanied by an increase in plasma beta-endorphin immunoreactivity. *Life Sci.*, 29:1249–1254.
60. Duggan, A. W. (1980): Enkephalins as transmitters in the central nervous system. *Circ. Res.*, 46:I149–I153.
61. Dunwiddie, T., Mueller, A., Palmer, M., Stewart, J., and Hoffer, B. (1980): Electrophysiological

interactions of enkephalins with neuronal circuitry in the rat hippocampus. I. Effects on pyramidal cell activity. *Brain Res.*, 184:311–330.

62. Dupont, A., Lepine, L., Langelier, P., Merand, Y., Rouleau, D., Vaudry, H., Gras, C., and Barden, N. (1980): Differential distribution of β-endorphin and enkephalins in rat and bovine brain. *Regulatory Peptides*, 1:43–52.

63. El-Sobky, A., Dostrovsky, J. O., and Wall, P. D. (1976): Lack of effect of naloxone on pain perception in humans. *Nature*, 263:783–784.

64. Feldberg, W., and Smyth, D. G. (1976): The C fragment of lipotropin—A potent analgesic. *J. Physiol.*, 260:30P.

65. Feldberg, W., and Smyth, D. G. (1977): C fragment of lipotropin—An endogenous potent analgesic peptide. *Br. J. Pharmacol.*, 60:445–453.

66. Fields, H. L., and Anderson, S. D. (1978): Evidence that raphe-spinal neurons mediate opiate and midbrain stimulation-produced analgesia. *Pain*, 5:333–349.

67. Fields, H. L., Basbaum, A. I., Clanton, C. H., and Anderson, S. D. (1977): Nucleus raphe magnus inhibition of spinal cord dorsal horn neurons. *Brain Res.*, 126:441–453.

68. Finley, J. C. W., Maderdrut, J. L., and Petrusz, P. (1981): The immunocytochemical localization of enkephalin in the central nervous system of the rat. *J. Comp. Neurol.*, 198:541–566.

69. Fletcher, J. E., Thomas, F. A., and Hill, R. G. (1980): β-Endorphin and parturition. *Lancet*, 1:310.

70. Fraioli, F., Moretti, C., Paolucci, D., Alicicco, E., Crescenzi, F., and Fortunio, G. (1980): Physical exercise stimulates marked concomitant release of β-endorphin and adrenocorticotropic hormone (ACTH) in peripheral blood in man. *Experientia*, 36:987–989.

71. Fratta, W., Yang, H.-Y., Majane, B., and Costa, E. (1979): Distribution of β-endorphin and related peptides in the hypothalamus and pituitary. *Neuroscience*, 4:1903–1908.

72. Frederickson, R. C. A. (1977): Enkephalin pentapeptides—A review of current evidence for a physiological role in vertebrate neurotransmission. *Life Sci.*, 21:23–42.

73. Fredrickson, R. C. A. (1978): Significance of endogenous opioids for regulation of nociceptive sensitivity in the normal and stressed conditions. In: *Characteristics and Function of Opioids*, edited by J. M. Van Ree and L. Terenius, pp. 135–141. Elsevier, Amsterdam.

74. Frederickson, R. C. A., and Norris, F. H. (1976): Enkephalin-induced depression of single neurons in brain areas with opiate receptors-antagonism by naloxone. *Science*, 194:440–442.

75. Frederickson, R. C. A., and Norris, F. H. (1978): Enkephalins as inhibitory transmitters modulating nociception. In: *Iontophoresis and Transmitter Mechanisms in the Mammalian Central Nervous System*, edited by R. W. Ryall and J. S. Kelly, pp. 320–322. Elsevier, Amsterdam.

76. Frederickson, R. C. A., and Geary, L. E. (1982): Endogenous opioid peptides: Review of physiological, pharmacological and clinical aspects. *Prog. Neurobiol.*, 19:19–69.

77. Frederickson, R. C. A., and Smithwick, E. L. (1979): Evidence for tonic activity of enkephalins in brain and development of systemically active analogues with clinical potential. In: *Endorphins in Mental Health Research*, edited by E. Usdin, W. E. Bunney, Jr., and N. S. Kline, pp. 352–365. Macmillan, Great Britain.

78. Frederickson, R. C. A., Burgis, V., and Edwards, J. D. (1977): Hyperalgesia induced by naloxone follows diurnal rhythm in responsivity to painful stimuli. *Science*, 198:756–758.

79. Frederickson, R. C. A., Nickander, R., Smithwick, E. L., Shuman, R., and Norris, F. H. (1976): Pharmacological activity of met-enkephalin and analogues in vitro and in vivo—Depression of single neuronal activity in specified brain regions. In: *Opiates and Endogenous Opioid Peptides*, edited by H. Kosterlitz, pp. 239–246. Elsevier, Amsterdam.

80. Frederickson, R. C. A., Parli, C. J., DeVane, G. W., and Hynes, M. D. (1983): Preclinical pharmacology of metkephamid (LY 127623), a net-enkephalin analogue. National Institute on Drug Abuse Research Monograph, edited by L. S. Harris 43:150–156.

81. Frederickson, R. C. A., Smithwick, E. L., and Henry, D. P. (1980): Opioid peptides as brain neurotransmitters with therapeutic potential: Basic and clinical studies. In: *Neuropeptides and Neural Transmission*, edited by C. Ajmore-Marsan and W. Traczyk, pp. 227–235. Raven Press, New York.

82. Frederickson, R. C. A., Smithwick, E. L., Shuman, R., and Bemis, K. G. (1981): Metkephamid, a systemically active analog of methionine enkephalin with potent opioid δ-receptor activity. *Science*, 211:603–605.

83. Fricker, L. D., and Snyder, S. H. (1982): Enkephalin convertase: Purification and characterization

of a specific enkephalin synthesizing carboxypeptidase localized to adrenal chromaffin granules. *Proc. Natl. Acad. Sci. U.S.A.*, 79:3886–3890.

84. Furui, T., Kageyama, N., Haga, T., Ichiyama, A., and Fukushima, M. (1980): Radioreceptor assay of methionine-enkephalin-like substance in human cerebrospinal fluid. *Pain*, 9:63–72.

85. Gacel, G., Fournie-Zaluski, M.-C., Fellion, E., and Roques, B. P. (1981): Evidence of the preferential involvement of μ receptors in analgesia using enkephalins highly selective for peripheral μ or δ receptors. *J. Med. Chem.*, 24:1119–1124.

86. Gahwiler, B. H. (1980): Excitatory action of opioid peptides and opiates on cultured hippocampal pyramidal cells. *Brain Res.*, 194:193–203.

87. Gallagher, D. W., and Pert, A. (1978): Afferents to brainstem nuclei in the rat as demonstrated by microiontophoretically applied horseradish peroxidase. *Brain Res.*, 144:257–275.

88. Ghazarossian, V. E., Dent, R. R., Otsu, K., Ross, M., Cox, B., and Goldstein, A. (1980): Development and validation of a sensitive radioimmunoassay for naturally occurring β-endorphin-like peptides in human plasma. *Anal. Biochem.*, 102:80–89.

89. Giesler, Jr., G. J., Gerhart, K. D., Yezierski, R. P., Wilcox, T. K., and Willis, W. D. (1981): Postsynaptic inhibition of primate spinothalamic neurons by stimulation in nucleus raphe magnus. *Brain Res.*, 204:184–188.

90. Gilbert, P. E., and Martin, W. R. (1976): The effects of morphine- and nalorphine-like drugs in the nondependent, morphine-dependent and cyclazocine-dependent chronic spinal dog. *J. Pharmacol. Exp. Ther.*, 198:66–82.

91. Gilles, G., Ratter, S., Grossman, A., Gaillard, R., Lowry, P. J., Besser, G. M., and Rees, L. H. (1980): Secretion of ACTH, LPH, and β-endorphin from human pituitary tumours in vitro. *Clin. Endocrinol.*, 13:197–205.

92. Gintzler, A. R., Levy, A., and Spector, S. (1976): Antibodies as a means of isolating and characterizing biologically active substances: Presence of a non-peptide morphine-like compound in the central nervous system. *Proc. Natl. Acad. Sci. U.S.A.*, 73:2132–2136.

93. Glowinski, J. (1981): In vivo release of transmitters in the cat basal ganglia. *Fed. Proc.*, 40:135–141.

93a. Glowinski, J., and Iversen, L. V. (1966): Regional studies of catecholamines in the rat brain-I. *J. Neurochem.*, 13:655.

94. Goldstein, A., and Ghazarossian, V. E. (1980): Immunoreactive dynorphin in pituitary and brain. *Proc. Natl. Acad. Sci. U.S.A.*, 77:6207–6210.

95. Goldstein, A., Tachibana, S., Lowney, L. I., Hunkapiller, M., and Hood, L. (1979): Dynorphin-(1-13), an extraordinarily potent opioid peptide. *Proc. Natl. Acad. Sci. U.S.A.*, 76:6666–6670.

96. Goland, R. S., Wardlaw, S. L., Stark, R. I., and Frantz, A. G. (1981): Human plasma β-endorphin during pregnancy, labor and delivery. *J. Clin. Endocrinol. Metab.*, 52:74–78.

97. Goodman, R. R., Snyder, S. H., Kuhar, M. J., and Young, W. S. III (1980): Differentiation of delta-opiate and mu-opiate receptor localizations by light microscopic autoradiography. *Proc. Natl. Acad. Sci. U.S.A.*, 77:6239–6243.

98. Gorenstein, C., and Snyder, S. H. (1979): Two distinct enkephalinases: Solubilization, partial purification and separation from angiotensin converting enzyme. *Life Sci.*, 25:2065–2070.

99. Gorenstein, C., and Snyder, S. H. (1980): Enkephalinases. *Proc. R. Soc. Lond. B* 210:123–132.

100. Gorenstein, C., and Snyder, S. H. (1980): Characterization of enkephalinases. In *Endogenous and Exogenous Opiate Agonists and Antagonists*, edited by E. Leong Way, pp. 345–348. Pergamon Press, New York.

101. Graf, L., Szekely, J. I., Ronai, A. Z., Dunai-Kovacs, Z., and Bajusz, S. (1976): Comparative study on analgesic effect of met⁵-enkephalin and related lipotropin fragments. *Nature*, 263:240–241.

102. Graf, L., Kenessey, A., Patthy, A., Grynbaum, A., Marks, N., and Lajtha, A. (1979): Cathepsin D generates γ-endorphin from β-endorphin. *Arch. Biochem. Biophys.*, 193:101–109.

103. Graffenried, B. von, del Pozo, E., Roubicek, J., Krebs, E., Poldinger, W., Burmeister, P., and Kerp, L. (1978): Effects of the synthetic enkephalin analogue FK 33 824 in man. *Nature*, 272:729–730.

104. Grevert, P., and Goldstein, A. (1977): Some effects of naloxone on behavior in the mouse. *Psychopharmacology*, 53:111–113.

105. Grevert, P., and Goldstein, A. (1977): Effects of naloxone on experimentally induced ischemic pain and on mood in human subjects. *Proc. Natl. Acad. Sci. U.S.A.*, 74:1291–1294.

106. Grevert, P., and Goldstein, A. (1978): Endorphins: Naloxone fails to alter experimental pain or mood in humans. *Science*, 199:1093–1095.
107. Gross, C., Pradelles, P., Humbert, J., Dray, F., Le Gal La Salle, G., and Ben-Ari, Y. (1978): Regional distribution of met-enkephalin within the amygdaloid complex and bed nucleus of the stria terminalis. *Neurosci. Lett.*, 10:193–196.
108. Gubler, U., Seeburg, P., Hoffmann, B. J., Gage, L. P., and Udenfriend, S. (1982): Molecular cloning establishes proenkephalin as precursor of enkepahlin-containing peptides. *Nature*, 295:206–208.
109. Guillemin, R., Vargo, T., Rossier, J., Minick, S., Ling, N., Rivier, C., Vale, W., and Bloom, F. (1977): β-endorphin and adrenocorticotropin are secreted concomitantly by the pituitary gland. *Science*, 197:1367–1369.
110. Hambrook, J. M., Morgan, B. A., Rance, M. J., and Smith, C. F. C. (1976): Mode of deactivation of the enkephalins by rat and human plasma and rat brain homogenates. *Nature*, 262:782–783.
111. Hartsuck, J. A., and Lipscomb, W. N. (1971): Carboxypeptidase A. In: *The Enzymes Vol. III*, edited by P. Bayer, pp. 1–56. Academic Press, New York.
112. Hayashi, M. (1978): Monkey brain arylamidase: II. Further characterization and studies on mode of hydrolysis of physiologically active peptides. *J. Biochem.*, 84:1363–1372.
113. Hayes, R. L., Newlon, P. G., Rosecrans, J. A., and Mayer, D. J. (1977): Reduction of stimulation-produced analgesia by lysergic acid diethylamide, a depressor of serotonergic neural activity. *Brain Res.*, 122:367–372.
114. Henderson, G., Hughes, J., and Kosterlitz, H. W. (1978): In vitro release of leu and met-enkephalin from the corpus striatum. *Nature*, 271:677–679.
115. Henry, J. L. (1975): Effects of morphine and meperidine in neurones in cat midbrain. *Fed. Proc.*, 34:757.
116. Herbert, E. (1981): Discovery of pro-opiomelanocortin—A cellular polyprotein. *Trends in Biochemical Sciences*, 6:184–188.
117. Hersh, L. B., and McKelvy, J. F. (1981): An aminopeptidase from bovine brain which catalyzes the hydrolysis of enkephalin. *J. Neurochem.*, 36:171–178.
118. Hersh, L. B., Smith, T. E., and McKelvy, J. F. (1980): Cleavage of endorphins to des-Tyr endorphins by homogeneous bovine brain aminopeptidase. *Nature*, 286:160–162.
119. Hexum, T. D., Hanbauer, I., Govoni, S., Yang, H.-Y. T., and Costa, E. (1980): Secretion of enkephalin-like peptides from canine adrenal gland following splanchnic nerve stimulation. *Neuropeptides*, 1:137–142.
120. Ho, W. K. K., Kwok, K. Y., and Lam, S. (1979): Characterization of a plasma factor having opiate and immunoactivity like β-endorphin. *Biochem. Biophys. Res. Commun.*, 87:448–454.
121. Hokfelt, T., Ljungdahl, A., Steinbusch, H., Verhofstad, A., Nilsson, G., Brodin, E., Pernow, B., and Goldstein, M. (1978): Immunohistochemical evidence of substance P-like immunoreactivity in some 5-hydroxytryptamine-containing neurons in the rat central nervous system. *Neuroscience*, 3:517–538.
122. Hokfelt, T., Lundberg, J. M., Schultzberg, M., Johansson, O., Ljungdahl, A., and Rehfeld, J. (1980): Coexistence of peptides and putative transmitters in neurons. In: *Advances in Biochemical Psychopharmacology*, edited by E. Costa and M. Trabucchi, pp. 1–23. Raven Press, New York.
123. Hokfelt, T., Lundberg, J. M., Skirboll, L., Johansson, O., Schultzberg, G. M., and Vincent, S. R. (1982): Co-existence of classical transmitters and peptides in neurons. In: *Co-transmission*, edited by A. C. Cuello, pp. 77–126. MacMillan, London.
124. Hollt, V., Przewlocki, R., and Herz, A. (1978): Radioimmunoassay of β-endorphin: Basal and stimulated levels in extracted rat plasma. *Naunyn Schmiedebergs Arch. Pharmacol.*, 303:171–174.
125. Hollt, V., Przewlocki, R., and Herz, A. (1978): β-endorphin-like immunoreactivity in plasma, pituitaries and hypothalamus of rats following treatment with opiates. *Life Sci.*, 23:1057–1066.
126. Hollt, V., Muller, O. A., and Fahlbusch, R. (1979): β-Endorphin in human plasma: Basal and pathologically elevated levels. *Life Sci.*, 25:37–44.
127. Hook, V. H., Eiden, L. E. E., and Brownstein, M. S. (1982): A carboxypeptidase processing enzyme for enkephalin precursors. *Nature*, 295:341–342.
128. Hosobuchi, Y., Adams, J. E., and Linchitz, R. (1977): Pain relief by stimulation of the central gray matter in humans and its reversal by naloxone. *Science*, 197:183–186.
129. Hosobuchi, Y., Rossier, J., Bloom, F. E., and Guillemenin, R. (1979): Stimulation of human

periaqueductal gray for pain relief increases immunoreactive β-endorphin in ventricular fluid. *Science*, 203:279–281.

130. Huang, W.-Y., Chang, R. C. C., Kastin, A. J., Coy, D. H., and Schally, A. V. (1979): Isolation and structure of pro-methionine-enkephalin: Potential enkephalin precursor from porcine hypothalamus. *Proc. Natl. Acad. Sci. U.S.A.*, 76:6177–6180.

131. Hughes, J. (1975): Isolation of an endogenous compound from the brain with pharmacological properties similar to morphine. *Brain Res.*, 88:295–308.

132. Hughes, J., Smith, T. W., Kosterlitz, H. W., Fothergill, L. A., Morgan, B. A., and Morris, H. R. (1975): Identification of two related pentapeptides from the brain with potent opiate agonist activity. *Nature*, 258:577–579.

133. Imura, H., and Nakai, Y. (1981): Endorphins in pituitary and other tissues. *Ann. Rev. Physiol.*, 43:265–278.

134. Iversen, L. V., Iversen, S. D., Bloom, F. E., Vargo, T., and Guillemin, R. (1978): Release of enkephalin from rat globus pallidus in vitro. *Nature*, 271:679–681.

135. Jacob, J. J., Tremblay, E. C., and Colombel, M. C. (1974): Facilitation des reactions nociceptives par la naloxone chez la souris et chez le rat. *Psychopharmacology*, 37:217–223.

136. Jacquet, Y. F., and Lajtha, A. (1973): Morphine action at central nervous system sites in rat: Analgesia or hyperalgesia depending on site and dose. *Science*, 182:490–492.

137. Jessen, K. R., Saffrey, M. J., van Noorden, S., Bloom, S. R., Polak, J. M., and Burnstock, G. (1980): Immunohistochemical studies of the enteric nervous system in tissue culture and *in situ*: Localization of vasoactive intestinal polypeptide (VIP), substance P and enkephalin immunoreactive nerves in the guinea pig gut. *Neuroscience*, 5:171–173.

138. Johansson, O., Hokfelt, T., Elde, R. P., Schultzberg, M., and Terenius, L. (1978): Immunohistochemical distribution of enkephalin neurons. *Adv. Biochem. Psychopharm.*, 18:51–70.

139. Kanagawa, K., Matsuo, H., and Igarashi, M. (1979): α-Neo-endorphin: A big leu-enkephalin with potent opiate activity from porcine hypothalami. *Biochem. Biophys. Res. Commun.*, 86:153–160.

140. Kendall, J., and Orwoll, E. (1980): Anterior pituitary hormones in the brain and other pituitary sites. In: *Frontiers in Neuroendocrinology*, edited by L. Martini and W. F. Ganong, vol. 6, pp. 33–65. Raven Press, New York.

141. Killian, A. K., Schuster, C. R., House, J. T., Sholl, S., Connors, M., and Wainer, B. H. (1981): A non-peptide morphine-like compound from brain. *Life Sci.*, 28:811–817.

142. Kiraly, I., Tapfer, M., Borsy, J., and Graf, L. (1981): Further evidence for the neuroleptic-like activity of γ-endorphin. *Peptides*, 2:9–12.

143. Knight, M., and Klee, W. A. (1979): Enkephalin generating activity of rat brain endopeptidases. *J. Biol. Chem.*, 254:10426–10430.

144. Knorring, L., Almay, B., Johansson, F., and Terenius, L. (1978): Pain perception and endorphin levels in cerebrospinal fluid. *Pain*, 5:359–365.

145. Kobayashi, R. M., Palkovits, M., Miller, R. J., Chang, K. J., and Cuatrecasas, P. (1978): Brain enkephalin distribution is unaltered by hypophysectomy. *Life Sci.*, 22:527–530.

146. Koida, M., Aono, J., Takenaga, K., Yoshimoto, T., Kimura, T., and Sakakibara, S. (1979): A novel enzyme in rat brain converting β-endorphin into methionine enkephalin: Affinity chromatography and specificity. *J. Neurochem.*, 33:1233–1237.

147. Kokka, N., and Fairhurst, A. S. (1977): Naloxone enhancement of acetic acid-induced writhing in rats. *Life Sci.*, 21:975–980.

148. Krieger, D. T., and Liotta, A. S. (1979): Pituitary hormones in brain: Where, How, and Why. *Science*, 205:366–372.

149. Krieger, D. T., Liotta, A., and Brownstein, M. J. (1977): Presence of corticotropin in brain of normal and hypophysectomized rats. *Proc. Natl. Acad. Sci. U.S.A.*, 74:648–652.

150. Krieger, D. T., Liotta, A., and Li, C. H. (1977): Human plasma immunoreactive β-lipotropin: Correlation with basal and stimulated plasma ACTH concentrations. *Life Sci.*, 21:1771–1778.

151. Krieger, D. T., Liotta, A., Nicholson, G., and Kizer, J. J. (1979): Brain ACTH and endorphin reduced in rats with monosodium glutamate-induced nuclear lesions. *Nature*, 278:562–563.

152. Kuhar, M. J., and Uhl, G. R. (1979): Histochemical localization of opiate receptors and the enkephalins. *Adv. Biochem. Psychopharmacol.*, 20:53–68.

153. Kumakura, K., Guidotti, A., Yang, H.-Y. T., Saiani, L., and Costa, E. (1980): A role for the opiate peptides that presumably coexist with acetylcholine in splanchnic nerves. *Adv. Biochem. Psychopharmacol.*, 22:571–580.

154. Kumakura, K., Karoum, F., Guidotti, A., and Costa, E. (1980): Modulation of nicotinic receptors by opiate receptor agonists in cultured adrenal chromaffin cells. *Nature*, 283:489–492.

155. Lakin, M. L., Miller, C. H., Stott, M. L., and Winters, W. D. (1981): Involvement of the pineal gland and melatonin in murine analgesia. *Life Sci.*, 29:2543–2551.

156. Larsson, L.-I., Childers, S., and Snyder, S. H. (1979): Met- and Leu-enkephalin immunoreactivity in separate neurons. *Nature*, 282:407–410.

157. Lasagna, L. (1965): Drug interaction in the field of analgesic drugs. *Proc. R. Soc. Med.*, 58:978–983.

158. Lee, H. K., Dunwiddie, T., and Hoffer, B. (1980): Electrophysiological interactions of enkephalins with neuronal circuitry in the rat hippocampus. II. Effects of interneuron excitability. *Brain Res.*, 184:331–342.

159. Levin, E. R., Sharp, B., Meyer, N., and Carlson, H. E. (1981): Morphine and naloxone: Effects on β-endorphin immunoreactivity in canine plasma and secretions from rat pituitaries. *Endocrinology*, 109:146–151.

160. Levine, J. D., Gordon, N. C., and Fields, H. L. (1978): The mechanism of placebo analgesia. *Lancet*, 2:654–657.

161. Levine, J. D., Gordon, N. C., Jones, R. T., and Fields, H. L. (1978): The narcotic antagonist naloxone enhances clinical pain. *Nature*, 272:826–827.

162. Levine, J. D., Gordon, N. C., and Fields, H. L. (1979): Naloxone dose-dependently produces analgesia and hyperalgesia in post-operative pain. *Nature*, 278:740–741.

163. Lewis, J. W., Cannon, J. .T., and Liebeskind, J. C. (1980): Opioid and nonopioid mechanisms of stress analgesia. *Science*, 208:623–625.

164. Lewis, R. V., Stein, S., Gerber, L., Rubinstein, M., and Udenfriend, S. (1978): High molecular weight opioid-containing proteins in striatum. *Proc. Natl. Acad. Sci. U.S.A.*, 75:4021–4023.

165. Lewis, R. V., Stern, A. S., Kimura, S., Rossier, J., Stein, S., and Udenfriend, S. (1980): An about 50,000-dalton protein in adrenal medulla: A common precursor of (met)- and (leu)-enkephalin. *Science*, 208:1459–1461.

166. Lewis, R. V., Stern, A. S., Rossier, J., Stein, S., and Udenfriend, S. (1979): Putative enkephalin precursors in bovine adrenal medulla. *Biochem. Biophys. Res. Commun.*, 89:822–829.

167. Liebeskind, J. C., Guilbaud, G., Besson, J.-M., and Oliveras, J.-L. (1973): Analgesia from electrical stimulation of the periaqueductal gray matter in the cat: Behavioral observations and inhibitory effects on spinal cord interneurons. *Brain Res.*, 50:441–446.

168. Lindberg, I., and Dahl, J. L. (1981): Characterization of enkephalin release from rat striatum. *J. Neurochem.*, 36:506–512.

169. Lindberg, I., Smythe, S. J., and Dahl, J. L. (1979): Regional distribution of enkephalin in bovine brain. *Brain Res.*, 168:200–204.

170. Lindberg, I., Yang, H.-Y. T., and Costa, E. (1982): An enkephalin-generating enzyme in bovine adrenal medulla. *Biochem. Biophys. Res. Commun.*, 106:186–193.

171. Lindblom, U., and Tegner, R. (1979): Are the endorphins active in clinical pain states. Narcotic antagonism in chronic pain patients. *Pain*, 7:65–68.

172. Lindeburg, T., Larsen, V., Kehlet, H., and Jacobsen, E. (1981): Respiratory, analgesic and endocrine responses to an enkephalin analogue in normal man. *Acta Anaesthesiol. Scand.*, 25:254–257.

173. Ling, G. S. F., and Pasternak, G. (1983): Receptor mechanisms of spinal and supraspinal analgesia. *Brain Res.*, 271:152–156.

174. Ling, N., Minick, S., Lazarus, L., Rivier, J., and Guillemin, R. (1977): Structure-activity relationships of enkephalin and endorphin analogs. In: *Peptides-Proceedings of the Fifth American Peptide Symposium*, edited by M. Goodman and J. Meienhofer, pp. 96–99. John Wiley and Sons, New York.

175. Liotta, A. S., and Krieger, D. T. (1980): In vitro biosynthesis and comparative post-translational processing of immunoreactive precursor corticotropin/β-endorphin by human placenta and pituitary cells. *Endocrinology*, 106:1504–1511.

176. Liotta, A. S., Suda, T., and Krieger, D. T. (1978): β-Lipotropin is the major opioid-like peptide of human pituitary and rat pars distalis: Lack of significant β-endorphin. *Proc. Natl. Acad. Sci. U.S.A.*, 75:2950–2954.

177. Liotta, A. S., Gildersleeve, D., Brownstein, M. J., and Krieger, D. T. (1979): Biosynthesis in vitro of immunoreactive 31,000 dalton corticotropin/β-endorphin-like materials by bovine hypothalamus. *Proc. Natl. Acad. Sci. U.S.A.*, 76:1448–1442.

178. Loh, H. H., Tseng, L. F., Wei, E., and Li, C. H. (1976): β-endorphin is a potent analgesic agent. *Proc. Natl. Acad. Sci. U.S.A.*, 83:2895–2898.

179. Lundberg, J. M., Hamberger, B., Schultzberg, M., Hokfelt, T., Cranberg, P.-O., Efendic, S., Terenius, L., Goldstein, M., and Luft, R. (1979): Enkephalin- and somatostatin-like immunoreactivity in human adrenal medulla and pheochromocytoma. *Proc. Natl. Acad. Sci. U.S.A.*, 76:4079–4083.

180. Lundberg, J. M., Hokfelt, T., Fahrenkrug, J., Nilsson, G., and Terenius, L. (1979): Peptides in the cat carotid body (glomus caroticum): VIP, enkephalin and substance P-like immunoreactivity. *Acta Physiol. Scand.*, 107:279–281.

181. Lundberg, J.M., Schultzberg, M., Hokfelt, T., Johansson, L., Sinhupak, R., Terenius, L., and Hamberger, B. (1979): Enkephalin in carotid body, SIF-cells, adrenal medulla and pheochromocytoma. *Acta Physiol. Scand. Suppl.*, 473:51.

182. Madden, IV, J., Akil, H., Patrick, R. L., and Barchas, J. D. (1977): Stress-induced parallel changes in central opioid levels and pain responsiveness in the rat. *Nature*, 265:358–360.

183. Mains, R. E., and Eipper, B. A. (1979): Synthesis and secretion of corticotropins, melanotropins, and endorphins by rat intermediate pituitary cells. *J. Biol. Chem.*, 254:7885–7894.

184. Mains, R. E., Eipper, B. A., and Ling, N. (1977): Common precursor to corticotropins and endorphins. *Proc. Natl. Acad. Sci. U.S.A.*, 74:3014–3018.

185. Malfroy, B., Swerts, J. P., Guyon, A., Roques, B. P., and Schwartz, J. C. (1978): High affinity enkephalin-degrading peptides in brain is increased after morphine. *Nature*, 276:523–526.

186. Malfroy, B., Swerts, J. P., Llorens, C., and Schwartz, J. C. (1979): Regional distribution of a high-affinity enkephalin-degrading peptidase (enkephalinase) and effects of lesions suggest localization in the vicinity of opiate receptors in brain. *Neurosci. Lett.*, 11:329–334.

187. Marks, N., Grynbaum, A., and Weidle, A. (1977): On the degradation of enkephalins and endorphins by rat and mouse brain extracts. *Biochem. Biophys. Res. Commun.*, 74:1552–1559.

188. Martin, W. R., Eades, C. G., Thompson, J. A., Huppler, R. E., and Gilbert, P. E. (1976): The effects of morphine- and nalorphine-like drugs in the nondependent and morphine-dependent chronic spinal dog. *J. Pharmacol. Exp. Ther.*, 197:517–532.

189. Mayer, D. J., and Price, D. D. (1976): Central nervous system mechanisms of analgesia. *Pain*, 2:379–404.

190. McGivern, R. F., and Berntson, G. G. (1980): Mediation of diurnal fluctuations in pain sensitivity in the rat by food intake patterns: Reversal by naloxone. *Science*, 210:210–211.

191. McGregor, W. H., Stein, L., and Beluzzi, J. D. (1978): Potent analgesic activity of the enkephalin-like tetrapeptide H-Tyr-D-Ala-Gly-Phe-NH$_2$. *Life Sci.*, 23:1371–1376.

192. Millan, M. J., Gramsch, C., Przewlocki, R., Hollt, V., and Herz, A. (1980): Lesions of the hypothalamic arcuate nucleus produce a temporary hyperalgesia and attenuate stress-evoked analgesia. *Life Sci.*, 27:1513–1523.

193. Millan, M. J., Przewlocki, R., Jerlicz, M., Gramsch, C. H., Hollt, V., and Herz, A. (1981): Stress-induced release of brain and pituitary β-endorphin: Major role of endorphins in generation of hyperthermia, not analgesia. *Brain Res.*, 208:325–338.

194. Miller, R. J. (1981): Peptides as neurotransmitters—Focus on the enkephalins and endorphins. *Pharmacol. Ther.*, 12:73–108.

195. Miller, R. J., Chang, K.-J., Cuatrecasas, P., and Wilkinson, S. (1977): The metabolic stability of the enkephalins. *Biochem. Biophys. Res. Commun.*, 74:1311–1318.

196. Morhland, J. S., and Gebhart, G. F. (1980): Effect of selective destruction of serotonergic neurons in nucleus raphe magnus on morphine-induced antinociception. *Life Sci.*, 27:2627–2632.

197. Morley, J. S. (1980): Structure-activity relationships of enkephalin-like peptides. *Ann. Rev. Pharmacol. Toxicol.*, 20:81–110.

198. Mullen, P. E., Jeffcoate, W. J., Linsell, C., Howard, R., and Rees, L. H. (1979): The circadian variation of immunoreactive lipotrophin and its relationship to ACTH and growth hormone in man. *Clin. Endocrinol.*, 11:533–539.

199. Naber, D., Cohen, R. M., Pickar, D., Kalin, N. H., Davis, G., Pert, C. B., and Bunney, W. E. Jr. (1981): Episodic secretion of opioid activity in human plasma and monkey CSF: Evidence for a diurnal rhythm. *Life Sci.*, 28:931–935.

200. Naber, D., Wirz-Justice, A., and Kafka, M. S. (1981): Circadian rhythm in rat brain opiate receptor. *Neurosci. Lett.*, 21:45–50.

201. Nakai, Y., Nakao, K., Oki, S., Imura, H., and Li, C. H. (1978): Presence of immunoreactive β-

endorphin in plasma of patients with Nelson's syndrome and Addison's disease. *Life Sci.*, 23:2293–2298.

202. Nakanishi, S., Inoue, A., Taii, S., and Numa, S. (1977): Cell-free translation product containing corticotropin and β-endorphin encoded by messenger RNA from anterior lobe and intermediate lobe of bovine pituitary. *FEBS Lett.*, 84:105–109.

203. Nakanishi, S., Inoue, A., Kita, T., Nakamura, M., Chang, A. C. Y., Cohen, S., and Numa, S. (1979): Nucleotide sequences of cloned cDNA for bovine corticotropin-β-lipotropin precursor. *Nature*, 278:423–427.

204. Nakanashi, S., Teranishi, Y., Noda, M., Notake, M., Watanabe, Y., Kakidani, H., Jingami, H., and Numa, S. (1980): The protein-coding sequence of bovine ACTH-β-LPH precursor gene is split near the signal region. *Nature*, 287:752–755.

205. Nakao, K., Nakai, Y., Oki, S., Horii, K., and Imura, H. (1978): Presence of immunoreactive β-endorphin in normal human plasma. *J. Clin. Invest.*, 62:1395–1398.

206. Nakao, K., Nakai, Y., Oki, S., Matsubara, S., Konishi, T., Nishitani, H., and Imura, H. (1980): Immunoreactive β-endorphin in human cerebrospinal fluid. *J. Clin. Endocrinol. Metab.*, 50:230–233.

207. Nakao, K., Oki, S., Tanaka, I., Horii, K., Nakai, Y., Furui, T., Fukushima, M., Kuwayama, A., Kageyama, N., and Imura, H. (1980): Immunoreactive β-endorphin and adrenocorticotropin in human CSF. *J. Clin. Invest.*, 66:1383–1390.

208. Nicoll, R. A., Alger, B. E., and Jahr, C. E. (1980): Enkephalin blocks inhibitory pathways in the vertebrate CNS. *Nature*, 287:22–25.

209. Noda, M., Furutani, Y., Takahashi, H., Toyosato, M., Hirose, T., Inayama, S., Nakanishi, S., and Numa, S. (1982): Cloning and sequence analysis of cDNA for bovine adrenal proenkephalin. *Nature*, 295:202–206.

210. North, R. A., (1979): Opiates, opioid peptides and single neurones. *Life Sci.*, 24:1527–1546.

211. Odagiri, E., Sherrell, B. J., Mount, C. D., Nicholson, W. E., and Orth, D. N. (1979): Human placental immunoreactive corticotropin, lipotropin and β-endorphin: Evidence for a common precursor. *Proc. Natl. Acad. Sci. U.S.A.*, 76:2027–2031.

212. Oleson, T. D., and Liebeskind, J. C. (1975): Relationship of neural activity in the raphe nuclei of the rat to brain stimulation-produced analgesia. *Physiologist*, 18:338.

213. Oleson, T. D., Kirkpatrick, D. B., and Goodman, S. J. (1980): Elevation of pain threshold to tooth shock by brain stimulation in primates. *Brain Res.*, 194:79–95.

214. Oliveras, J.-L., Besson, J.-M., Guilbaud, G., and Liebeskind, J. C. (1974): Behavioral and electrophysiological evidence of pain inhibition from midbrain stimulation in the cat. *Exp. Brain Res.*, 20:32–44.

215. Oliveras, J.-L., Redjemi, F., Guilbaud, G., and Besson, J.-M., (1975): Analgesia induced by electrical stimulation of the inferior centralis of the raphe in the cat. *Pain*, 1:139–145.

216. Osborne, H., and Herz, A. (1980): K⁺-evoked release of met-enkephalin from rat striatum in vitro: Effect of putative neurotransmitters and morphine. *Naunyn Schmiedebergs Arch. Pharmacol.*, 310:203–209.

217. Osborne, H., Hollt, V., and Herz, A. (1978): Potassium-induced release of enkephalins from rat striatal slices. *Eur. J. Pharmacol.*, 48:219–221.

218. Pasternak, G. W., Childers, S. R., and Snyder, S. H. (1980): Opiate analgesia: Evidence for mediation by a subpopulation of opiate receptors. *Science*, 208:514–516.

219. Palmer, M. R., and Hoffer, B. J. (1980): Catecholamine modulation of enkephalin-induced electrophysiological responses in cerebral cortex. *J. Pharmacol. Exp. Ther.*, 213:205–215.

220. Patey, G., DeLaBaume, S., Schwartz, J.-C., Gros, C., Roques, B., Fourne-Zaluski, M.-C., and Soroca-Lucas, E. (1981): Selective protection of met-enkephalin released from brain slices by enkephalinase inhibition. *Science*, 212:1153–1155.

221. Pert, A. (1976): Behavioral pharmacology of d-alanine²-methionine-enkephalin amide and other long-acting opiate peptides. In: *Opiates and Endogenous Opioid Peptides*, edited by H. W. Kosterlitz, pp. 87–94. Elsevier, Amsterdam.

222. Pert, A., and Yaksh, T. (1974): Localization of the antinociceptive action of morphine in primate brain. *Pharmacol. Biochem. Behav.*, 3:133–138.

223. Pert, C. B., Pert, A., Chang, J.-K., and Fong, B. T. W. (1976): [D-Ala²]-Met-Enkephalinamide: A potent, long-lasting synthetic pentapeptide analgesic. *Science*, 194:330–332.

224. Polak, J. M., Sullivan, S. N., Bloom, S. R., Facer, P., and Pearse, A. G. E. (1977): Enkephalin-like immunoreactivity in the human gastrointestinal tract. *Lancet*, 1:972–975.

225. Proudfit, H. K. (1980): Reversible inactivation of raphe magnus neurons: Effects of nociceptive threshold and morphine-induced analgesia. *Brain Res.*, 201:459–464.
226. Procacci, P., Della Corte, M., Zoppi, M., Romano, S., Maresca, M., and Voegelin, M. R. (1972): Pain threshold measurements in man. In: *Recent Advances on Pain (Pathophysiology and Clinical Aspects*, edited by J. J. Bonica, P. Procacci, and C. A. Pagni, pp. 105–147. Charles C Thomas, Springfield, Ill.
227. Przewlocki, R., Hollt, V., and Herz, A. (1978): Release of β-endorphin from rat pituitary in vitro. *Eur. J. Pharmacol.*, 51:179–183.
228. Richardson, D. E., and Akil, H. (1977): Pain reduction by electrical brain stimulation in man: 1. Acute administration in periaqueductal and periventricular sites. *J. Neurosurg.*, 47:178–183.
229. Richardson, D. E., and Akil, H. (1977): Pain reduction by electrical brain stimulation in man. Part 2. Chronic self-administration in the periventricular gray matter. *J. Neurosurg.*, 47:184–194.
230. Richter, J. A., Wesche, D. L., and Frederickson, R. C. A. (1979): K^+-Stimulated release of leu- and met-enkephalin from rat striatal slices: Lack of effect of morphine and naloxone. *Eur. J. Pharmacol.*, 56:105–113.
231. Roberts, J. L., and Herbert, E. (1977): Characterization of a common precursor to corticotropin and β-lipotropin: Cell-free synthesis of the precursor and identification of corticotropin peptide in the molecule. *Proc. Natl. Acad. Sci. U.S.A.*, 74:4826–4830.
232. Roemer, D., Buscher, H. H., Hill, R. C., Pless, J., Bauer, W., Cardinaux, F., Closse, A., Hauser, D., and Huguenin, R. (1977): A synthetic enkephalin analogue with prolonged parenteral and oral analgesic activity. *Nature*, 268:547–549.
233. Roques, B. P., Fournie-Zaluski, M. C., Soroca, E., Lecomte, J. M., Malfroy, B., Llorens, C., and Schwartz, J.-C. (1980): The enkephalinase inhibitor thiorphan shows antinociceptive activity in mice. *Nature*, 288:286–288.
234. Rosenfeld, J. P., and Rice, P. E. (1979): Diurnal rhythms in nociceptive thresholds of rats. *Physiol. Behav.*, 23:419–420.
235. Ross, M., Berger, P. A., and Goldstein, A. (1979): Plasma β-endorphin immunoreactivity in schizophrenia. *Science*, 205:1163–1164.
236. Rossier, J. (1981): Enkephalin biosynthesis, the search for a common precursor. *Trends in Neurosciences*, 4:94–97.
237. Rossier, J., French, E. D., Rivier, C., Ling, N., Guillemin, R., and Bloom, F. E. (1977): Foot-shock induced stress increases β-endorphin levels in blood but not brain. *Nature*, 270:618–620.
238. Rossier, J., Vargo, T. M., Minick, S., Ling, N., Bloom, F. E., and Guillemin, R. (1977): Regional dissociation of β-endorphin and enkephalin contents in rat brain and pituitary. *Proc. Natl. Acad. Sci. U.S.A.*, 74:5162–5165.
239. Rossier, J., French, E., Gros, C., Minick, S., Guillemin, R., and Bloom, F. E. (1979): Adrenal-ectomy, dexamethasone or stress alters opioid peptide levels in rat anterior pituitary but not intermediate lobe or brain. *Life Sci.*, 25:2105–2112.
240. Rossier, J., Trifaro, J. M., Lewis, R. V., Lee, R. W. H., Stern, A., Kimura, S., Stein, S., and Udenfriend, S. (1980): Studies with [^{35}S]methionine indicate that the 22,000-dalton met-enke-phalin-containing protein in chromaffin cells is a precursor of met-enkephalin. *Proc. Natl. Acad. Sci. U.S.A.*, 77:6889–6891.
241. Ruda, M. A. (1975): Autoradiographic study of the efferent connections of the midbrain central gray in the cat. *Anat. Rec.*, 181:468–469.
242. Sar, M., Stumpf, W. E., Miller, R. J., Chang, K.-J., and Cuatrecasas, P. (1978): Immunohisto-chemical localization of enkephalin in rat brain and spinal cord. *J. Comp. Neurol.*, 182:17–38.
243. Sarne, Y., Azov, R., and Weissman, B. A. (1978): A stable enkephalin-like immunoreactive substance in human CSF. *Brain Res.*, 151:399–403.
244. Sarne, Y., Gothilf, Y., and Weissman, B. A. (1980): Humoral endorphin: Endogenous opiate in blood cerebrospinal fluid and brain. In: *Endogenous and Exogenous Opiate Agonists and Antag-onists*, edited by E. Leong Way, pp. 317–320. Pergamon Press, New York.
245. Sarne, Y., Weissman, B. A., Keren, O., and Urca, G. (1981): Humoral endorphin: A new endogenous factor with opiate-like activity. *Life Sci.*, 28:673–680.
246. Satoh, M., Akaike, A., and Takagi, H. (1979): Excitation by morphine and enkephalin of single neurons of nucleus reticularis paragigantocellularis in the rat: A probable mechanism of analgesic action of opioids. *Brain Res.*, 169:406–410.
247. Satoh, M., Akaike, A., Nakazawa, T., and Takagi, H. (1980): Evidence for involvement of

separate mechanisms in the production of analgesia by electrical stimulation of the nucleus reticularis paragigantocellularis and nucleus raphe magnus in the rat. *Brain Res.*, 194:525–529.

248. Sawada, S., and Yamamoto, C. (1981): Postsynaptic inhibitory actions of catecholamines and opioid peptides in the bed nucleus of the stria terminalis. *Exp. Brain Res.*, 41:264–270.

249. Sawynok, J., and Labella, F. S. (1981): GABA and baclofen potentiate the K^+-evoked release of met-enkephalin from rat striatal slices. *Eur. J. Pharmacol.*, 70:103–110.

250. Sawynok, J., Pinsky, C., and Labella, F. S. (1979): Minireview on the specificity of naloxone as an opiate antagonist. *Life Sci.*, 25:1621–1632.

251. Sawynok, T., Labella, F. S., and Pinsky, C. (1980): Effects of morphine and naloxone on the K^+-stimulated release of met-enkephalin from slices of rat corpus striatum. *Brain Res.*, 189:483–493.

252. Schild, H. O. (1947): pA, a new scale for the measurement of drug antagonism. *Br. J. Pharmacol. Chemother.*, 2:189–206.

253. Schnebli, H. P., Phillips, M. A., and Barclay, R. K. (1979): Isolation and characterization of an enkephalin-degrading aminopeptidase from rat brain. *Biochem. Biophys. Acta*, 569:89–98.

254. Schultzberg, M., Hokfelt, T., Lundberg, J. M., Terenius, L., Elfvin, L.-G., and Elde, R. (1978): Enkephalin-like immunoreactivity in nerve terminals in sympathetic ganglia and adrenal medulla and in adrenal medullary gland cells. *Acta Physiol. Scand.*, 103:475–477.

255. Schultzberg, M., Lundberg, J. M., Hokfelt, T., Terenius, L., Brandt, J., Elde, R., and Goldstein, M. (1978): Enkephalin-like immunoreactivity in gland cells and nerve terminals of the adrenal medulla. *Neuroscience*, 3:1169–1186.

256. Schultzberg, M., Hokfelt, T., Terenius, L., Elfvin, L.-G., Lundberg, J. M., Brandt, J., Elde, R. P., and Goldstein, M. (1979): Enkephalin immunoreactive nerve fibres and cell bodies in sympathetic ganglia of the guinea-pig and rat. *Neuroscience*, 4:249–270.

257. Schultzberg, M., Hokfelt, T., Nilsson, G., Terenius, L., Rehfeld, J. F., Brown, M., Elde, R., Goldstein, M., and Said, S. J. (1980): Distribution of peptide—and catecholamine—containing neurons in the gastrointestinal tract of the rat and guinea pig: Immunohistochemical studies with antisera to substance P, VIP, enkephalins, somatostatin, gastric/CCK, neurotensin and dopamine-β-hydroxylase. *Neuroscience*, 5:689–744.

258. Shah, Y., and Dostrovsky, J. O. (1980): Electrophysiological evidence for a projection of the periaqueductal gray matter to nucleus raphe magnus in cat and rat. *Brain Res.*, 193:534–538.

259. Shanks, M. F., Clement-Jones, V., Linsell, C. J., Mullen, P. E., Rees, L. H., and Besser, G. M. (1981): A study of 24-hour profiles of plasma met-enkephalin in man. *Brain Res.*, 212:403–409.

260. Simantov, R. (1978): Basal and potassium stimulated, calcium dependent, endorphin release from pituitary cells. *Life Sci.*, 23:2503–2508.

261. Simmons, W. H., and Ritzman, R. L. (1980): An inhibitor of opioid peptide degradation produces analgesia in mice. *Pharmacol. Biochem. Behav.*, 13:715–718.

262. Sjolund, B., and Eriksson, M. (1976): Electro-acupuncture and endogenous morphines. *Lancet*, 2:1085.

263. Sjolund, B., Terenius, L., and Eriksson, M. (1977): Increased cerebrospinal fluid levels of endorphins after electro-acupuncture. *Acta Physiol. Scand.*, 100:382–384.

264. Smyth, D. G., Massey, D. E., Zakarian, S., and Finnie, M. D. A. (1979): Endorphins are stored in biologically active and inactive forms: Isolation of α-N-acetyl peptides. *Nature*, 279:252–254.

265. Snyder, S. H. (1980): Brain peptides as neurotransmitters. *Science*, 209:976–983.

266. Spector, S., Shorr, J., Finberg, J., and Foley, K. (1979): Presence of a non-peptide morphine-like compound in human CSF and urine. In: *Endorphins in Mental Health Research*, edited by E. Usdin, W. E. Bunney, Jr., and N. S. Kline, pp. 569–575. MacMillan, London.

267. Stacher, G., Bauer, P., Steinringer, H., Schreiber, E., and Schmierer, G. (1979): Effects of the synthetic enkephalin analogue FK 33-824 on pain threshold and pain tolerance in man. *Pain*, 7:159–172.

268. Stern, A. S., Lewis, R. V., Kimura, S., Rossier, J., Gerber, L. D., Brink, L., Stein, S., and Udenfriend, S. (1979): Isolation of the opioid heptapeptide met-enkephalin [Arg^6, Phe^7] from bovine adrenal medullary granules and striatum. *Proc. Natl. Acad. Sci. U.S.A.*, 76:6680–6683.

269. Stern, A. S., Lewis, R. V., Kimura, S., Rossier, J., Stein, S., and Udenfriend, S. (1980): Opioid hexapeptides and heptapeptides in adrenal medulla and brain: Possible implications on the biosynthesis of enkephalins. *Arch. Biochem. Biophys.*, 205:606–613.

270. Stine, S. M., Yang, H.-Y. T., and Costa, E. (1980): Inhibition of in situ metabolism of [³H]met-enkephalin and potentiation of met-enkephalin analgesia by captopril. *Brain Res.*, 188:295–299.

271. Stubbs, W. A., Jones, A., Edwards, C. A. W., Delitala, D., Jeffcoate, W. J., and Ratter, S. J. (1978): Hormonal and metabolic responses to an enkephalin analogue in normal man. *Lancet*, 2:1225–1227.

272. Suda, T., Liotta, A. S., and Krieger, D. T. (1978): β-Endorphin is not detectable in plasma from normal human subjects. *Science*, 202:221–223.

273. Suhar, A., and Marks, N. (1979): Purification and properties of cathespin B: Evidence for cleavage of pituitary lipotropins. *Eur. J. Biochem.*, 101:23–30.

274. Sullivan, S., Akil, H., and Barchas, J. D. (1978): In vitro degradation of enkephalin: Evidence for cleavage at the gly-phe bond. *Commun. Psychopharmacol.*, 2:525–531.

275. Sullivan, S., Akil, H., Blacker, D., and Barchas, J. D. (1980): Enkephalinase: Selective inhibitors and partial characterization. *Peptides*, 1:31–35.

276. Swerts, J. P., Perdrisot, R., Malfroy, B., and Schwartz, J. C. (1979): Is 'enkephalinase' identical with angiotensin-converting enzyme? *Eur. J. Pharmacol.*, 53:209–210.

277. Swerts, J. P., Perdrisot, R., Patey, G., De La Baume, S., and Schwartz, J. C. (1979): 'Enkephalinase' is distinct from brain angiotensin converting enzyme. *Eur. J. Pharmacol.*, 57:279–281.

278. Takagi, H., Satoh, M., Akaike, A., Shibata, T., Yajima, H., and Ogawa, H. (1978): Analgesia by enkephalins injected into the nucleus reticularis gigantocellularis of the rat medulla oblongata. *Eur. J. Pharmacol.*, 49:113–116.

279. Terenius, L., and Wahlstrom, A. (1975): Search for an endogenous ligand for the opiate receptor. *Acta Physiol. Scand.*, 94:74–81.

280. Terenius, L., Wahlstrom, A., Lindstrom, L., and Widerlof, E. (1976): Increased CSF levels of endorphins in chronic psychosis. *Neurosci. Lett.*, 3:157–162.

281. Terenius, L., Wahlstrom, A., and Johansson, L. (1979): Endorphins in human cerebrospinal fluid and their measurement. In: *Endorphins in Mental Health Research*, edited by E. Usdin, W. E. Bunney, Jr., and N. S. Kline, pp. 553–560. MacMillan, London.

282. Traficante, L. J., Rotrosen, J., Siekierski, J., Tracer, H., and Gershon, S. (1980): Enkephalin inactivation by N-terminal tyrosine cleavage: Purification and partial characterization of a highly specific enzyme from human brain. *Life Sci.*, 26:1697–1706.

283. Traficante, L. J., Rotrosen, J., Siekierski, J., Tracer, H., and Gershon, S. (1980b): Antibiotics as inhibitors of enkephalin degradation. *Pharmacol. Res. Commun.*, 10:575–580.

284. Troy, C. M., and Musacchio, J. M. (1981): Bovine chromaffin granules contain an enzyme and a precursor which generate met-enkephalin in vitro. *Abstr. Soc. Neurosci.*, 11:91.

285. Tsou, K., and Jang, C. S. (1964): *Sci. Sin.*, 13:1099.

286. Uhl, G. R., Kuhar, M. J., and Snyder, S. H. (1978): Enkephalin-containing pathway: Amygdaloid afferents in the stria terminalis. *Brain Res.*, 149:223–228.

287. Urca, G., Frenk, H., Liebeskind, J. C., and Taylor, A. N. (1977): Morphine and enkephalin: Analgesic and epileptic properties. *Science*, 197:83–86.

288. Vale, W., Spiess, J., Rivier, C., and Rivier, J. (1981): Characterization of a 41-residue ovine hypothalamic peptide that stimulates secretion of corticotropin and β-endorphin. *Science*, 213:1394–1397.

289. Vaught, J. L., Rothman, B. B., and Westfall, T. C. (1982): Mu and delta receptors: Their role in analgesia and in the differential effects of opioid peptides on analagesia. *Life Sci.*, 30:1443–1455.

290. Vavrek, R. J., Hsi, L.-H., York, E. J., Hall, M. E., and Stewart, J. M. (1981): Minimum structure opioids—Dipeptide and tripeptide analogs of the enkephalins. *Peptides*, 2:303–308.

291. Vermes, I., Mulder, G. H., Smellik, P. G., and Tilders, F. J. H. (1980): Differential control of β-endorphin/β-liprotropin secretion from anterior and intermediate lobes of the rat pituitary gland in vitro. *Life Sci.*, 27:1761–1768.

292. Vidal, C., and Jacob, J. (1980): The effect of medial hypothalamus lesions on pain control. *Brain Res.*, 199:89–100.

293. Vogel, Z., and Altstein, M. (1979): The effect of puromycin on the biological activity of leu-enkephalin. *FEBS Lett.*, 98:44–48.

294. Wagner, G. W., and Dixon, J. E. (1981): Inhibitors of rat brain aminopeptidase. *J. Neurochem.*, 37:709–713.

295. Wagner, G. W., Tavianini, M. A., Herrmann, K. M., and Dixon, J. E. (1981): Purification and characterization of an enkephalin aminopeptidase from rat brain. *Biochemistry*, 20:3884–3890.

296. Wahlstrom, A., Johansson, L., and Terenius, L. (1976): Characterization of endorphins (endogenous morphine-like factors) in human csf and brain extracts. In: *Opiates and Endogenous Opioid Peptides*, edited by H. Kosterlitz, pp. 49–56. Elsevier, Amsterdam.

297. Wardlaw, S. L., and Frantz, A. G. (1979): Measurement of β-endorphins in human plasma. *J. Clin. Endocrinol. Metab.*, 48:176–180.
298. Wardlaw, S. L., Stark, R. I., Baxi, L., and Frantz, A. G. (1979): Plasma β-endorphin and β-lipotropin in the human fetus at delivery: Correlation with arterial pH and pCO_2. *J. Clin. Endocrinol. Metab.*, 79:888–891.
299. Watson, S. J., Akil, H., Richard, C. W., and Barchas, J. D. (1978): Evidence for two separate opiate peptide neuronal systems. *Nature*, 275:226–228.
300. Watson, S. J., Akil, H., Ghazarossian, V. E., and Goldstein, A. (1981): Dynorphin immunocytochemical localization in brain and peripheral nervous system: Preliminary studies. *Proc. Natl. Acad. Sci. U.S.A.*, 78:1260–1263.
300a. Watson, S. J., and Barchas, J. D. (1979): *Mechanisms of Pain and Analgesic Compounds*, edited by R. F. Beers, Jr., and E. G. Bassett. Raven Press, New York.
301. Weber, E., Roth, K. A., and Barchas, J. D. (1981): Colocalization of α-neoendorphin and dynorphin immunoreactivity in hypothalamic neurons. *Biochem. Biophys. Res. Commun.*, 103:951–958.
302. Weidemann, E., Saito, T., Linfoot, J. A., and Li, C. H. (1979): Specific radioimmunoassay of human β-endorphin in unextracted plasma. *J. Clin. Endocrinol. Metab.*, 49:478–480.
303. Wesche, D. L., and Frederickson, R. C. A. (1979): Diurnal differences in opioid peptide levels correlated with nociceptive sensitivity. *Life Sci.*, 24:1861–1868.
304. Wesche, D. L., and Frederickson, R. C. A. (1980): Diurnal difference in enkephalin levels correlated with nociceptive sensitivity. In: *Endogenous and Exogenous Opiate Agonists and Antagonists*, edited by E. Long Way, pp. 463–466. Pergamon Press, New York.
305. Wesche, D. L., and Frederickson, R. C. A. (1981): The role of the pituitary in the diurnal variation in tolerance to painful stimuli and brain enkephalin levels. *Life Sci.*, 29:2199–2205.
306. Wesche, D. L., and Frederickson, R. C. A. (1981): Diurnal rhythm in response to noxious stimuli-increase of met-enkephalin in globus pallidus. In: *Advances in Endogenous and Exogenous Opioids*, edited by H. Takayi, p. 30, p. 90 *(Abstr.)*. International Narcotic Research Conference, Japan.
307. Wesche, D., Hollt, V., and Herz, A. (1977): Radioimmunoassay of enkephalins: Regional distribution in rat brain after morphine treatment and hypophysectomy. *Naunyn Schmiedebergs Arch. Pharmacol.*, 301:79–82.
308. Willer, J. C., Dehen, H., and Cambier, J. (1981): Stress-induced analgesia in humans: Endogenous opioids and naloxone-reversible depression of pain reflexes. *Science*, 212:689–691.
309. Wilson, S. P., Chang, K.-J., and Viveros, O. H. (1980): Synthesis of enkephalins by adrenal medullary chromaffin cells: Reserpine increases incorporation of radiolabeled amino acids. *Proc. Natl. Acad. Sci. U.S.A.*, 77:4364–4368.
310. Wolstencroft, J. H., West, D. C., and Gent, G. P. (1978): Actions of morphine and opioid peptides on neurones in the reticular formation, raphe nuclei and the periaqueductal gray. In: *Iontophoresis and Transmitter Mechanisms in the Mammalian Central Nervous System*, edited by R. W. Ryall and J. S. Kelly, pp. 341–343. Elsevier, Amsterdam.
311. Wood, P. L., Charleson, S. E., Lane, D., and Hudgin, R. L. (1981): Multiple opiate receptors: Differential binding of μ- κ- and δ-agonists. *Neurophamacology*, 20:1215–1220.
312. Woolf, C. J., Barrett, G. D., Mitchell, D., and Myers, R. A. (1977): Naloxone-reversible peripheral electroanalgesia in intact and spinal rats. *Eur. J. Pharmacol.*, 45:311–314.
313. Yaksh, T. L. (1979a): Central nervous system sites mediating opiate analgesia. In: *Advances in Pain Research and Therapy*, Vol. 3, edited by J. J. Bonica, J. C. Liebeskind, and D. G. Albe-Fessard, pp. 411–425. Raven Press, New York.
314. Yaksh, T. L. (1979): Direct evidence that spinal serotonin and noradrenaline terminals mediate the spinal antinociceptive effects of morphine in the periaqueductal gray. *Brain Res.*, 160:180–185.
315. Yaksh, T. L., and Rudy, T. A. (1978): Narcotic analgesics: CNS sites and mechanisms of action as revealed by intracerebral injection techniques. *Pain*, 4:299–359.
316. Yaksh, T. L., DuChateau, J. C., and Rudy, T. A. (1976): Antagonism by methysergide and cinanserin of the antinociceptive action of morphine administered into the periaqueductal gray. *Brain Res.*, 104:367–372.
317. Yaksh, T. L., Huang, S.P., Rudy, T. A., and Frederickson, R. C. A. (1977): The direct and specific opiate-like effect of Met⁵-enkephalin and analogues on the spinal cord. *Neuroscience*, 2:593–596.
318. Yaksh, T. L., Wang, J.-Y., and Howe, J. R. (1982): The pharmacology of spinal pain modulatory systems. In: *Recent Advances in the Management of Pain*, Raven Press, New York *(in press)*.
319. Yamaguchi, H., Liotta, A., and Krieger, D. (1980): Simultaneous determination of human plasma

immunoreactive β-lipotropin, γ-lipotropin and β-endorphin using immune-affinity chromatography. *J. Endocrinol. Metab.*, 51:1002–1008.

320. Zakarian, S., and Smyth, D. (1979): Distribution of active and inactive forms of endorphins in rat pituitary and brain. *Proc. Natl. Acad. Sci. U.S.A.*, 76:5972–5976.

321. Zieglgansberger, W., French, E. D., Siggins, G. R., and Bloom, F. E. (1979): Opioid peptides may excite hippocampal pyramidal neurons by inhibiting adjacent inhibitory interneurons. *Science*, 205:414–417.

322. Zimmerman, E. A., Liotta, A., and Krieger, D. T. (1978): β-Lipotropin in brain: Localization in hypothalamic neurons by immunoperoxidase technique. *Cell Tissue Res.*, 186:393–398.

Analgesics: Neurochemical, Behavioral, and Clinical Perspectives, edited by M. Kuhar and G. Pasternak. Raven Press, New York © 1984

Multiple Opiate Receptors

Robert R. Goodman and Gavril W. Pasternak

The Cotzias Laboratory of Neuro-Oncology, Memorial Sloan-Kettering Cancer Center, Departments of Neurology and Pharmacology, Cornell University Medical College, New York, NY 10021

Originally proposed near the turn of the century (20,30,38,75), the receptor theory of drug action was based upon a number of observations: rigid structural requirements for pharmacological activity, including stereospecificity; the existence of specific antagonists; the observation of dose-dependent actions with a maximal response, or a "saturation" of pharmacological response with increasing drug dosage; and, in some cases, the existence of cross tolerance and dependence. It was proposed that drug action resulted from binding to a specific recognition site, or receptor. In contrast to enzymes, drugs dissociated from their receptor unchanged, permitting a single molecule to interact with many receptors. However, the complexity of this approach increased sharply with the realization that a single compound could interact with more than one type of receptor site. Furthermore, different pharmacological actions produced by a single compound often appeared to be mediated through these different receptor subtypes. First described with the muscarinic and nicotinic receptors for acetylcholine (26), the concept of multiple receptors for transmitters has now been demonstrated for many systems. This concept has become a cornerstone in pharmaceutical development. As a result of extensive studies, pharmacologists have often been able to develop compounds selective for a specific subtype of receptor, whose actions were far more limited and specific than those of the original ligand, which bound to more subclasses of receptor.

Studies of opiate pharmacology over the past 50 years have suggested the existence of opiate receptors, fulfilling the criteria listed above. Extensive structure-activity studies involving hundreds of compounds established firm stereochemical structural requirements for opioid activity (127), and suggested chemically defined requirements for an opiate binding site (2). Opiate antagonists, such as naloxone, were also developed (6,7,33,82). Bioassays measuring *in vivo* analgesia (4,27,48,117,140,165) or opioid inhibition of the electrically-induced contraction of the guinea pig ileum (47,115,116) clearly showed dose-dependent effects with a well-defined maximal response. Opiate tolerance, the need to use increasing dosages to maintain a given pharmacological effect with chronic administration, was associated with physical dependence, manifested by specific withdrawal symptoms after either opiate abstinence or administration of an antagonist (84,85). Cross tolerance and cross dependence between opiates (136) was very specific and was not seen with nonopiate agents.

BIOCHEMICAL DEMONSTRATION AND CHARACTERIZATION OF OPIATE BINDING SITES

Technical difficulties delayed the demonstration of specific opiate binding sites until 1973 (121,122,143,151), despite a number of earlier attempts. Using the important criteria of stereospecificity (42), these classic studies clearly established a high potency of opiates for these binding sites and the stereospecificity corresponding to their pharmacological actions *in vivo*. A number of other criteria were also examined to further support the relevancy of these binding sites. The binding sites were localized to gray matter regions of the brain, and more specifically, to those areas known to be involved with opioid action (74,118; Table 1). Subcellular studies revealed an association of the binding sites with synaptosomal membranes (120). An important study also demonstrated an excellent correlation between the binding characteristics of opiates in the nerve plexus of the guinea pig ileum and their potency in the guinea pig ileum contraction assay (25; Fig. 1).

The binding sites were also characterized biochemically. Early studies clearly established the importance of both proteins and lipids (111). Since then the role of lipids has been examined far more extensively (18,19,24,77,80). A number of compounds have received consideration, including cerebroside sulfate, phosphatidylserine, phosphatidylinositol and phosphatidylethanolamine. Of the reported studies, those implicating a role for cerebroside sulfate have been the most convincing. In addition to binding opiates (18), cerebroside sulfate also has been associated with analgesia and opiate actions. Jimpy mice, leucodystrophic mutants deficient in brain cerebroside sulfate, were less sensitive to morphine analgesia than their normal littermate controls (77). In addition, administration of antibodies directed to cerebroside sulfate into the periaqueductal gray antagonized morphine's actions (24). This complex biochemical aspect of opiate binding sites has been extensively reviewed (19,80).

Many studies have described differences between the binding of opiate agonists and antagonists (16,110,112,113,119,158; Table 2). These have involved a number of ions as well as protein modifying reagents, proteolytic enzymes, and even temperature. Although the mechanisms producing these actions remain unclear, this ability to discriminate biochemically between agonists and antagonists may provide the means to understand their molecular basis of opiate action.

Finally, as techniques evolved and binding sensitivity improved, a new opioid binding site with far greater affinity ($K_D < 1$ nM) for opiates was described (112). This novel high affinity binding site was the first biochemical suggestion of receptor heterogeneity, and has proven very important in our understanding of opiate action, as discussed later in this chapter.

TABLE 1. *Regional distribution of opiate receptor binding in the monkey brain*

Region	^{3}H-Dihydromorphine binding (fmoles/mg protein)
Cortex	
Frontal pole	11.9
Temporal gyrus	6–11
Precentral gyrus	3.4
Postcentral gyrus	2.8
Occipital pole	2.3
White matter areas	
Corpus callosum	<2
Corona radiata	<2
Optic chiasm	<2
Fornix	<2
Limbic cortex	
Amygdala (anterior/posterior)	65.1/34.1
Hippocampus	12.5
Hypothalamus	23.2
Mammillary bodies	5
Thalamus (medial/lateral)	24.6/7.8
Caudate	9–19
Putamen	11.7
Globus pallidus	7.7
Midbrain	
Colliculi (superior/inferior)	10.6/6.7
Raphe area	8.2
Interpeduncular nuclear	13.7
Periaqueductal gray	31.1
Pons (ventral)	1.4
Cerebellum	<2
Medulla (lower)	5.8

From Kuhar et al. (74).

IN VIVO PHARMACOLOGIC EVIDENCE FOR MULTIPLICITY OF OPIATE RECEPTORS

Studies of nalorphine, the N-allyl derivative of morphine, provided the first suggestion for multiple types of opiate receptors (51,52,126). Although a potent analgesic when given alone (76), nalorphine antagonized morphine's effects when the two were given together (29,156,157). However, it was then observed that at a fixed morphine dose, concurrent low doses of nalorphine antagonized analgesia, whereas larger doses of nalorphine restored it (60). These results led Martin (85) to propose the theory of "Receptor Dualism." This theory postulated two receptors, one for morphine, and the other for nalorphine. Martin suggested that a drug could be a strong agonist, a partial agonist, or an antagonist at either of these receptors. Thus, nalorphine would be an antagonist at the morphine site, and an agonist at the nalorphine site. Martin's theory of opiate receptor dualism was subsequently supported by clinical studies (66).

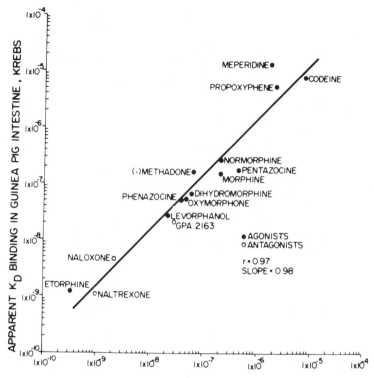

FIG. 1. Comparison of the potency of opiates in inhibiting the guinea pig ileum contraction assay and opiate receptor binding in the guinea pig ileum. The potency of many opiates in the electrically stimulated guinea pig ileum contraction bioassay was determined and compared to their affinity for opiate binding sites in the ileum preparation. (From Creese and Snyder, ref. 26.)

In the early 1970s, it became apparent to Martin that this two receptor theory did not adequately explain the actions of cyclazocine and pentazocine, two partial agonists of the benzomorphan series (1,50,67,68,91). Their actions, in clinical studies, differed from those of morphine (36,90) and of N-allylnormetazocine (SKF 10,047). Three different syndromes were then identified in single-dose studies with various opiates in the chronic spinal dog (41,87–89,92,93). Briefly, their experimental method utilized dogs that were spinally transected 1 to 17 months before testing various opiates. Effects on the flexor reflex, skin twitch reflex, pupil diameter, temperature, respiration, and pulse were determined, as well as many signs of withdrawal with weighting factors to minimize variance. These syndromes then were attributed to three distinct opiate receptors (mu, kappa, and sigma) (Table 3). Morphine is the prototype agonist for the mu receptor, causing miosis, bradycardia, hypothermia, decreased respiration rate, depression of nociceptive responses, and indifference to environmental stimuli. The partial agonists were found to cause two other distinct syndromes. Ketocyclazocine, a benzomorphan, and prototypic kappa agonist, caused miosis, depressed flexor reflex and sedation,

TABLE 2. *Discrimination of opiate agonist and antagonist binding*

Treatment	Agonist binding	Antagonist binding
Ions		
Monovalent		
Sodium	Decrease	Increase
Potassium	Slight decrease	Slight decrease
Lithium	Decrease	Increase
Divalent		
Magnesium	Increase	Little change
Manganese	Increase	Little change
Calcium	Little change	Little change
Enzymes		
Trypsin	Decrease	Little change
Chymotrypsin	Decrease	Little change
Reagents		
N-ethylmaleimide	Decrease	Little change
Iodoacetamide	Decrease	Little change
GTP	Decrease	Little change

TABLE 3. *Opiate actions in the chronic spinal dog*

	Mu (Morphine)	Kappa (Ketocyclazocine)	Sigma (SKF 10,047)
Pupil	Miosis	Miosis	Mydriasis
Respiratory rate	Stimulation then depression	No change	Stimulation
Heart rate	Bradycardia	No change	Tachycardia
Body temperature	Hypothermia	No change	No change
Affect	Indifference	Sedation	Delerium
Nociceptive reflexes			
Flexor	Decrease	Decrease	Modest decrease
Skin twitch	Decrease	No effect	No effect

From Iwamoto and Martin (64).

but unlike morphine, did not markedly alter pulse rate, temperature, respiratory rate, or the skin twitch reflex. SKF 10,047, a potent hallucinogen in man and an effective morphine antagonist with little analgesic activity (69,117), was the prototypic sigma agonist which, unlike morphine and ketocyclazocine, caused mydriasis, tachycardia, hyperthermia, tachypnea, and mania. This syndrome was felt to be quite similar to apomorphine effects, and it was suggested that a dopaminergic mechanism might be involved. The effects of all three agonist types were antagonized by naltrexone.

Further studies involved the effects of these drugs on the morphine-dependent and cyclazocine-dependent chronic spinal dog (41,88). An earlier study had shown that ketocyclazocine neither suppressed nor precipitated abstinence in the morphine-dependent monkey (147). These studies were reproduced in the chronic spinal dog, and further differences described. The abstinence syndromes for morphine and cyclazocine were qualitatively different, and ethylketocyclazocine (a kappa agonist) suppressed only that of cyclazocine. Also, naltrexone precipitated abstinence 20-fold less potently in cyclazocine-dependent than in morphine-dependent dogs. A number of opiates were then classified as agonists, partial agonists, or antagonists at each of these potential receptors. For example, pentazocine was classified as a weak mu antagonist, strong kappa agonist, and strong sigma agonist; nalorphine a mu antagonist and a partial kappa and sigma agonist; and buprenorphine a partial mu agonist only. Martin then proposed that the mu receptor mediated a supraspinal type of analgesia, euphoria, and an important part of morphine-type physical dependence; the kappa receptor mediated spinal analgesia, sedation, anesthesia, and many of the signs of cyclazocine dependence, and the sigma receptor mediated dysphoria and respiratory stimulation (86).

The recent development of behavioral assays which discriminate mu, kappa, and sigma agonists may greatly facilitate the future study of these various classes of opiates (23). In contrast to morphine, cyclazocine and pentazocine caused side-to-side head movements and pivoting on the hind feet in rodents, which were resistant to naloxone antagonism (21,133). In mice, the Straub tail is seen with morphine but not cyclazocine, pentazocine, ketocyclazocine and ethylketocyclazocine (21,164). A recent review by Iwamoto and Martin (64) summarized the involvement of distinct dopaminergic mechanisms in mediating mu, kappa, and sigma opiate effects in motility. Although both morphine and cyclazocine increase locomotor activity in many mouse strains, only morphine is easily antagonized by naloxone (100,144,150). In contrast, pentazocine (32) and ethylketocyclazocine (143,150) depress locomotor activity in mice. Thus, the evidence suggested that mu agonists increased motility via a different mechanism than sigma agonists, and that kappa agonists decreased motility through yet a third mechanism.

EVIDENCE FOR DISTINCT MORPHINE AND ENKEPHALIN RECEPTORS

After the discovery of the enkephalins (61,62,95,107,109,142,152), most investigators felt they had found "the brain's own morphine." The enkephalins (Tyr-Gly-Gly-Phe-Leu and Tyr-Gly-Gly-Phe-Met) were two related peptides whose potent analgesic actions could be blocked by naloxone and showed cross tolerance with morphine (5,70). However, as investigations into the pharmacology of the enkephalins progressed, it soon became apparent that significant differences existed between the peptides and the alkaloids. Comparison of the potencies of opiates and enkephalins in the mouse vas deferens and guinea pig ileum bioassays, coupled with displacement studies of receptor binding, led to the initial proposal for two distinct opioid receptors (81). Met^5-enkephalin and leu^5-enkephalin were far more potent in the mouse vas deferens, whereas morphine was more effective in the guinea pig ileum. In addition, 16-fold greater doses of naloxone were required to antagonize enkephalin than to reverse normorphine in the mouse vas deferens assay.

Binding studies in brain homogenates revealed dramatic selectivity in the binding of ^{3}H-naloxone and ^{3}H-leu[5]-enkephalin; morphine inhibited ^{3}H-naloxone binding far better than enkephalins, whereas ^{3}H-enkephalin binding was more sensitive to displacement by enkephalins than morphine. These results were soon reproduced (12,141). Modifying the enkephalin structure could also alter the selectivity of a peptide for the mouse vas deferens and guinea pig ileum bioassays. These results provided very strong evidence to support the proposal for mu (morphine-preferring) receptors located in the guinea pig ileum and delta (enkephalin-preferring) receptors in the mouse vas deferens. Extensive structure-activity analysis of mu/delta receptors (35,71) utilizing these two bioassays has associated mu specificity with shorter enkephalin sequences and removal of the terminal carboxy group, replacement of the aromatic Phe[4] residue with a lipophilic alkyl-chain; and the introduction of a hydrophobic D-amino acid as the second residue. Delta receptor activity was enhanced by lengthening the sequence; maintaining an aromatic moiety in the fourth position; promoting the fit of the Phe[4] side-chain into a subsite apparently specific for delta sites, and placing a hydrophilic side-chain in position 2. The most selective delta agonist, ^{3}H-Tyr-D-Ser-Gly-Phe-Leu-Thr, presumably labeled only delta receptors at concentrations up to 20 nM. In general, the mu receptor prefers compact hydrophobic compounds and the delta receptor larger hydrophilic ones.

The separation of mu and delta agonist activities also was reported by Schulz et al. (134,135). They produced differential tolerance in the mouse vas deferens preparation to mu and delta drugs. Tolerance to the mu agonist sufentanyl (800-fold) did not alter the response to the delta agonist D-Ala[2]-D-Leu[5]-enkephalin (DADL), and, conversely, tolerance to DADL (1,000-fold) did not alter sensitivity to sufentanyl. Thus, in the mouse vas deferens, the pharmacological activity of mu and delta agonists seemed to be mediated via distinct receptor mechanisms.

Binding studies presented the first evidence that mu and delta opiate receptors are physically distinct within the CNS (11,12). Two radiolabeled enkephalins with differing pharmacological properties were used: ^{125}I-D-Ala[2]-D-Leu[5]-enkephalin (^{125}I-DADL), which was felt to be selective for delta sites, and the ^{125}I-labeled Sandoz analogue (FK33, 824) which preferentially labeled mu sites (Table 4). The results were quite similar to those described earlier (91) and suggested pharmacologically distinct binding sites. Similar studies also demonstrated that morphine's displacement of ^{125}I-DADL was biphasic. Morphine displaced about 30% of ^{125}I-DADL binding with an IC_{50} value of 0.3 nM whereas the remainder of the binding had an IC_{50} value of about 45 nM. These results implied that ^{125}I-DADL bound to a site to which morphine had high affinity and another site to which morphine bound poorly. These biphasic displacements were soon to become important in our understanding of opioid binding sites (see next section). Chang et al. (15) later described the actions of guanyl nucleotides and cations on mu and delta receptors. GTP depressed the affinity of mu agonists far more than delta agonists, whereas sodium ions lowered the binding of both classes equally.

Differential protection experiments also suggested two separate binding sites (131). Dihydromorphine protected ^{3}H-dihydromorphine binding (mu sites) from

TABLE 4. *Inhibition of ^{125}I-opioid binding*

Compound	IC$_{50}$ (nM)	
	^{125}I-DADL (delta)	^{125}I-FK33, 824 (mu)
Morphine	35 ± 5	0.4 ± 0.2
Oxymorphone	21 ± 6	0.3 ± 0.1
Nalorphine	8.0 ± 1.2	0.3 ± 0.1
Butorphanol	1.7 ± 0.3	0.4 ± 0.2
Oxilorphan	1.0 ± 0.1	0.3 ± 0.1
Pentazocine	67 ± 20	9.3 ± 0.7
Cyclazocine	1.2 ± 0.3	0.3 ± 0.1
Naloxone	15 ± 8	1.1 ± 0.2
FK33, 824	14 ± 5	1.2 ± 0.4
D-Ala^2-Met^5-enkephalin	2.1 ± 0.2	5.3 ± 1.3
D-Ala^2-Leu^5-enkephalin	1.5 ± 0.1	4 ± 0.2
Met^5-enkephalin	4.4 ± 0.9	8 ± 2
Leu^5-enkephalin	3.0 ± 0.3	20 ± 5
DADL	1.6 ± 0.2	4 ± 0.2

From Chang et al. (11).

phenoxybenzamine six times more potently than DADL, whereas DADL protected ^{3}H-DADL binding 20 times more potently than dihydromorphine.

One of the strongest pieces of evidence implying distinct sites was the localization of mu and delta receptors to different brain regions as demonstrated with ^{125}I-DADL (enkephalin-selective) and ^{125}I-FK33, 824 (morphine-selective) binding. Approximately equal numbers of each receptor type were found in frontal cortex, striatum, and sensomotor cortex. However, the amount of ^{125}I-FK33, 824 binding in the hippocampus, brainstem, thalamus, and hypothalamus was from twofold to fivefold higher than ^{125}I-DADL. Goodman et al. (46), using *in vitro* autoradiography techniques (166), found similar differences. Mu receptors were specifically labeled with ^{125}I-FK33, 824, whereas delta sites were labeled with ^{125}I-DADL, both in the presence and absence of FK33, 824 (1 nM) to eliminate any mu binding of ^{125}I-DADL. Significant differences between the localization of mu and delta sites were found, particularly in the rostral CNS. Adjacent sections (Fig. 2A) showed high concentrations of delta sites only in layers II, III, and IV of the frontal cortex and diffusely in the corpus striatum (especially ventrolaterally), with low concentrations in layers I and IV of the cortex, the hippocampus, thalamus, and hypothalamus. In contrast, high concentrations of mu sites occurred in a number of regions: layers I and IV of the frontal cortex, the subcallosal streak, clusters in the corpus striatum, the pyramidal cell layer of the hippocampus and especially in the thalamus and hypothalamus (Fig. 2B). Other areas containing predominantly mu sites were the periaqueductal gray, interpeduncular nucleus, inferior colliculus, and midbrain median raphe, whereas regions with high delta densities included the amygdala, nucleus accumbens, olfactory tubercle, and pontine nuclei. A number of areas contained significant concentrations of both mu and delta sites: layer VI of the frontal cortex, the nucleus tractus solitarius, vagal fibers, the nucleus ambiguus, and the substantia gelatinosa of the spinal cord and trigeminal tract. These localizations have been independently confirmed (28). Knowledge of these different localizations may allow the differentiation of mu and delta actions through experiments using regional administration of different types of opiates.

HIGH AND LOW AFFINITY OPIATE BINDING: MU_1, MU_2, AND DELTA SITES

The previous section clearly illustrates many of the differences between opiate and enkephalin actions and binding sites. However, they do not explain similarities, such as the cross-tolerance between both morphine and enkephalin analgesia (5,70). These pharmacological results suggested the existence of a common site binding for both classes of compounds. Early ^{3}H-opiate binding experiments revealed a type of opiate receptor duality quite distinct from the mu and delta subtypes discussed above. Using ^{3}H-naloxone and ^{3}H-dihydromorphine of high specific activities, Pasternak and Snyder (112) labeled a novel opiate binding site in rat brain whose affinity ($K_D < 1nM$) for the ^{3}H-ligand was over 10-fold greater than that previously reported. Initially demonstrated by curvilinear Scatchard plots resolvable into two components, the existence of this site has now been supported by many additional experimental approaches. Biochemically, this high affinity site appears to be distinct, based on its greater sensitivity to inhibition by sodium ions, reagents, and some proteolytic enzymes, from the other subtypes of sites (94,110,111).

In addition, its regional localization within the brain (164), developmental appearance (114,169), and distribution across species (8) further differentiated the high affinity component from the other, lower affinity binding sites.

The development of selective antagonists for these high affinity sites further established their existence, as well as helping understand their *in vivo* pharmacological actions, as described later in this chapter. Two of these compounds, naloxazone and naloxonazine (Fig. 3), have been extensively studied (39,49,96,101–106,108, 167,168,169). Both drugs effectively and irreversibly inhibited the high affinity binding component of a variety of radiolabeled opiates and enkephalin derivatives, suggesting that they all bound with highest affinity to a common site. This concept of a common site has also been supported by extensive displacement studies.

Although a common site for enkephalins and opiates did explain the analgesic cross-tolerance between them, the question of the selective sites for morphine and the enkephalins, as presented in the previous section, was not resolved (11,12,17,81). The above studies focused upon the high affinity binding component. Could the lower affinity ($K_D < 15$ nM) binding correspond to these selective sites? This possibility was examined by performing displacements (similar to those studied by Chang and Cuatrecasas (12)) in tissue whose high affinity sites had been eliminated. Displacements of ^{3}H-dihydromorphine (mu) and ^{3}H-D-Ala^2-D-Leu^5-enkephalin (delta) binding performed with tissue, whose high affinity binding had been previously blocked by naloxazone, demonstrated that mu drugs, such as morphine, were up to eightfold more potent on ^{3}H-dihydromorphine, whereas enkephalins, such as D-

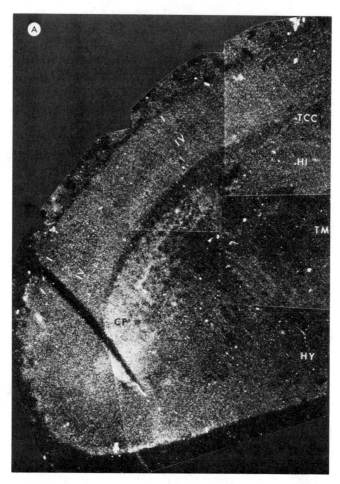

FIG. 2. Distribution of delta and mu opiate receptors as shown by dark field micrographs of adjacent coronal sections of cerebral cortex. Bar = 1,000 μm. **A,** Selective labeling of delta receptors by 0.2 nM of ^{125}I-DADL in the presence of 1 nM of FK33, 824. **B,** Mu receptors labeled by 0.2 nM of ^{125}I FK33, 824. Note the high mu receptor **(B)** densities (seen as white) in laminae I and IV of the cerebral cortex and in the subcallosal streak and clusters in the caudate-putamen (CP).

Ala^2-D-Leu^5-enkephalin were up to 6-fold more effective against ^{3}H-D-ala^2-D-leu^5-enkephalin. These results implied that the morphine-selective and enkephalin-selective sites corresponded to the lower affinity binding component, and led to a new classification of morphine and enkephalin binding sites (Table 5). Both opiates and enkephalins apparently bound with highest affinity ($K_D < 1$ nM) to a common site which is naloxazone and naloxonazine sensitive, termed the mu$_1$ (high affinity) site, whereas the low affinity ^{3}H-dihydromorphine site (mu$_2$) preferentially bound morphine-like drugs, and the low affinity ^{3}H-D-Ala^2-D-Leu^5-enkephalin site (delta) selectively bound enkephalins. The kappa opiate ethylketocyclazocine and the sigma

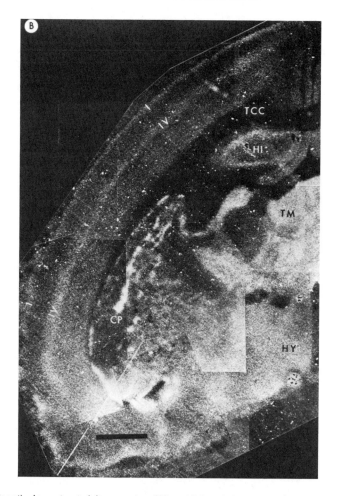

FIG. 2. *(cont)* In contrast, delta receptors **(A)** are highest in laminae II, III and V of the cerebral cortex and more diffusely, particularly ventrolaterally, in the caudate-putamen. Labeling of mu receptors in the pyramidal cell layer of the hippocampus (HI) can be seen **(B)**, but little labeling of delta receptors in the hippocampus is seen **(A)**. (Note that the overall intensity of the labeling in the CP is similar in **A** and **B**.) Comparison of the intensity of labeling in the hypothalamus (HV) and the dorsomedial (TM) and ventral thalamus with that in the CP shows that these areas are greatly enriched in mu receptors.

drug SKF 10,047 also bound with highest affinity to the mu_1 site. However, their lower affinity binding ($K_D < 15$ nM) has unique pharmacological properties and may correspond to kappa and sigma sites (160), as discussed in detail later in this chapter.

Many other irreversible opiates have proven quite useful in opiate receptor research. Chlornaltrexamine (CNA), a potent opioid receptor alkylating agent, is a long-lasting narcotic antagonist which probably works through alkylation of

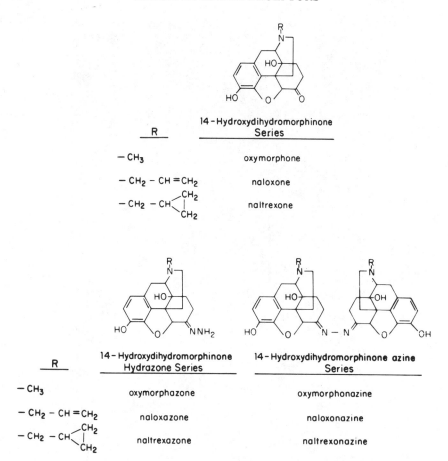

FIG. 3. Structures of some 14 hydroxydihydromorphinone derivatives.

receptors (128,129). The nonequilibrium antagonism of morphine's actions by CNA also supported an irreversible mechanism of action. A similar derivative of oxymorphone, chloroxymorphamine (COA), was a potent irreversible narcotic agonist in the guinea pig ileum assay (10). The actions of CNA and COA did not seem to be selective for a subtype of opiate receptors (9). Both drugs inactivated the delta receptors in NG108-5 neuroblastoma cells (31). Recently, the fumarate methyl ester derivatives of naltrexone (FNA) and oxymorphone (FOA) were found to be reversible agonists in the guinea pig ileum assay (130,148). It was interesting that FNA acted as an irreversible morphine antagonist, whereas FOA did not. In contrast to CNA, FNAs antagonism was very selective in that it antagonized pure mu agonists (e.g., morphine), but had little or no effect on the putative kappa agonists (nalorphine, pentazocine, and ethylketocyclazocine). These results further support the existence of opiate receptor heterogeneity.

TABLE 5. *Classification of morphine and enkephalin sites in the CNS*

	Approximate K_D Values (nM)		
	Mu_1	Mu_2	Delta
Morphine			
Saturation studies	0.4	11	–
Displacement studies	<1	8	71
D-Ala^2-D-Leu^5-enkephalin			
Saturation studies	0.5	–	5
Displacement studies	<1	50	8

From Wolozin and Pasternak (161).

RECEPTOR MECHANISMS IN OPIOID ANALGESIA

The demonstration of cross-tolerance between the analgesic actions of enkephalins and morphine (5) implied a common analgesic receptor in contrast to the selective sites present in the guinea pig ileum and mouse vas deferens (81). Recent work has indicated that the analgesic actions of enkephalins, β-endorphin, and morphine are mediated in large part through the mu_1 sites to which both the enkephalins and morphine bind with the highest affinity (53,78,101–106,114,169). The selective *in vivo* blockade of mu_1 sites in adult rats and mice with either naloxazone or naloxonazine markedly inhibited the analgesic properties of a series of opiates and opioid peptides (Table 6). As the mu_1 sites returned to normal levels over a period of three days, morphine's analgesic potency also increased to control levels. Similar correlations between mu_1 sites and analgesia were seen in developmental studies (Table 7; 114,169). Mu_1 sites have a later appearance in the rat brain than either mu_2 or delta. At 2 days of age, when the levels of mu_1 binding were only 22% of the adult levels, morphine's ED_{50} was 56 mg/kg. By 14 days of age, the density of mu_1 sites had increased nearly threefold with a corresponding increase in morphine's analgesic potency (ED_{50}, 1.4 mg/kg). Thus, two separate experimental models have suggested a role of mu_1 sites in opiate and opioid analgesia.

Earlier, the concept of receptor dualism was presented (60,85). On the basis of interactions between morphine and its corresponding mixed agonist-antagonist, nalorphine, Martin concluded that two classes of receptors were involved in opioid analgesia. Although the results described above implicated a role of mu_1 sites, other studies have confirmed the concept of multiple analgesic receptors. Although the blockade of mu_1 sites did shift the dose-response curves of the various drugs for analgesia to the right, sufficient doses of the drug were still analgesic. One possibility was that the agents were working through residual mu_1 sites. However, if this were true, a similar shift for all the drugs would be expected. This was not the case (Table 6). Compounds with high affinity for delta sites, such as D-Ala^2-D-Leu^5-enkephalin, were shifted far less than drugs with a poor affinity for delta sites, such as morphine. These results suggested that delta sites could mediate

TABLE 6. *Effect of mu$_1$ site blockade on opiate and opioid peptide analgesia; opioid actions in naloxone and naloxozone-treated mice*

Opioid	Control group	Naloxazone group	Shift
Morphine (SC)[a]			
Analgesic ED$_{50}$ (writhing)	0.21 ± 0.03 mg/kg	2.7 ± 0.1 mg/kg	12.8
Analgesic ED$_{50}$ (tail flick)	6.1 ± 0.1 mg/kg	70.3 ± 4.0 mg/kg	11.5
Ketocyclazocine (SC)[a]			
Analgesic ED$_{50}$ (writhing)	0.08 ± 0.005 mg/kg	0.47 ± 0.002 mg/kg	5.9
Analgesic ED$_{50}$ (tail flick)	7.4 ± 0.4 mg/kg	55 ± 0.4 mg/kg	7.4
SKF 10,047 (N-allylnormetazocine)			
Analgesic ED$_{50}$ (writhing)	0.62 ± 0.09 mg/kg	2.8 ± 1.1 mg/kg	4.5
D-ala^2-D-leu^5-enkephalin (icv)[b]			
Analgesic ED$_{50}$ (tail flick)	1.1 μg	3.9 μg	3.5
β$_h$-endorphin (1 μg, icv)[b]			
% analgesic at 30 min (tail flick)	100% (N = 6)	0% (N = 6)	

Mice were given either naloxone (control) or naloxazone (both at 200 mg/kg) and tested with the above drugs 20–24 hr later (78,101,106). Twenty-four hr after, naloxone mice were as sensitive as untreated mice.
[a]SC = subcutaneous.
[b]icv = intracerebroventricular.

TABLE 7. *Developmental aspects of morphine pharmacology*

	2-Day old rats	14-Day old rats
Binding site density of ^{3}H-Morphine		
(% adult)		
High affinity (mu$_1$)	22 ± 7%	61 ± 5%
Low affinity (mu$_2$)	72 ± 16%	88 ± 4%
Analgesia		
Morphine sulfate ED$_{50}$	56 mg/kg	1.4 mg/kg
Respiratory rate depression		
Morphine sulfate ID$_{50}$	2.5 mg/kg	9.3 mg/kg
Ratio (analgesia/respiratory depression)	22.4	0.15

From Zhang and Pasternak (169).

analgesia, though at higher drug doses than those activating the mu$_1$ sites. These conclusions confirmed earlier studies with a unique enkephalin derivative, Met-kephamid, suggesting a role for delta receptors in analgesia (37).

Additional studies also investigated the role of spinal transection on opioid analgesia (78). In brief, spinal transection in the mouse had virtually the same effect as the mu$_1$ blockade. Therefore it was concluded that mu$_1$ analgesia was mediated supraspinally whereas spinal mechanisms involved delta sites. These studies, however, were performed in mice. Evidence is mounting that significant species differences may exist. Thus, extrapolation to other species, including man, is difficult. Many investigators, working with other types of animals have suggested that other classes of receptors, particularly kappa (162), might also be involved with analgesia. Further work will be needed to completely understand these analgesic systems.

RECEPTOR MECHANISMS IN OTHER OPIOID ACTIONS

Many other opioid actions have been studied, particularly with the involvement of mu_1 sites. As noted previously, the guinea pig ileum is the prototypic mu bioassay. With the subsequent suggestion of multiple classes of mu receptors, it was necessary to determine whether it was mu_1 or mu_2. It was expected that mu_2 sites were involved, because morphine was more effective than the enkephalins. In a series of experiments, Gintzler and Pasternak *(in preparation)* found that naloxonazine had no irreversible actions in the ileum either in the bioassay or binding studies, implying that mu_1 sites were not involved. *In vivo* mu_1 blockade has also been used to examine the effects of morphine on prolactin and growth hormone release (146), catalepsy (103), opioid actions on acetylcholine and dopamine turnover (163), sedation (101), and respiratory depression (79,169). The classification of these actions is given in Table 8.

Of these actions, respiratory depression is the most important. In the developmental studies, respiratory depression, as measured by respiratory rate, appeared to be dissociated from analgesia (168). While morphine was 40-fold less potent as an analgesic in 2-day old than in 14-day old rats, it depressed respiratory rates equally well in both age groups (Table 7). Similar conclusions were obtained from studies examining the effects of *in vivo* blockade of mu_1 sites on analgesia and respiratory depression, measured by blood gases (Table 9; 79). Although blockade of mu_1 sites *in vivo* by naloxonazine eliminated any analgesic response by morphine (3.5 mg/kg i.v.), respiratory depression was unaffected. Thus, the receptors mediating respiratory depression do not appear to be mu_1. The receptors actually involved with respiratory depression remain unknown. Developmental studies (169) found a similar potency of morphine and enkephalins in depressing respiratory rates. Similarly, Ward and Holaday (155) have recently reported that both mu and

TABLE 8. *Association of opioid actions with mu_1 sites*

Mu₁ mediated	Not mu₁ mediated
Supraspinal analgesia (low drug doses)	Analgesia (higher drug doses, delta in
Prolactin release	mouse; may vary between species)
Catalepsy	Growth hormone release
Modulation of acetylcholine turnover in	Lethality
hippocampus and parietal cortex	Respiratory depression (mu₂ and/or delta)
Morphine-induced hypothermia	Sedation
	Inhibition of gastrointestinal motility (mu)
	Modulation of dopamine turnover in
	striatum (mu₂ and/or delta)
	Reversal of endotoxic shock (delta)
	Morphine-induced bradycardia (mu₂)

TABLE 9. *Effects of mu₁ blockade on morphine analgesia and respiratory depression*

	Base line	After morphine	Change	
Control				
Tail flick latencies	3.0 ± 0.2 sec	9.2 ± 0.8 sec	+207%	$p < 0.001$
Arterial blood				
pH	7.46 ± 0.02	7.38 ± 0.02	−0.08	$p < 0.02$
pO₂	89.2 ± 1.5 mm Hg	72.7 ± 4.3 mm Hg	−16.5 mm Hg	$p < 0.01$
pCO₂	37.2 ± 1.2 mm Hg	48.9 ± 3.5 mm Hg	+11.7 mm Hg	$p < 0.01$
Naloxonazine treated (mu₁ blockade)				
Tail flick latencies	3.0 ± 0.1 sec	3.4 ± 0.4 sec	+13%	ns
Arterial blood				
pH	7.46 ± 0.01	7.42 ± 0.03	−0.04	ns
pO₂	87.1 ± 0.7 mm Hg	64.3 ± 4.8 mm Hg	−22.8 mm Hg	$p < 0.002$
pCO₂	37.3 ± 1.3 mm Hg	46.9 ± 2.6 mm Hg	+9.6 mm Hg	$p < 0.01$

delta antagonists can reverse respiratory depression in rats. Thus, mu_2 and/or delta sites may mediate this action.

KAPPA RECEPTORS

Soon after Martin presented his evidence for kappa opiates, further evidence for a putative kappa receptor was demonstrated in other bioassay systems (63,81). Those studies found that several putative kappa agonists were relatively more potent in the guinea pig ileum than in the mouse vas deferens assay, as compared to a variety of other opiate agonists. Furthermore, the benzomorphan (kappa) agonists were relatively resistant to naloxone antagonism, suggesting that the guinea pig ileum contained significant numbers of receptors, which were more sensitive to the benzomorphans (kappa) than morphine, possibly a result of a kappa receptor. Schulz et al. (135) demonstrated selective tolerance between mu and kappa agonists in the guinea pig ileum (GPI). The development of approximately 80-fold tolerance to mu agonists (normorphine, fentamyl, and FK33, 824) caused little or no tolerance to kappa agonists [ethylketocyclazocine, MR 2034 and (5,9-dimethyl,2'5)-5,-9-dimethyl-2'-hydroxy-2(methoxy-propyl)-6,7-benzomorphan] and vice versa. These results provided strong evidence for pharmacologically distinct kappa sites in the peripheral bioassay systems.

A specific bioassay for kappa-receptor agonists has been reported (97) using the depression of electrically-evoked contractions of the rabbit vas deferens. Only putative kappa agonists were active, including bremazocine, ethylketazocine, ketocyclazocine, and cyclazocine (in order of decreasing potency). Although reversible by naloxone, high doses of the antagonist were required. Compounds inactive at concentrations up to 0.1 mM included the mu agonists (morphine and FK33, 824), a sigma agonist (SKF 10,047), delta agonists (Met⁵-enkephalin, Leu⁵-enkephalin,

D-Ala[2]Met[5]-enkephalin, and D-ala[2]-D-leu[5]-enkephalin) and β-endorphin. Bremazo-cine, a kappa benzomorphan derivative (132), is a potent centrally-acting analgesic in the mouse and monkey, which was relatively resistant to naloxone antagonism, did not cause respiratory depression or Straub tail, and was not self-administered by monkeys. Bremazocine-tolerant rats were not cross-tolerant to morphine, but morphine-tolerant animals were tolerant to bremazocine, and the withdrawal syndrome in bremazocine-dependent monkeys precipitated by naloxone was milder and more kappa-like than that seen in morphine-dependent monkeys. The rabbit vas deferens appears to possess only kappa sites and may prove a useful screening test.

Another *in vivo* pharmacological assay suggestive of multiple opiate receptors is discriminative stimulus testing. A recent review by Herling and Woods (54) summarized the discriminative stimulus evidence in rat, squirrel monkey, rhesus monkey, and pigeon which supports the concept of opiate receptor heterogeneity. Rats trained to discriminate the mu agonists morphine (3,40,55,58) and fentanyl (22,98) give drug appropriate responses to many putative mu agonist and analgesics, including methadone, meperidine, heroin, codeine, oxymorphone, levorphanol, profadol, etonitazene, phenazacine, propoxyphene, and butorphanol (40,57,98,133–139,159). Many of these compounds also produce morphine-like subjective effects in man (65). A number of mixed agonist-antagonist analgesics (ketazocine, nalorphine, cyclazocine, nalbuphine, oxilorphan and SKF 10,047), most of which have been characterized as kappa and/or sigma agonists, failed to produce morphine-appropriate responses (57,98,99,138,139). These findings were supported by similar studies in rhesus monkeys trained to recognize codeine and etorphine (54). Appropriate responses were generated by many mu agonists, but not cyclazocine, pentazocine, ethylketocyclazocine, and SKF 10,047.

Demonstrating kappa sites through binding studies in the brain proved more difficult owing to the ability of kappa drugs to bind to a number of receptor classes. A number of studies noted only similarities between the kappa agonist ethylketo-cyclazocine and mu-like ligands (13,17,56,123). Other studies (14,72,101,125,145,160) clearly demonstrated that ^{3}H-ethylketocyclazocine bound to more than one site, based on both Scatchard and displacement experiments. The high affinity ^{3}H-ethylketocyclazocine binding site ($K_D < 1$ nM) corresponded to the mu_1 site described previously (101,161), whereas the lower affinity included a kappa site (160). The selective ability of kappa drugs to protect ^{3}H-ethylketocyclazocine binding from phenoxybenzamine alkylation (73) also provided strong evidence for a selective kappa site. A major problem with ^{3}H-ethylketocyclazocine binding was the strong mu-like character of the drug (56,72,101). In fact, unlabeled ethylketocyclazocine displaced mu_2 (^{3}H-dihydromorphine) and delta (^{3}H-D-ala[2]-D-leu[5]-enkephalin) sites as potently as it displaced ^{3}H-ethylketocyclazocine binding (Table 10; 160). However, the poor ability of unlabeled morphine and D-Ala[2]-D-Leu[5]-enkephalin to inhibit ^{3}H-ethylketocyclazocine binding indicated that ^{3}H-ethylketo-cyclazocine did, indeed, bind to an additional site other than mu_2 or delta.

The use of multiphasic displacements as evidence for a kappa site was strengthened significantly through the use of computer analysis (125). In elegant studies, a unique site (R_3) was described which appeared specific for benzomorphans. In addition, dynorphin, a novel, extremely potent opioid peptide discovered by Goldstein and co-workers (43), was proposed as the ligand for this site.

The strongest evidence for kappa receptors was provided by two independent investigations that utilized *in vitro* autoradiography to demonstrate a unique localization of kappa receptors in guinea pig brain. This species was chosen because binding studies in rats found kappa sites to represent only about 10% of all opiate receptor binding, whereas they were about 40% in guinea pigs (73). One study examined the binding of a new kappa type agonist ^{3}H-bremazocine (34), while the other used ^{3}H-ethylketazocine (44,45). Both studies found a uniquely high concentration of kappa sites in laminae V and VI of the cerebral cortex. Interestingly, this localization may relate to the unique sedative effects associated with kappa type agonists.

Further compelling evidence for a separate kappa site is a recent study that reported distinct high-affinity binding sites for ^{3}H-ethylketocyclazocine in a neuroblastoma-brain hybrid cell line (94). This cell line (NCB-20) contained two distinct binding sites for ^{3}H-ethylketocyclazocine, one corresponding to the delta site previously described in similar hybrid cell lines (NG108-15; 11) and another one with unique pharmacological properties. The lack of both mu_1 and mu_2 sites in these cells makes the interpretation of the data far more simple. Naloxone bound poorly to this binding site as did etorphine (both $IC_{50} > 100$ nM). Therefore, some discrepancies between this site and those described in the brain remain. The unique binding may represent a pharmacologically relevant opiate receptor, but further correlation to pharmacological opiate actions will be necessary.

THE SIGMA OPIATE RECEPTOR

Martin's studies with SKF 10,047 suggested a unique opiate receptor which he classified as sigma (88). Although an early study with ^{3}H-SKF 10,047 suggested that a portion of its binding was distinct from the mu sites (145), no clear demonstration of a distinct sigma site was demonstrated. Most other studies were unable to distinguish a sigma site distinct from the kappa site (15,125). However, like most other ^{3}H-opioids, ^{3}H-SKF 10,047 bound to more than one site (104).

Although ^{3}H-SKF 10,047 bound with the highest affinity to the mu_1 site, the lower affinity binding component (K_D 6 nM) possessed unique pharmacological properties (104,160). ^{3}H-SKF 10,047 binding was potently inhibited by both unlabeled SKF 10,047 and ethylketocyclazocine (Table 10), but not morphine or enkephalin. The similar potency of unlabeled SKF 10,047 and ethylketocyclazocine raised the possibility of a common benzomorphan site. However, ketocyclazocine, another kappa drug, clearly differentiated between the two. Ketocyclazocine displaced ^{3}H-ethylketocyclazocine binding fivefold more potently than ^{3}H-SKF 10,047 binding. Also the regional binding of ^{3}H-SKF was different from that of ^{3}H-

TABLE 10. *Inhibition of opiate receptor binding in naloxazone treated tissue*

Drug	IC$_{50}$ (nM)				
	[^{3}H]dihydromorphine	[^{3}H]ethylketocyclazocine	[^{3}H]SKF 10,047	[^{3}H]D-Ala^2-D-Leu^5-enkephalin	
Morphine	13.1 ± 2.8	82 ± 39	143 ± 39	276 ± 92	ns
Ketocyclazocine	130 ± 36	37.6 ± 3.7	193 ± 41	155 ± 40	$F_{3,8}$ = 4.16 $p < 0.01$
Ethylketocyclazocine	12.3 ± 3.6	11.9 ± 3.6	25.5 ± 8.7	18.3 ± 0.9	$F_{3,8}$ = 9.75 ns
N-Allylnormetazocine (SKF 10,047)	38.8 ± 13	20.2 ± 7.2	24.5 ± 12	51.8 ± 24	$F_{3,8}$ = 1.63 ns
Cyclazocine	6.4 ± 1.0	3.7 ± 0.9	4.5 ± 2.0	5.8 ± 0.6	$F_{3,12}$ = 0.88 ns
Pentazocine	101 ± 26	89.8 ± 27.1	119 ± 19	178 ± 37	$F_{3,8}$ = 0.98 ns
Nalorphine	7.4 ± 0.6	15.0 ± 1.3	16.0 ± 1.0	61.2 ± 5.6	$F_{3,8}$ = 1.96 $p < 0.001$
D-Ala^2-D-leu^5-enkephalin	323 ± 91	448 ± 43	371 ± 65	20.4 ± 2.6	$F_{3,8}$ = 70.6 $p < 0.01$

Tissue was treated with naloxazone to eliminate the mu$_1$ (high affinity binding), and extensively washed. Binding was measured with the stated ^{3}H-ligands (2 nM) and IC$_{50}$ values determined.
From Wolozin et al. (160).

ethylketocyclazocine (160). The recent binding studies by McLawhon et al. (94), in the neuroblastoma-brain hybrid cell line NCB-20, also found evidence for a unique ^{3}H-SKF 10,047 (sigma) receptor. However, the lack of specificity of SKF 10,047 binding, evidenced by its high affinity to mu_1, mu_2, delta, and potential kappa sites, makes the interpretation of binding experiments difficult.

Numerous studies have suggested an association between the actions of phencyclidine (PCP) and SKF 10,047. Despite technical difficulties (83), binding studies with ^{3}H-phencyclidine (^{3}H-PCP) identified a specific receptor in the rat brain (K_D 200 nM) whose binding of a series of PCP analogs correlated well with their pharmacological activities, and with a subcellular and regional localization consistent with that expected for the PCP receptor (153,154,171). The relationship of the PCP receptors to a sigma opiate receptor was suggested by the ability of SKF 10,047 to displace ^{3}H-PCP binding and subsequently supported by discriminative stimulus testing in the rat (59,149). The first study found that animals trained to recognize cyclazocine recently identified ketocyclazocine and SKF 10,047 far better than ethylketocyclazocine, pentazocine, and levallorphan (149). Ketamine (a PCP-analog) and PCP mimicked the discriminative effects of cyclazocine, whereas mescaline, d-amphetamine, and LSD did not. In addition, the dose-response curve of cyclazocine could be shifted to the right by naltrexone, but not completely blocked. In subsequent studies, rats trained to identify ketamine generalized to cyclazocine, SKF 10,047 and dextrorphan, but not ethylketocyclazocine, ketocyclazocine, pentazocine, or dextromethorphan (59). ^{3}H-Cyclazocine labeled a site with many of the characteristics expected from these PCP studies, although with far lower affinity than to any of the opioid sites described earlier (170), including the potential sigma receptor (104,160). Based on these findings, it has been suggested that the PCP site may be a sigma receptor (171). If this is true, it could reflect a different site from that described above (160). The SKF 10,047 binding site, which may correspond to the PCP site, has more than a 10-fold lower affinity for SKF 10,047 (K_D70 nM) than the other SKF 10,047 selective site described by Wolozin et al. (K_D6 nM) (160). In addition, it shows poor stereoselectivity and is displaced by a PCP derivative. The site described by Wolozin et al. shows strict stereoselectivity and is not displaced by a PCP derivative. Thus, the exact relationship of the PCP site and opioid sites remains uncertain and several sites selective for SKF 10,047 may exist.

CONCLUSION

The pharmacological and biochemical evidence for the multiplicity of opiate receptors is now quite convincing. Correlating the biochemically defined subtypes of site with the vast variety of opioid-mediated actions is still at an early stage. Strong evidence exists that all opiates (mu, kappa, and sigma) and enkephalins bind with the highest affinity to a common site, which mediates their supraspinal analgesic actions (101–106,114). There also appears to be a series of sites which bind selectively morphine-like (mu_2), enkephalin (delta), ketocyclazocine-like (kappa), and SKF 10,047-like (sigma) drugs. A major difficulty for the study of multiple opiate receptors has been the lack of drugs with strong specificity for specific receptor subtypes, particularly the kappa and sigma types. Knowledge of the actions of these receptors is important. As we gain understanding and we can assign specific actions to selected binding sites, we may be able to develop more selective drugs lacking many of the side effects of those currently used.

REFERENCES

1. Archer, S., Albertson, N. F., Harris, L. S., Pierson, A. K., Bird, J. G., Keats, A. S., Telford, J., and Papadopoulos, C. N. (1962): Narcotic antagonists as analgesics. *Science*, 137:541–543.
2. Beckett, A. H., and Casy, A. F. (1965): Analgesics and their antagonists: Biochemical aspects and structure-activity relationships. In: *Progress in Medicinal Chemistry, Vol. 4*, edited by G. P. Ellis and G. B. West, pp. 171–218. Butterworth Ltd., London.
3. Belleville, R. E. (1964): Control of behavior by drug-produced internal stimuli. *Psychopharmacologia*, 5:95–105.
4. Bianchi, C., and Francheschini, J. (1954): Experimental observations on Haffner's method for testing analgetic drugs. *Br. J. Pharmacol. Chemother.*, 9:280–284.
5. Blassig, J. F., and Herz, A. (1976): Tolerance and dependence induced by morphine-like peptides in rats. *Naunyn-Schmiedebergs Arch. Pharmacol.*, 294:297–300.
6. Blumberg, H., Dayton, H. B., George, M., and Rapaport, D. N. (1961): N-allylnoroxymorphone: A potent narcotic antagonist. *Fed. Proc.*, 20:311.
7. Blumberg, H., Dayton, H. B., and Wolf, P. S. (1966): Counteraction of narcotic antagonist analgesics by the narcotic antagonist naloxone. *Proc. Soc. Exp. Biol.*, 123:755–758.
8. Buatti, M. C., and Pasternak, G. W. (1981): Multiple opiate receptors: Phylogenetic differences. *Brain Res.*, 281:400–405.
9. Caruso, T. P., Larson, D. L., Portoghese, P. S., and Takemori, A. E. (1980): Pharmacological studies with an alkylating narcotic agonist, chloroxymorphamine and antagonist, chlornaltrexamine. *J. Pharmacol. Exp. Ther.*, 213:539–544.
10. Caruso, T. P., Takemori, A. E., Larson, D. L., and Portoghese, P. S. (1979): Chloroxymorphamine, an opioid receptor site directed alkylating agent having narcotic agonist activity. *Science*, 204:316–318.
11. Chang, K.-J., Cooper, B. R., Hazum, E., and Cuatrecasas, P. (1979): Multiple opiate receptors: different regional distribution in the brain and differential binding of opiates and opioid peptides. *Mol. Pharmacol.*, 16:91–104.
12. Chang, K.-J., and Cuatrecasas, P. (1979): Multiple opiate receptors: enkephalins and morphine bind to receptors of different specificity. *J. Biol. Chem.*, 254:2610–2618.
13. Chang, K.-J., Hazum, E., and Cuatrecasas, P. (1980): Possible role of distinct morphine and enkephalin receptors in mediating actions of benzomorphan drugs (putative kappa and sigma agonists). *Proc. Natl. Acad. Sci. U.S.A.*, 77:4469–4473.
14. Chang, K.-J., Hazum, E., and Cuatrecasas, P. (1981): Novel opiate binding sites selective for benzomorphan drugs. *Proc. Natl. Acad. Sci. U.S.A.*, 78:4141–4145.
15. Chang, K.-J., Hazum, E., Killian, A., and Cuatrecasas, P. (1981): Interactions of ligands with morphine and enkephalin receptors are differentially affected by guanine nucleotide. *Mol. Pharmacol.*, 20:1–7.
16. Childers, S. R., and Snyder, S. H. (1980): Differential regulation by guanine nucleotides of opiate agonist and antagonist receptor interactions. *J. Neurochem.*, 34:583–593.
17. Childers, S. R., Creese, I., Snowman, A. M., and Snyder, S. H. (1979): Opiate receptor binding affected differentially by opiates and opioid peptides. *Eur. J. Pharmacol.*, 55:11–18.
18. Cho, T. M., Cho, J. S., and Loh, H. H. (1979): Physicochemical basis of opiate-cerebroside sulfate interaction and its application to receptor theory. *Mol. Pharmacol.*, 16:393–405.
19. Cho, T. M., Law, P. Y., and Loh, H. A. (1979): A proposed mode of action for narcotic agonists and antagonists. In: *Advances in Biochemistry Psychopharmacology, Vol. 20: Neurochemical Mechanisms of Opiates and Endorphins*, edited by H. H. Loh and D. H. Ross, pp. 69–101. Raven Press, New York.
20. Clark, A. J. (1933): *The Mode of Action of Drugs on Cells*. Williams & Wilkins Co., Baltimore.

21. Collier, H. O. J., and Schneider, C. (1969): Profiles of activity in rodents of some narcotic and narcotic antagonist drugs. *Nature*, 224:610–612.
22. Colpaert, F. C., Lal, H., Niemegeers, C. J. E., and Janssen, P. A. J. (1975): Investigations on drug produced and subjectively experienced discriminative stimuli. 1. The fentanyl cue, a tool to investigate subjectively experienced narcotic drug actions. *Life Sci.*, 16:705–716.
23. Cowan, A. (1981): Simple *in vivo* tests that differentiate prototype agonists at opiate receptors. *Life Sci.*, 28:1559–1570.
24. Craves, F., Leybin, L., Loh, H. H., Zalc, B., and Baumann, N. (1979): Cerebroside sulfate antibodies inhibit the effects of morphine and β-endorphin. *Science*, 207:75–76.
25. Creese, I., and Snyder, S. H. (1975): Receptor binding and pharmacological activity of opiates in the guinea-pig intestine. *J. Pharmacol. Exp. Ther.*, 194:205–291.
26. Dale, H. H. (1914): The action of certain esters and ethers of choline and their relation to muscarine. *J. Pharmacol. Exp. Ther.*, 6:147–190.
27. D'Amour, F. F., and Smith, D. L. (1941): A method for determining loss of pain sensation. *J. Pharmacol. Exp. Ther.*, 72:74–79.
28. Duka, T., Schubert, P., Wuster, M., Stoiber, R., and Herz, A. (1981): A selective distribution pattern of different opiate receptors in certain areas of rat brain as revealed by *in vitro* autoradiography. *Neurosci. Lett.*, 21:119–124.
29. Eckenhoff, J. E., Elder, J. D., and King, B. D. (1951): The effect of N-allylnormorphine in treatment of opiate overdose. *Am. J. Med. Sci.*, 222:115–117.
30. Ehrlich, P. (1913): Chemotherapeutics: Scientific principles, methods and results. *Lancet*, 2:445–451.
31. Fantozzi, R., Mulliken-Kilpatrick, D., and Blume, A. J. (1981): Irreversible inactivation of the opiate receptors in the neuroblastoma × glioma hybrid NG108-15 by chlornaltrexamine. *Mol. Pharmacol.*, 20:8–15.
32. Fidecka, S., Malec, D., and Langwinski, R. (1978): Central action of narcotic analgesics. II. Locomotor activity and narcotic analgesics. *Pol. J. Pharmacol. Pharm.*, 30:5–16.
33. Foldes, F. F., Lunn, J. N., Moore, J., and Brown, I. M. (1963): N-allyloxymorphone: a new potent narcotic antagonist. *Am. J. Med. Sci.*, 245:23–30.
34. Foote, R. W. and Maurer, R. (1982): Autoradiographic localization of opiate kappa-receptors in the guinea-pig brain. *Eur. J. Pharmacol.*, 85:99–103.
35. Fournie-Zaluski, M. C., Gacel, G., Maigret, B., Premilat, S., and Roques, B. P. (1981): Structural requirements for specific recognition of mu or delta opiate receptors. *Mol. Pharmacol.*, 20:484–491.
36. Fraser, H. F., and Rosenberg, D. E. (1964): Studies on the human addiction liability of 2-hydroxy-5,9-dimethyl-2-(3,3-dimethylallyl)-6,7-benzomorphan (WIN 20-228). *J. Pharmacol. Exp. Ther.*, 143:149–156.
37. Frederickson, R. C. A., Smithwick, E. L., Shuman, R., and Bemis, K. G. (1981): Metkephamid, a systematically active analog of methionine enkephalin with potent opioid delta receptor activity. *Science*, 211:603–605.
38. Gaddum, J. H. (1937): The quantitative effects of antagonistic drugs. *J. Physiol.*, 89:7–9.
39. Galletta, S., Ling, G. S. F., and Pasternak, G. W. (1982): Receptor binding and analgesic properties of oxymorphazone. *Life Sci.*, 31:1389–1392.
40. Gianutsos, G., and Lal, H. (1975): Effect of loperamide, haloperidol and methadone in rats trained to discriminate morphine from saline. *Psychopharmacology (Berlin)*, 41:267–270.
41. Gilbert, P. E., and Martin, W. R. (1976): The effects of morphine- and nalorphine-like drugs in the nondependent, morphine-dependent and cyclazocine-dependent chronic spinal dog. *J. Pharmacol. Exp. Ther.*, 198:66–82.
42. Goldstein, A., Lowney, L. I., and Pal, B. K. (1971): Stereospecific and nonspecific interactions of the morphine congener levorphanol in subcellular fractions of mouse brain. *Proc. Natl. Acad. Sci. U.S.A.*, 68:1742–1747.
43. Goldstein, A., Tachibana, S., Lowney, L. I., Hunkapiller, M., and Hood, L. (1979): Dynorphin-(1-12), an extraordinarily potent opioid peptide. *Proc. Natl. Acad. Sci. U.S.A.*, 76:6666–6670.
44. Goodman, R. R. and Snyder, S. H. (1982): Autoradiographic localization of kappa opiate receptors to deep layers of the cerebral cortex may explain unique sedative and analgesic effects. *Life Sci.*, 31:1291–1294.
45. Goodman, R. R., Snyder, S. H. (1982): Kappa opiate receptors localized by autoradiography to

deep layers of cerebral cortex: Relation to sedative effects. *Proc. Natl. Acad. Sci. U.S.A.*, 79:5703–5707.

46. Goodman, R. R., Snyder, S. H., Kuhar, M. J., and Young, W. S., III (1980): Differentiation of delta and mu opiate receptor localizations by light microscopic autoradiography. *Proc. Natl. Acad. Sci. U.S.A.*, 77:6239–6243.

47. Gyang, E. A., and Kosterlitz, H. W. (1966): Agonist and antagonist actions of morphine-like drugs on the guinea-pig isolated ileum. *Br. J. Pharmacol. Chemother.*, 27:514–527.

48. Haffner, F. (1929): Experimentille prufung schmerzstillenden. *Mittel. Dtsch. Med. Wochenschr.*, 55:731–733.

49. Hahn, E. F., Carroll-Buatti, M., and Pasternak, G. W. (1982): Irreversible opiate agonists and antagonists: The 14 hydroxydihydromorphine azines. *J. Neurosci.*, 2:572–576.

50. Harris, L. S., and Pierson, A. K. (1964): Some narcotic antagonists in the benzomorphan series. *J. Pharmacol. Exp. Therap.*, 143:141–148.

51. Hart, E. R. (1941): N-allylnorcodeine and N-allylnormorphine, two antagonists of morphine. *J. Pharmacol. Exp. Therap.*, 72:19.

52. Hart, E. R., and McCawley, W. L. (1944): The pharmacology of N-allylnormorphine as compared with morphine. *J. Pharmacol. Exp. Therap.*, 82:339–348.

53. Hazum, E., Chang, K.-J., Cuatrecasas, P., and Pasternak, G. W. (1981): Naloxazone irreversibly inhibits the high affinity binding of [^{125}I]D-ala^2-D-leu^5-enkephalin. *Life Sci.*, 28:2973–2979.

54. Herling, S., and Woods, J. H. (1981): Mini-symposium. IV. Discriminative stimulus effects of narcotics: Evidence for multiple receptor-mediated actions. *Life Sci.*, 28:1571–1584.

55. Hill, H. E., Jones, B. E., and Bell, E. C. (1971): State dependent control of discrimination by morphine and pentabarbital. *Psychopharmacology (Berlin)*, 22:305–313.

56. Hiller, J. M., and Simon, E. J. (1979): ^{3}H-ethylketocyclazocine binding: Lack of evidence for a separate kappa receptor in rats CNS. *Eur. J. Pharmacol.*, 60:389–390.

57. Hirschhorn, I. D., and Rosecrans, J. A. (1974): Morphine and Δ^9-tetrahydrocannabinol: Tolerance to the stimulus effects. *Psychopharmacology (Berlin)*, 36:243–253.

58. Hirschhorn, I. D., and Rosecrans, J. A. (1976): Generalization of morphine and lysergic acid diethylamide (LSD) stimulus properties to narcotic and analgesics. *Psychopharmacology (Berlin)*, 47:65–69.

59. Holtzman, S. G. (1980): Phencyclidine-like discriminative effects of opioids in the rat. *J. Pharmacol. Exp. Ther.*, 214:614–619.

60. Houde, R. W., and Wallenstein, S. L. (1956): Clinical studies of morphine-nalorphine combinations. *Fed. Proc.*, 15:440–441.

61. Hughes, J. (1975): Isolation of an endogenous compound from the brain with pharmacological properties similar to morphine. *Brain Res.*, 88:295–308.

62. Hughes, J., Smith, T. W., Kosterlitz, H. W., Fothergill, L. A., Morgan, B. A., and Morris, H. R. (1975): Identification of two related pentapeptides from the brain with potent opiate agonist activity. *Nature*, 258:577–579.

63. Hutchinson, M., Kosterlitz, H. W., Leslie, F. M., Westerfield, A. A., and Terenius, L. (1975): Assessment in the guinea-pig ileum and mouse vas deferens of benzomorphans which have strong antinociceptive activity but do not substitute for morphine in dependent monkey. *Br. J. Pharmacol.*, 55:541–546.

64. Iwamoto, E. T., and Martin, W. R. (1981): Multiple opioid receptors. *Med. Res. Rev.*, 1:411–440.

65. Jasinski, D. R. (1977): Assessment of the abuse potentiality of morphine like drugs (methods used in man). In: *Drug Addiction I: Morphine, Sedative/Hypnotic and Alcohol Dependence*, edited by W. R. Martin, pp. 197–258. Springer-Verlag, Berlin.

66. Jasinski, D. R., Martin, W. R., and Haertzen, C. A. (1967): The human pharmacology and abuse potential of N-allylnoroxymorphone (naloxone). *J. Pharmacol. Exp. Ther.*, 157:420–426.

67. Jasinski, D. R., Martin, W. R., and Hoeldtke, R. D. (1970): Effects of short and long term administration of pentazocine in man. *Clin. Pharmacol. Ther.*, 11:385–403.

68. Jasinski, D. R., Martin, W. R., and Sapira, J. D. (1968): Antagonism of the subjective, behavioral, pupillary, and respiratory depressant effects of cyclazocine by naloxone. *Clin. Pharmacol. Ther.*, 9:215–222.

69. Keats, A. S., and Telford, J. (1964): Naloxone antagonists as analgesics. Clinical aspects. In: *Molecular Modification in Drug Design, Advances in Chemistry Series 45*, edited by R. F. Gould, pp. 170–176. American Chemical Society, Washington.

70. Kosterlitz, H. W., and Hughes, J. (1977): Opiate receptors and endogenous opioid peptides in

tolerance and dependence. In: *Alcohol Intoxication and Withdrawal*, (M. Gross, ed.) Plenum, N.Y. pp 141–154.

71. Kosterlitz, H. W., Lord, J. A. H., Paterson, S. J., and Weterfield, A. A. (1980): Effect of changes in the structure of enkephalins and of narcotic analgesic drugs on their interactions with mu and delta-receptors. *Br. J. Pharmacol.*, 68:332–342.

72. Kosterlitz, H. W., and Paterson, S. J. (1980): Characterization of opioid receptors in nervous tissue. *Proc. R. Soc. Lond.*, 210:113–122.

73. Kosterlitz, H. W., Paterson, S. J., and Robson, L. E. (1981): Characterization of the kappa-subtype of the opiate receptor in the guinea-pig brain. *Br. J. Pharmacol.*, 73:939–949.

74. Kuhar, M. J., Pert, C. B., and Snyder, S. H. (1973): Regional distribution of opiate receptor binding in monkey and human brain. *Nature*, 245:447–451.

75. Langley, J. N. (1909): On the contraction of muscle, chiefly in relation to the presence of "receptive" substances. Part IV. The effect of curare and of some other substances on the nicotine response of the sartorius and gastrocnemius muscles of the frog. *J. Physiol.*, 39: 235–295.

76. Lasagna, L., and Beecher, H. K. (1954): The analgesic effectiveness of nalorphine and nalorphine-morphine combinations in man. *J. Pharmacol. Exp. Ther.*, 112:356–363.

77. Law, P. Y., Harris, R. A., Loh, H. H., and Way, B. L. (1978): Evidence for the involvement of cerebroside sulfate in opiate receptor binding: Studies with Azure A and Jimpy mutant mice. *J. Pharmacol. Exp. Ther.*, 207:458–468.

78. Ling, G. S. F., and Pasternak, G. W. (1983): Spinal and supraspinal opioid analgesia in the mouse: the role of subpopulation of opioid binding sites. *Brain Res.*, 271:152–156.

79. Ling, G. S. F., Spiegel, K., Nishimura, S., and Pasternak, G. W. (1983): Dissociation of morphine's analgesic and respiratory depressant actions. *Europ. J. Pharmacol.*, 86:487–488.

80. Loh, H. A., and Law, P. Y. (1980): The role of membrane lipids in receptor mechanisms. *Ann. Rev. Pharmacol. Toxicol.*, 20:201–234.

81. Lord, J. H., Waterfield, A. A., Hughes, J., and Kosterlitz, H. W. (1977): Endogenous opioid peptides: Multiple agonists and receptors. *Nature*, 267:495–499.

82. Lunn, J. N., Foldes, F. F., Moore, J., and Brown, I. M. (1961): The influence of N-allylnoroxymorphone on the respiratory effects of oxymorphone in anaesthetized man. *Pharmacologist*, 3:66.

83. Maayani, S., and Weinstein, H. (1980): "Specific binding" of ^{3}H-phencyclidine: Artifacts of the rapid filtration method. *Life Sci.*, 26:2011–2022.

84. Martin, W. R. (1963): Analgesic and antipyretic drugs: Strong analgesics. In: *Physiological Pharmacology, Vol. 1—The Nervous System*, Part A: Central Nervous System Drugs, edited by W. S. Root and F. G. Hofman, pp. 275–312. Academic Press Inc., New York.

85. Martin, W. R. (1967): Opioid antagonists. *Pharmacol. Rev.*, 19:463–521.

86. Martin, W. R. (1979): History and development of mixed opioid agonists, partial agonists and antagonists. *Br. J. Clin. Pharmacol.*, 7:2735–2795.

87. Martin, W. R., Eades, C. G., Fraser, H. F., and Wikler, A. (1964): Use of hindlimb reflexes of the chronic spinal dog for comparing analgesics. *J. Pharmacol. Exp. Ther.*, 144:8–11.

88. Martin, W. R., Eades, C. G., Thompson, J. A., Huppler, R. E., and Gilbert, P. E. (1976): The effects of morphine- and nalorphine-like drugs in the nondependent and morphine-dependent chronic spinal dog. *J. Pharmacol. Exp. Ther.*, 197:517–532.

89. Martin, W. R., Eades, C. G., Thompson, W. O., Thompson, J. A., and Flanary, H. G. (1974): Morphine physical dependence in the dog. *J. Pharmacol. Exp. Ther.*, 189:759–771.

90. Martin, W. R., Fraser, H. F., Gorodetzky, C. W., and Rosenberg, D. E. (1965): Studies of the dependence-producing potential of the narcotic antagonist 2-cyclopropylmethyl-2'-hydroxy-5,9-dimethyl-6,7-benzomorphan (cyclazocine, WIN-20,740,ARC II-C-3). *J. Pharmacol. Exp. Therap.*, 150:426–436.

91. May, E. L., and Ager, J. H. (1959): Structures related to morphine. XI. Analogs and a diastereoisomer of 2'-hydroxy-2,5,9-trimethyl-6,7-benzomorphan. *J. Org. Chem.*, 24:1432–1435.

92. McClane, T. K., and Martin, W. R. (1967a): Effects of morphine, nalorphine, cyclazocine and naloxone on the flexor reflex. *Int. J. Neuropharmacol.*, 6:89–98.

93. McClane, T. K., and Martin, W. R. (1967b): Antagonism of the spinal cord effects of morphine and cyclazocine by naloxone and thebaine. *Int. J. Neuropharmacol.*, 6:325–327.

94. McLawhon, R. W., West, R. E., Jr., Miller, R. J., and Dawson, G. (1981): Distinct high affinity binding sites for benzomorphan drugs and enkephalin in a neuroblastom-brain hybrid cell line. *Proc. Natl. Acad. Sci. U.S.A.*, 78:4309–4313.

95. Miller, R. J., and Cuatrecasas, P. (1979): Enkephalins and endorphins *Vitam. and Horm.*, 36:297–382.
96. Nishimura, S., and Pasternak, G. W. (1983): Biochemical characterization of opioid binding site subtypes. *Mol. Pharmacol., (in press).*
97. Oka, T., Negishi, K., Suda, M., Matsumiya, T., Inazu, T., and Ueki, M. (1981): Rabbit vas deferens: A specific bioassay for opioid kappa-receptor agonists. *Eur. J. Pharmacol.*, 73:235–236.
98. Overton, D. A., and Batta, S. K. (1979): Investigation of narcotics and antitussives using drug discrimination techniques. *J. Pharmacol. Exp. Therap.*, 211:401–408.
99. Palumbo, P. A., and Winter, J. C. (1979): Discriminative stimulus properties of morphine, keto-cyclazocine, and SKF 10,047. *Fed. Proc.*, 38:855.
100. Parker, R. B. (1974): Mouse locomotor activity: Effect of morphine, narcotic antagonists, and the interaction of morphine and narcotic antagonists. *Psychopharmacology (Berlin)*, 38:15–23.
101. Pasternak, G. W. (1980): Multiple opiate receptors: [³H]Ethylketocyclazocine receptor binding and ketocyclazocine analgesia. *Proc. Natl. Acad. Sci. U.S.A.*, 77:3691–3694.
102. Pasternak, G. W. (1981): Opiate, enkephalin and endorphin analgesia: Relations to a single subpopulation of opiate receptors. *Neurology*, 31:1311–1315.
103. Pasternak, G. W. (1982): High and low affinity binding sites: Relationship to mu and delta sites. *Life Sci.*, 31:1303–1306.
104. Pasternak, G. W., Carroll-Buatti, M., and Spiegel, K. (1981): The binding and analgesic properties of sigma opiate, SKF 10,047. *J. Pharmacol. Exp. Ther.*, 219:192–198.
105. Pasternak, G. W., Childers, S. R., and Snyder, S. H. (1980): Opiate analgesia: Evidence for mediation by a subpopulation of opiate receptors. *Science*, 208:514–516.
106. Pasternak, G. W., Childers, S. R., and Snyder, S. H. (1980): Naloxazone, a long-acting opiate antagonist: effects on analgesia in intact animals and on opiate receptor binding in vitro. *J. Pharmacol. Exp. Ther.*, 214:455–462.
107. Pasternak, G. W., Goodman, R., and Snyder, S. H. (1975): An endogenous morphine-like factor in mammalian brain. *Life Sci.*, 16:1765–1769.
108. Pasternak, G. W., and Hahn, E. F. (1980): Long acting opiate agonists and antagonists: 14-hydroxydiphydromorphinone hydrazones. *J. Med. Chem.*, 23:674–676.
109. Pasternak, G. W., Simantov, R., and Snyder, S. H. (1976): Characterization of an endogenous morphine-like factor (enkephalin) in mammalian brain. *Mol. Pharmacol.*, 12:504–513.
110. Pasternak, G. W., Snowman, A., and Snyder, S. H. (1975): Selective enhancement of ³H-opiate agonist binding by divalent cations. *Mol. Pharmacol.* 11:735–744.
111. Pasternak, G. W., and Snyder, S. H. (1974): Opiate receptor binding: effects of enzymatic treatments. *Mol. Pharmacol.*, 10:183–193.
112. Pasternak, G. W., and Snyder, S. H. (1975): Identification of novel high affinity opiate receptor binding in rat brain. *Nature*, 253:563–565.
113. Pasternak, G. W., Wilson, H. A., and Snyder, S. H. (1975): Differential effects of protein-modifying reagents on receptor binding of opiate agonists and antagonists. *Mol. Pharmacol.*, 11:340–351.
114. Pasternak, G. W., Zhang, A. Z., and Tecott, L. (1980): Developmental differences between high and low affinity opiate binding sites: their relationship to analgesia and respiratory depression. *Life Sci.*, 27:1185–1190.
115. Paton, W. D. M. (1955): The response of the guinea-pig ileum to electrical stimulation. *J. Physiol.*, 127:40–41.
116. Paton, W. D. M. (1957): The action of morphine and related substances on contraction and on acetylcholine output of coaxially stimulated guinea-pig ileum. *Br. J. Pharmacol.*, 12:119–127.
117. Pearl, J., and Harris, L. S. (1966): Inhibition of writhing by narcotic antagonists. *J. Pharmacol. Exp. Ther.*, 154:319–323.
118. Pert, A., and Yaksh, T. L. (1974): Sites of morphine induced analgesia in the primate brain: Relation to pain pathways. *Brain Res.*, 80:135–140.
119. Pert, C. B., Pasternak, G. W., and Snyder, S. H. (1973): Opiate agonists and antagonists discriminated by receptor binding in brain. *Science*, 182:1359–1361.
120. Pert, C. B., Snowman, A. M., and Snyder, S. H. (1974): Localization of opiate receptor binding in synaptic membranes of rat brain. *Brain Res.*, 70:184–188.
121. Pert, C. B., and Snyder, S. H. (1973): Opiate receptor: Demonstration in nervous tissue. *Science*, 179:1011–1014.

122. Pert, C. B., and Snyder, S. H. (1973b): Properties of specific opiate receptor binding in rat brain. *Proc. Natl. Acad. Sci. U.S.A.*, 70:2243–2247.

123. Pert, C. B., Snyder, S. H., and May, E. L. (1976): Opiate receptor interactions of benzomorphans in rat brain homogenates. *J. Pharmacol. Exp. Ther.*, 196:316–322.

124. Pfeiffer, A., and Herz, A. (1981): Evidence for a kappa-binding site in rat brain homogenate. *Neurosci. Lett. (Suppl. 7)*, 184.

125. Pfeiffer, A., and Herz, A. (1981): Demonstration and distribution of an opiate binding site in rat brain with high affinity for ethylketocyclazocine and SKF 10,047. *Biochem. Biophys. Res. Comm.*, 101:38–44.

126. Pohl, J. (1915): Uber das N-allylnorcodein, einen antagonisten des morphins. *Z. Exp. Pathol. Ther.*, 17:370–382.

127. Portoghese, P. S. (1970): Relationships between stereostructure and pharmacological activity. *Ann. Rev. Pharm.*, 10:51–76.

128. Portoghese, P. S., Larson, D. L., Jiang, J. B., Caruso, T. P., and Takemori, A. E. (1979): Synthesis and pharmacologic characterization of alkylating analogue (chloranhereximine) of naltrexone with ultralong-lasting narcotic antagonist properties. *J. Med. Chem.*, 22:168–173.

129. Portoghese, P. S., Larson, D. L., Jiang, J. B,, Takemori, A. E., and Caruso, T. P. (1978): 6B-[N,N-Bis(2-chloroethyl)amino]-17-(cyclopropylmethyl)-4,5d-epoxy-3,14-dihydroxymorphinan (chlornaltrexamine), a potent opioid receptor alkylating agent with ultralong narcotic antagonist activity. *J. Med. Chem.*, 21:598–599.

130. Portoghese, P. S., Larson, D. L., Sayre, L. M., Fries, D. S., and Takemori, A. E. (1980): A novel opioid receptor site directed alkylating agent with irreversible narcotic antagonistic and reversible agonistic activities. *J. Med. Chem.*, 23:233–234.

131. Robson, L. E., and Kosterlitz, H. W. (1979): Specific protection of the binding sites of D-Ala²-D-Leu⁵-enkephalin (delta-receptors) and dihydromorphine (mu-receptors). *Proc. R. Soc. Lond.*, 205:425–432.

132. Romer, D., Buscher, H., Hill, R. C., Maurer, R., Petcher, T. J., Welle, H. B. A., Bakel, H. C. C. K., and Akkerman, A. M. (1980): Bremazocine: A potent, long-acting opiate kappa-agonist. *Life Sci.*, 27:971–978.

133. Schneider, C. (1968): Behavioural effects of some morphine antagonists and hallucinogens in the rat. *Nature*, 220:586–587.

134. Schulz, R., Wuster, M., Krenss, H., and Herz, A. (1980): Selective development of tolerance without dependence in multiple opiate receptors of mouse vas deferens. *Nature*, 285:242–243.

135. Schulz, R., Wuster, M., Rubini, P., and Herz, A. (1981): Functional opiate receptors in the guinea-pig ileum: their differentiation by means of selective tolerance development. *J. Pharmacol. Exp. Ther.*, 219:547–550.

136. Seevers, M. H., and Deneau, G. A. (1963): Physiological aspects of tolerance and physical dependence. In: *Physiological Pharmacology, Vol. 1—The Nervous System*, Part A: Central Nervous System Drugs, edited by W. S. Root and F. G. Hofman, pp. 565–640. Academic Press Inc., New York.

137. Shannon, H. E., and Holtzman, S. G. (1976): Evaluation of the discriminative effects of morphine in the rat. *J. Pharmacol. Exp. Ther.*, 198:54–65.

138. Shannon, H. E., and Holtzman, S. G. (1977): Further evaluation of the discriminative effects of morphine in the rat. *J. Pharmacol. Exp. Ther.*, 201:55–66.

139. Shannon, H. E., and Holtzman, S. G. (1979): Morphine training dose: a determinant of stimulus generalization to narcotic antagonists in the rat. *Psychopharmacology (Berlin)*, 61:239–244.

140. Siegmund, E., Cadmus, R., and Lee, G. (1957): A method for evaluating both non-narcotic and narcotic analgetics. *Proc. Soc. Exp. Biol. Med.*, 95:729–731.

141. Simantov, R., Childers, S. R., and Snyder, S. H. (1978): The opiate receptor binding interactions of ³H-methionine enkephalin, an opiate peptide. *Eur. J. Pharmacol.*, 47:319–331.

142. Simantov, R., and Snyder, S. H. (1976): Morphine-like peptides in mammalian brain: Isolation, structure elucidation, and interactions with the opiate receptor. *Proc. Natl. Acad. Sci. U.S.A.*, 73:2515–2519.

143. Simon, E. J., Hiller, J. M., and Edelman, I. (1973): Stereospecific binding of the potent narcotic analgesic ³H-etorphine to rat brain homogenates. *Proc. Natl. Acad. Sci. U.S.A.*, 70:1947–1949.

144. Smith, C. B., and Sheldon, M. I. (1973): Effects of narcotic analgesic drugs on brain noradrenergic

mechanisms. In: *Agonist and Antagonist Actions of Narcotic Analgesic Drugs*, edited by H. W. Kosterlitz, H. O. J. Collier, and J. E. Villarreal, pp. 164–175. University Park Press, Baltimore.

145. Snyder, S. H., and Goodman, R. R. (1980): Multiple neurotransmitter receptors. *J. Neurochem.*, 35:5–15.

146. Spiegel, K., Kourides, I., and Pasternak, G. W. (1982): Prolactin and growth hormone release by morphine in the rat: Different receptor mechanisms. *Science*, 217:745–747.

147. Swain, H. H., and Seevers, M. H. (1974): Evaluation of new compounds for morphine-like physical dependence in the rhesus monkey. Presented to Committee on Problems of Drug Dependence, National Research Council, Mexico City.

148. Takemori, A. E., Larson, D. L., and Portoghese, P. S. (1981): The irreversible narcotic antagonistic and reversible agonistic properties of the fumaramate methylester derivative of naltrexone. *Eur. J. Pharmacol.*, 70:445–451.

149. Teal, J. J., and Holtzman, S. G. (1979): Discriminative stimulus effects of cyclazocine in the rat. *J. Pharmacol. Exp. Therap.*, 212:368–376.

150. Tepper, P., and Woods, J. H. (1978): Changes in locomotor activity and naloxone-induced jumping in mice produced by WIN35,197-2 (ethylketazocine) and morphine. *Psychopharmacology (Berlin)*, 58:125–129.

151. Terenius, L. (1973): Characteristics of the "receptor" for narcotic analgesics in synaptic plasma membrane fractions from rat brain. *Acta Pharmacol. Toxicol.*, 33:377–384.

152. Terenius, L., and Wahlstrom, A. (1975): Search for an endogenous ligand for the opiate receptor. *Acta Physiol. Scand.*, 94:74–81.

153. Vincent, J. P., Kartalovski, B., Geneste, P., Kamenka, J. M., and Lazdunski, M. (1979): Interaction of phencyclidine ("angel dust") with a specific receptor in rat brain membranes. *Proc. Natl. Acad. Sci. U.S.A.*, 76:4678–4683.

154. Vincent, J. P., Vignon, J., Kartalovski, B., and Lazdunski, M. (1980): Binding of phencyclidine to rat brain membranes: Technical aspect. *Eur. J. Pharmacol.*, 68:73–77.

155. Ward, S. J., and Holaday, J. W. (1982): Relative involvement of mu and delta opioid mechanisms in morphine-induced depression of respiration in rats. *Proc. Soc. Neurosci.*, 8:388.

156. Weijland, J., and Erickson, A. E. (1942): N-allylnormorphine. *J. Am. Chem. Soc.*, 64:869–890.

157. Wikler, A., Fraser, H. F., and Isbell, H. (1953): N-allylnormorphine. Effects of single doses and precipitation of acute "abstinence syndromes" during addiction to morphine, methadone or heroin in man. *J. Pharmacol. Exp. Ther.*, 109:8–29.

158. Wilson, H. A., Pasternak, G. W., and Snyder, S. H. (1975): Differentiation of opiate agonist and antagonist receptor binding by protein modifying reagents. *Nature*, 253:448–450.

159. Winter, J. C. (1975): The stimulus properties of morphine and ethanol. *Psychopharmacology (Berlin)*, 44:209–214.

160. Wolozin, B. L., Nishimura, S., and Pasternak, G. W. (1982): The binding of kappa and sigma opiates in rat brain. *J. Neurosci.*, 2:708–713.

161. Wolozin, B. L., and Pasternak, G. W. (1981): Classification of multiple morphine and enkephalin binding sites in the central nervous system. *Proc. Natl. Acad. Sci. U.S.A.*, 78:6181–6185.

162. Wood, P. L., Rackham, A., and Richard, J. (1981): Spinal analgesia: Comparison of the mu agonist morphine and the kappa agonist ethylketazocine. *Life Sci.*, 28:2119–2125.

163. Wood, P. L., Richard, J. W., and Thakur, M. (1982): Mu opiate isoreceptors: differentiation with kappa agonists. *Life Sci.*, 31:2313–2317.

164. Woods, J. H., Smith, C. B., Medzihradsky, F., and Swain, H. H. (1979): Preclinical testing of new analgesic drugs. In: *Mechanisms of Pain and Analgesic Compounds*, edited by R. F. Beers, Jr., and E. G. Bassett, pp. 429–445. Raven Press, New York.

165. Woolfe, D., and MacDonald, A. D. (1944): The evaluation of the analgesic action of pethidine hydrochloride (Demerol). *J. Pharmacol. Exp. Ther.*, 80:300–307.

166. Young, W. S., III, and Kuhar, M. J. (1979): A new method for receptor autoradiography: [^{3}H]Opioid receptors in rat brain. *Brain Res.*, 179:255–270.

167. Zhang, A.-Z., Chang, J.-K., and Pasternak, G. W. (1981): The actions of naloxazone on the binding and analgesic properties of morphiceptin (NH$_2$Tyr-Pro-Phe-Pro-CONH$_2$), a selective mu-receptor ligand. *Life Sci.*, 28:2829–2836.

168. Zhang, A.-Z., and Pasternak, G. W. (1980): mu and delta-opiate receptors: Correlation with high and low affinity opiate binding sites. *Europ. J. Pharmacol.*, 67:323–324.

169. Zhang, A.-Z., and Pasternak, G. W. (1981): Ontogeny of opioid pharmacology and receptors: high and low affinity site differences. *Europ. J. Pharmacol.*, 73:29–40.
170. Zukin, R. S., and Zukin, S. R. (1981): Demonstration of [³H]cyclazocine binding to multiple opiate receptor sites. *Mol. Pharmacol.*, 20:246–254.
171. Zukin, S. R., and Zukin, R. S. (1979): Specific [³H]phencyclidine binding in rat central nervous system. *Proc. Natl. Acad. Sci. U.S.A.*, 76:5372–5376.

Analgesics: Neurochemical, Behavioral, and Clinical Perspectives, edited by M. Kuhar and G. Pasternak. Raven Press, New York © 1984.

Anatomical Substrates of Pain and Pain Modulation and Their Relationship to Analgesic Drug Action

Allan I. Basbaum

Department of Anatomy, University of California, San Francisco, San Francisco, California 94143

Numerous reviews of the anatomical organization underlying the generation and control of pain have been published. Therefore, this chapter will focus on those areas where the most recent and most important observations have been made. Emphasis will be placed on those areas that bear on the mechanism of action of a variety of analgesic drugs. Particular attention will be paid to the spinal dorsal horn, where several technological breakthroughs in anatomical and physiological methodology have significantly extended our understanding of its organization. This is particularly important, because a variety of drugs have now been shown to exert a powerful analgesic action when injected intrathecally, i.e., directly into the subarachnoid space of the spinal cord.

FROM THE PERIPHERY TO THE CENTRAL NERVOUS SYSTEM

Until recently, and to some extent even to this day, there remained a heated discussion concerning the specificity or lack of specificity in somatosensory pathways. For example, the prevailing view in the 19th century was that different peripheral fiber types are qualitatively distinguishable. That is, it was proposed that stimulation of one fiber type always generated pain, whereas stimulation of others transmit heat, cold, touch, etc. Each afferent fiber was also thought to have a morphologically distinct receptor, which was sensitive to a particular stimulus modality.

The opposite view (pattern theory) holds that there is absolutely no specificity within the peripheral or central nervous system, and that any sensation or perception results from a particular pattern of firing generated across fibers by any given stimulus. The cornea is always cited as the best evidence for pattern theory, because only one morphological receptor type is found, namely the free nerve ending. Nevertheless, qualitatively different sensations can be elicited from corneal stimulation.

Whether a given stimulus activates a "labeled line," from periphery through the central nervous system, ultimately leading to a particular perception, is still unknown. For the periphery, however, there is now strong evidence for a considerable degree of fiber specificity. Many fibers have been physiologically characterized; many of these are very selective for the type of stimulus that excites them. With some exception, noxious stimuli excite small myelinated, A delta, and unmyelinated, C fibers. Within the A delta and C fiber ranges, there are subclasses of peripheral nociceptors. In the myelinated range, the A delta high threshold mechanoreceptor responds to high intensity mechanical stimulation, and is much less responsive, if at all, to chemical or thermal nociceptive inputs (26). In the unmyelinated range is the C polymodal nociceptor (22). This fiber is sensitive to a variety of potentially painful stimuli, including mechanical, thermal, and chemical stimuli. It has been suggested that the acute, "first" and diffuse, burning, "second" pain reflects activity in A delta and C fibers nociceptors, respectively. This is consistent with the conduction velocity differences in the two fiber types; nevertheless, the contribution of second and third order cells to first and second pain must be considered.

It should be pointed out that not all C fibers are nociceptors. Thus, in the cat, approximately 40% of the C fibers respond to low threshold mechanical stimulation. In the primate, only 10% of the C fibers are sensitive to low intensity stimuli. The fact that C fibers are not uniformly responsive to noxious stimuli emphasizes that studies using electrical stimulation of peripheral nerves must be interpreted with caution; an electrically evoked C volley activates both nociceptive and non-nociceptive inputs. Thus, recordings of the responses from second order cells, or of dorsal root potentials that are generated by C fibers, may reflect the modality of the C fiber stimulated more than the diameter of the fiber. This may explain some of the disagreements in the literature concerning the central effects of C fiber stimulation.

One promising approach to a better characterization of peripheral nerve fibers is the use of antibodies to identify the peptides which they contain. Although many studies concentrate on the peptide content of the dorsal horn, which derives from primary afferent fibers, it must be emphasized that a given dorsal root ganglion cell emits peptidergic axons both centrally and peripherally. Much of the peptide synthesized in the dorsal root ganglion is transported to the peripheral process. Because small diameter dorsal root ganglion cells (many of which are nociceptors) contain different peptides, it is likely that the peripheral nociceptors may be distinguishable on the basis of their peptide content. For example, high concentrations of substance P have been demonstrated in peripheral terminals in the skin and in the tooth pulp (92). The latter is of particular interest because it has been suggested that stimulation of tooth pulp afferents only generates pain.

Unfortunately, we have little information about the functional significance of peripheral peptides. They are presumably released on stimulation, and may modify the sensitivity of the afferent terminal. Alternatively, some action on local circulation can be envisioned, which, in turn, would modify the sensitivity of the peripheral receptors. One can imagine that topical application of enzymatically resistant peptide compounds, or drugs which antagonize these peptides, may dramatically modify nociceptive inputs to the spinal cord. It would be of interest to determine transmitter receptor characteristics, if any, in the region of the peripheral terminals.

The contribution of peptides in the peripheral branch of sensory axons may bear on the mechanism of pain from inflammation. For years, emphasis was placed on the "pain producing" substances that have been isolated from inflamed tissue. That these were peptides, e.g., bradykinin, is consistent with the hypothesis that neuronal peptides contribute to the inflammatory process. Conceivably "antipeptide" agents could exert a peripheral action.

Although it has been generally taught that peripheral nerve damage results in degeneration only of the distal process of the peripheral nerve, many studies indicate that this is incorrect (49,53). Gunnar Grant first demonstrated that peripheral nerve section, in fact, results in significant degenerative changes of primary afferents *within* the spinal dorsal horn. Many of these changes are reversible. There is also convincing evidence for dramatic changes in the central terminals after peripheral nerve damage. For example, peripheral axotomy results in a significant decrease in substance P levels in the dorsal horn (74). The fact that central changes do occur has proven particularly valuable, for example, to studies using capsaicin, the active ingredient in paprika. When capsaicin is applied to the skin, it generates a severe burning sensation with subsequent analgesia in the injected area. Correlated with the behavioral change is a significant decrease in peptide levels of the dorsal horn (40,73). These decreases are presumed to result from a massive discharge of the primary afferent fibers, and release of the putative peptide transmitter (113). If the capsaicin is administered neonatally, there is an irreversible loss of primary afferent fibers, generally restricted to the small diameter range (70,71). Since recent studies illustrated peripheral nerve transport of opiate binding sites, (Nincovic, *personal communication*) one can imagine a peripheral enkephalin-substance P interaction comparable to that reported at the central branch of dorsal root ganglion cells in the cord (72). These data raise the important possibility that the pain that often follows peripheral nerve damage is in part the result of changes in the dorsal horn as well as in the periphery (116).

These observations may also explain why treatment of peripheral neuralgias is often so unsatisfactory. Treatment focused on reducing the afferent barrage, e.g., by sympathectomy or intra-arterial injection of guanethidine (117) are helpful, but this may not get at the problem resulting from the deafferented dorsal horn neurons. Obviously the consequences of peripheral nerve damage are far more severe than was originally assumed.

THE SPINAL DORSAL HORN

Perhaps the most extensive and significant breakthroughs in our understanding of transmission systems that contribute to pain concerns the organization of the spinal dorsal horn. Several new techniques have been instrumental in opening up this area. First, individual cells of the superficial dorsal horn, including the smallest cells of the substantia gelatinosa, have been intracellularly recorded from and filled with the electron dense marker, horseradish peroxidase (HRP). This permits a precise correlation of structure and function heretofore impossible. Moreover, ultrastructural studies of these functionally identified neurons have lent new insight into the synaptic interactions that underlie processing within the dorsal horn. Finally, immunohistochemical characterization of the dorsal horn has provided a wealth of pharmacological information previously unavailable. Although the latter studies have underscored the complexity of the dorsal horn, they nevertheless indicate that anatomical subsets can be recognized, and thus functional correlations can be determined.

In general, the dorsal horn can be divided into three segments, each of which is cytoarchitecturally laminated (105). The superficial dorsal horn includes the marginal zone, or lamina I, and the substantia gelatinosa, lamina II. The marginal zone is a thin band which caps the dorsal horn. It contains a variety of neuronal types, among which is the large Waldeyer cell, whose dendrites cap the dorsal horn (47). Many marginal neurons are at the origin of long ascending pathways; some project to the reticular formation, some to the cerebellum, and others to the thalamus. Many interconnect distant spinal segments, with long propriospinal axons. Most importantly, almost all marginal neurons are nociceptors (32,82).

The substantia gelatinosa (SG), long refractory to both anatomical and physiological studies, has now been more accurately characterized (30). Several categories of neurons have been described within the SG (59). Of these, two are most prominent. First is the stalk cell (21,48), a small neuron whose cell body is located at the I-II border. Its dendrites descend through the layers of the SG; many penetrate ventrally into lamina III. The stalk cell axon characteristically arborizes within the marginal zone. It has been proposed that this neuron is an excitatory interneuron transmitting high threshold mechanoreceptive input into the marginal zone (100). A second prominent SG neuron is the islet cell, which is found both in the inner and outer layers of the SG (20,48). Seen in sagittal section, it has a fusiform cell body; its dendrites course longitudinally through the SG. Its axon courses within the confines of its own dendritic tree. Ultrastructural analysis of electrophysiologically characterized and HRP-filled islet cells indicates that its dendrites contain synaptic vesicles, and are presynaptic to other elements of the neuropile (51) (Fig. 1). Moreover, the presynaptic islet cell dendrites bear strong similarity to the GABAergic synapses identified in immunohistochemical preparations using antibodies directed against glutamic acid decarboxylase, the biosynthetic enzyme for GABA (9,18). Thus, some islet cells may be GABAergic. On the other hand, morphological similarities between islet cells and enkephalin-immunoreactive SG neurons have also been reported (44). Thus, it is unlikely that islet cells are pharmacologically distinct, and thus are presumably not functionally homogeneous.

On the basis of its afferent input and physiological organization, the SG appears to contain at least two layers. The outer layer receives high threshold inputs, and includes small neurons responsive both to noxious and non-noxious inputs. The inner layer receives small diameter fiber, low threshold inputs, and contains cells responsive predominantly to non-nociceptive inputs (20,21,31,82). A population of

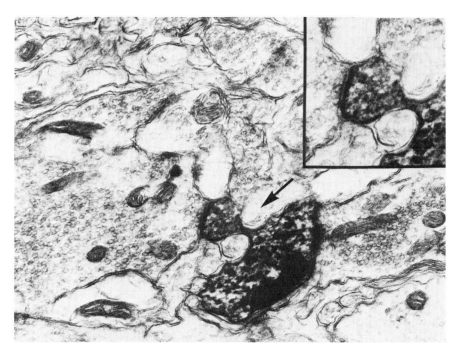

FIG. 1. Electron micrograph demonstrating labeled dendrites from intracellularly filled islet cell in lamina II of the cat dorsal horn. Spine appendage (inset) contains vesicles, and thus is a presynaptic "dendrite." A comparable structure has been reported for GAD-immunoreactive terminals. (Courtesy of Gobel, ref. 51.)

SG neurons are unusual in that they are spontaneously active and are profoundly inhibited by natural stimulation (31,59). Since these SG neurons have properties just the opposite of others within the same regions, i.e., are inhibited by natural stimulation, they have been referred to as inverse neurons.

The second region of the dorsal horn, located ventrally to the SG, has been given various names, but in this discussion will be referred to as the nucleus proprius. It includes laminae III, IV, and V of Rexed. In Nissl stained preparations, in which only the cell bodies and proximal dendrites are identified, it is difficult to distinguish the three layers. There is a tendency for cell size to increase more ventrally. Many of the neurons of the nucleus proprius are at the origin of major ascending spinal pathways, including spinocervical, spinoreticular, and spinothalamic tracts. Golgi preparations indicate that some of the dendrites of these neurons penetrate the SG, and thus would come under the influence of neurons of the superficial dorsal horn. In general, however, the neurons of the nucleus proprius arborize ventral to the SG.

Anatomical characterization of the remainder of the spinal grey, laminae VI, VII, and the more ventral horn is much less detailed. Nevertheless, these regions probably contribute to the transmission of nociceptive messages. Specifically, many neurons of lamina VII respond to high threshold inputs and are at the origins of ascending spinal pathways. Their precise role in nociception will be discussed later.

To some extent the physiological characterization of dorsal horn neurons originally described by Wall (115) and later by Christensen and Perl (32) can be predicted on the basis of studies of the afferent input to the dorsal horn. Early studies using silver degeneration methods could not distinguish between functionally identified inputs, and, in fact, had difficulty distinguishing between inputs from large and small diameter fibers. However, recent studies have reported important differences in their central projection. It is now generally accepted that the larger diameter fibers of the dorsal root take a medial course as they enter the spinal cord, before they penetrate through the superficial layers of the dorsal horn. Very few large diameter fibers terminate with the SG; the vast majority arborize in the nucleus proprius and more ventrally (80,81,101). In contrast, the fine fibers enter over the lateral aspect of the dorsal horn, and arborize extensively within laminae I and II (102). A collateral branch of the small fiber curves around the dorsal horn and terminates more ventrally in the region of lamina V and near the lateral aspect of the central canal. Characterization of the projection of single fibers, physiologically identified, and stained intercellularly with HRP has revealed further detail (81) (Fig. 2). For example, the A delta high threshold mechanoreceptor arborizes in the marginal zone and more ventrally in lamina V. Some Aδ axons also send collaterals to the SG (50). It has been suggested that C fibers arborize predominantly in the SG, not in lamina I, but it has not been possible to record from C fibers, and thus, the information is inferential. Other studies indicate that a class of very fine fibers distributes to lamina I as well as to the SG (52). By analyzing several studies, it can be concluded that high threshold fibers distribute predominantly to lamina I

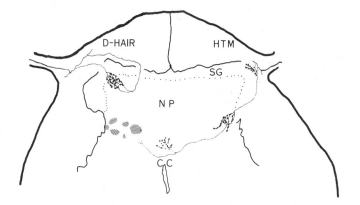

FIG. 2. Schematic diagram illustrating the differential projection of physiologically identified primary afferent fibers. The projection of a D hair (non-nociceptive) afferent to the nucleus proprius is indicated on the *left*. The projection of an Aδ high threshold mechanoreceptor to laminae I and V and to the region of the central canal is illustrated on the right. (From ref. 95a, with permission.)

and to the outer part of the substantia gelatinosa. It is of interest that some afferent fibers in the ventral root arborize in the SG as well (83). Since the ventral root afferents are predominantly C fibers (33), their projection is consistent with that of dorsal root C fibers. Questions that remain are whether deeper (laminae V and VII) nociceptors receive monosynaptic input from high threshold afferents or whether there is a cascade of input from neurons of the superficial dorsal horn.

The original characterization of nucleus proprius dorsal horn neurons has not changed significantly. Wall (115) first demonstrated that a physiological laminar organization could be recognized in the dorsal horn. He reported that in any given electrode penetration through the dorsal horn, there is a characteristic order in which response properties are found. Just beneath the SG, neurons respond predominantly, if not exclusively, to non-noxious inputs. They have relatively small receptive fields. Many of these neurons, in lamina III and particularly lamina IV, are at the origin of the spinocervical tract. More ventrally, in the region of lamina V, one finds neurons with convergent inputs from low and high threshold fibers. In addition, visceral afferent fibers converge onto these neurons. This convergent of mechanoreceptive and visceral input has been offered as an explanation for referred pain, in which pain from the viscera is referred to a somatic structure. Ventrally to lamina V, one characteristically finds neurons with convergent inputs from skin and from proprioceptive structures.

With rare exception, all of the neurons in the superficial dorsal horn and the nucleus proprius have ipsilateral receptive fields. In contrast, cells located more ventrally, in laminae VII and VIII often have very complex receptive fields (39,90). These may be bilateral and often include inhibitory components. Laminae VII and VIII neurons are also particularly susceptible to the anesthetic state, and thus have proven difficult to characterize. Nevertheless, recent anatomical and physiological studies indicate that many are of the origin of spinoreticular and spinothalamic axons, have nociceptive inputs, and thus probably contribute to the transmission of nociceptive messages.

PEPTIDES

Immunohistochemical studies reveal that the majority of biologically active peptides, which have been characterized, are found in relatively high concentrations in the superficial dorsal horn. Most important is that the different compounds have somewhat independent and characteristic domains. Some derive from primary afferent fibers, others derive from neurons intrinsic to the dorsal horn, and a third peptide population derives from axon terminals whose cell bodies are located in the brainstem. The functional significance of each of these peptides is only beginning to be understood. Several, however, have undergone extensive biochemical, electrophysiological, and behavioral analyses, revealing an important contribution to the transmission and control of nociceptive messages. Other chapters in this book go into significant detail about peptide distributions; therefore, this chapter will only highlight some of the anatomical differences found in the spinal cord.

SUBSTANCE P

With respect to pain, substance P, an 11 amino acid peptide is probably the best characterized and most significant. It is found in small diameter primary afferent fibers that terminate densely within the superficial dorsal horn, lamina I, and the outer SG (10,61). Given the physiological properties of afferent fibers projecting to the neurons of the superficial dorsal horn, it has been hypothesized that substance P is a transmitter for nociceptors. Iontophoretic application of substance P excites nociceptors of the dorsal horn (58). Moreover, high intensity stimulation of peripheral nerves, which excites Aδ and C fibers, releases substance P into the spinal CSF (125). Ultrastructural studies demonstrate that substance P is localized in large dense core vesicles of primary afferent terminals, which are presynaptic to second order neurons (10). Of particular interest are the studies using capsaicin. Systemic or intrathecal administration of capsaicin produces a massive discharge of primary afferent fibers, which is followed by a decrease in immunoreactive substance P in the superficial dorsal horn (124). In the adult, the peptide loss is reversible. If administered to neonates, this decrease is irreversible and correlates with a loss of small diameter dorsal root ganglion cells (71). More importantly, the peptide disappearance correlates with a loss of thermal pain sensitivity (124). Apparently, capsaicin selectively destroys or temporarily abolishes a population of C fibers that contribute to noxious heat sensibility.

If it is true that substance P is a nociceptive transmitter, then several therapeutic approaches can be envisioned. Antagonists to substance P have been recently synthesized (98); these presumably act by displacing substance P from the postsynaptic receptor. If substance P antagonists could be administered intrathecally to humans, then a regionally specific antinociceptive compound might be available. Alternatively, any compound that could destroy the substance P containing fibers (like capsaicin) might offer an effective method of pain relief. The latter approach is, of course, far more destructive, and thus probably far less selective.

ENKEPHALIN

With the discovery of endogenous opioid compounds, considerable advances were made in our understanding of the mechanism of exogenous opiate action. Although the endorphins have a wide distribution through the central nervous system, several loci are consistent with their contribution to pain control mechanisms. Perhaps the most interesting and clinically relevant location is the superficial dorsal horn. Early biochemical studies demonstrated significant opiate binding in the dorsal horn and on primary afferent fibers. While the studies that reported a decrease in spinal cord binding after rhizotomy (76) have been interpreted as the result of transneuronal damage to second order neurons, other studies conclusively establish that opiate binding sites are found on primary afferent fibers (8,38,60). Significant binding, however, remains after rhizotomy, indicating that receptors are also found on spinal neurons. Thus, opiates probably act both pre and postsynaptically to block the discharge of spinal nociceptors.

Immunohistochemical studies reveal dense enkephalin-like immunoreactivity in laminae I and II, more ventrally in laminae V, VII, and near the central canal (44,63). As described above, these regions contain cells responsive to noxious inputs; thus, the enkephalin terminals are ideally situated to postsynaptically modulate nociceptive transmission. On the other hand, Duggan et al. (35) demonstrated that inhibition of nucleus proprius nociceptors was produced by microinjecting opiates into the SG; injection near the soma was less effective and less selective. The latter results could be interpreted in two ways. Conceivably, the opiate binding sites are located on distal dendrites of nucleus proprius nociceptors. Alternatively, the opiate may act presynaptically on the fine fiber primary afferent fibers which terminate superficially.

Early studies concluded that all enkephalin immunoreactivity derives from local neurons, but recent studies indicate that some bulbospinal fibers are also enkephalin-containing (65). The vast majority of spinal enkephalin, however, derives from spinal neurons. Early studies also indicated that most enkephalin neurons are found in the SG (63); a subsequent study in the cat emphas' ed the large contribution of marginal neurons which are enkephalin-immunoreactive (44) (Fig. 3). The former observations were consistent with a modulatory role of the SG interneurons and were, in fact, offered as evidence in favor of the Gate Control Theory of pain (89, *see* below). In contrast, because marginal neurons are generally thought to be projection neurons, the possibility was raised that the "pain transmission neuron" is enkephalin-containing. Moreover, because most, if not all, marginal neurons are nociceptive, these data provided evidence for a local negative feedback circuit which is turned on by a noxious stimulus, and which modulates the output of the projection neuron.

The mechanism of spinal action of opiates in general, and of enkephalin in particular, is still controversial. In some cases, opiates exert a clear inhibitory postsynaptic effect, hyperpolarizing the postsynaptic membrane (97). Biochemical studies of opiate effects on substance P released from primary afferent fibers (72), however, led to the hypothesis that opiates presynaptically control the release of substance P, perhaps by altering Ca^{++} permeability. The presynaptic hypothesis was consistent both with the biochemical data and with the evidence for significant numbers of binding sites on primary afferent fibers. Unfortunately, ultrastructural studies have failed to find axoaxonic relationships in which enkephalin terminals are presynaptic to primary afferent fibers (7,45,48,68) (Fig. 4). The possibility that spinal enkephalin neurons exert a presynaptic control via a "neurohumoral" mechanism has been raised.

The clinical significance of the opiate binding and opiate peptide content of the dorsal horn reflects the recent observation that intrathecal or epidural morphine is a remarkably potent and specific analgesic. The presence of a direct spinal action of morphine was originally described in the rat, cat, and primate (126,127), more recently, it has been used effectively in humans. In fact, in some settings it is routinely used to control postoperative pain in cesarean section patients. The advantages of this approach are obvious. When administered locally, morphine

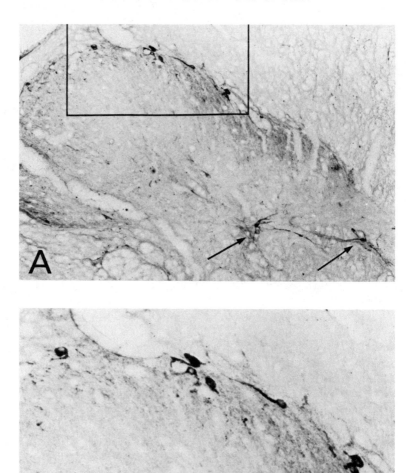

FIG. 3. Immunocytochemical localization of enkephalin-immunoreactive cells and terminals in the superficial dorsal horn of the cat. Cells predominate in laminae I and V (arrows). Higher magnification of marginal neurons is seen in B. (From Glazer and Basbaum, ref. 44.)

exerts a very selective action on nociceptors. Two point discrimination is intact; muscle tone is not altered. The diverse opiate effects produced by systemic injection, e.g., respiratory depression, can also be avoided. Perhaps most significantly, any unexpected consequences of the drug can be overcome by administering the opiate antagonist, naloxone. Thus, intrathecal morphine offers an effective, selective and safe approach to pain control. Presumably intrathecal opiates act by binding to the opiate binding site in the dorsal horn. Thus, morphine could postsynaptically

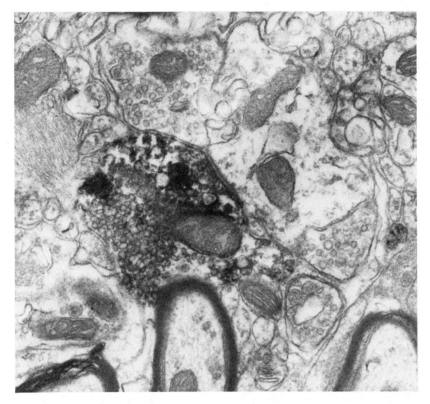

FIG. 4. Ultrastructural localization of immunoreactive enkephalin terminal presynaptic to un-labeled dendrite. This is a predominant enkephalin synaptic relationship in the superficial dorsal horn. A possible enkephalin axoaxonic relationship is also evident, but synaptic specializations were not seen.

block second order nociceptors, or it may act presynaptically by blocking the release of "nociceptive neurotransmitters."

OTHER PEPTIDES

Although most attention has focused on substance P and enkephalin, a variety of other peptides have been localized to the superficial dorsal horn. Although the function of these is less well understood, preliminary studies suggest that some contribute either to nociception or to the control of nociceptive inputs. For example, neurotensin terminals are most densely concentrated in lamina IIi of the superficial dorsal horn. They derive predominantly, if not, exclusively, from neurons within the substantia gelatinosa (69,108). Iontophoresis of neurotensin selectively excites spinal nociceptors (91). On the other hand, somatostatin, exerts a predominantly inhibitory effect on nociceptors (103). Since early studies reported that spinal somatostatin derives from a population of small diameter dorsal root ganglion cells, none of which overlap with substance P (61), its inhibitory effect was surprising. These data raised the possibility that primary afferent fibers can exert a direct inhibitory action on second order neurons, a mechanism previously considered unlikely. More recently, however, studies in which higher doses of colchicine were adminstered to the spinal cord, revealed a population of somatostatin cell bodies within lamina IIi (69). Thus, the inhibitory action of iontophoretic somatostatin probably mimics that produced by somatostatin release from local interneurons. The possibility that a single primary afferent fiber contains an inhibitory transmitter, which coexists with a more traditional excitatory transmitter, cannot be ruled out. This is particularly true because recent studies emphasize that coexistence of neurotransmitters is a relatively common occurrence in the central nervous system (46,58,64).

The list of dorsal horn peptides continues to grow. It includes bombesin, cholecystokinin, vasoactive intestinal polypeptide, and avian pancreatic polypeptide hormone (69). Of particular interest is the presence of immunoreactive oxytocin in the superficial dorsal horn (111). The peptide apparently derives from spinally-projecting hypothalamic neurons. Although its function is unknown, the possibility of direct hypothalamic control of spinal nociceptors must be considered.

Many of the peptides described above, although found in primary afferent fibers and second order neurons are also located in bulbospinal neurons. This includes substance P, enkephalin, somatostatin, and thyrotropin releasing hormone (TRH)-containing cells. In many of these neurons, the biogenic amine, serotonin, coexists (62). The functional significance of the coexistence of peptides and amines is unclear. Nevertheless, the fact that stimulation of many of these bulbospinal neurons generates analgesia makes them a fascinating focus of study.

Nonpeptidergic elements in the dorsal horn also contribute to the control of nociception. These include GABA, norepinephrine, and 5HT. The former has been best characterized by demonstrating immunoreactive glutamic acid decarboxylase (GAD), the biosynthetic enzyme for GABA (9,18). Both physiological and anatomical studies indicate that GABA exerts both pre and postsynaptic control of nociceptors. Conceivably, the synaptic interaction between GABAergic terminals, neurons, and nociceptors underlies the analgesic action of baclofen, a compound which, to some extent, mimics GABA (122). The contribution of the biogenic amines to pain control will be discussed later.

ASCENDING PATHWAYS

Although considerable new information is available concerning the organization of the spinal dorsal horn, those pathways necessary or sufficient for conveying the spinal input to higher centers are still unclear. Much of our information reflects the clinical fact that anterolateral cordotomy (i.e., a lesion of the anterolateral quadrant of the cord) is an effective surgical procedure for pain relief. Although it is generally taught that this operation cuts spinothalamic tract fibers, and thus severs "pain" inputs, this is an oversimplified picture. Anterolateral cordotomy cuts far more than spinothalamic tract fibers (23,24); spinorecticular, spinotectal, and numerous propriospinal fibers are simultaneously destroyed. It has, in fact, been argued that spinoreticular fibers are more significant to chronic pain than are spinothalamic tract axons.

Although we do not know the importance of individual pathways to clinical pain states, there is much new anatomical and physiological information about the cells of origin and central distribution of spinothalamic and spinoreticular pathways. Perhaps most significantly, it has been demonstrated that the spinothalamic tract is not a pure "pain" pathway. For example, as defined by retrograde transport or by antidromic activation from the thalamus, spinothalamic tract (STT) neurons have been localized to most laminae of the cord (6,27,41,42,114,120,121). Not surprisingly, many respond to noxious inputs; nevertheless, consistent with their location in laminae III and IV, many are responsive solely to non-noxious tactile stimulation. Others located near lamina VI respond to non-noxious joint manipulation. A large number are located in the ventral horn and overlap the distribution of many spinoreticular neurons.

More detailed studies of the central projection of dorsal versus ventral horn spinothalamic tract neurons revealed an interesting segregation. Neurons of dorsal horn laminae I, IV, and V predominantly project to the lateral thalamus (6,41–43). Given the response properties of neurons in these laminae, it has been proposed that these STT neurons convey localized "pain" sensations. In contrast, some cells of lamina I and almost all spinothalamic tract neurons found in laminae VII and VIII project to the intralaminar nuclei of the medial thalamus, particularly the central lateral nucleus. As described above, many neurons in the ventral horn have wide receptive fields, with complex excitatory and inhibitory components. The diffuse character of chronic pain would be more consistent with it being generated from activity in cells with large, poorly defined receptive fields. On this basis alone, one might predict that the medial thalamus is more concerned with the generation of chronic pain, and that the lateral thalamus is more concerned with the transmission of the discrete characteristics of a noxious stimulus. Arguments to the contrary, however, have been raised (*see* below).

Given the properties of spinoreticular neurons, it is clear that their contribution to the perception of chronic pain is important. Spinoreticular neurons derive predominantly from the ventral parts of the dorsal horn and from the ventral horn, particularly laminae VII and VIII (1,39). The receptive field, of most medullary reticular neurons are large, and bilateral; most respond to noxious stimulation. Stimulation within the reticular formation also elicits pain behavior in animals (28). For example, animals will work to avoid reticular stimulation. Thus, the spinoreticular and spinoreticulomedial thalamic systems are probably important elements in the generation of chronic pain.

Since it is difficult, if not impossible, to selectively cut the spinothalamic or the spinoreticular pathways, it is difficult to establish their individual roles. Certainly anterolateral cordotomy cuts both systems. It is of interest, however, that mesencephalic tractotomy, a relatively selective lesion of the lateral spinothalamic tract, at the midbrain-thalamic junction, often results in loss of localized pain sensation with preserved diffuse pain. These data are consistent with a major contribution of the medial thalamic projecting spinothalamic and spinoreticular systems to the generation of chronic pain.

It must be emphasized that the task of the clinician is to treat chronic, not acute (e.g., pin prick) pain. Thus, one must be especially careful in the choice of a pain test when assessing the analgesic potency of drugs. Demonstrating that acute pain is abolished, or that neurons responsive to pinch or pin prick are inhibited by a particular drug, may in no way predict the clinical value of the treatment. Since it is much easier to administer and to control the intensity of acute noxious stimuli, most studies use them. Nevertheless, new pain tests, which more closely model chronic pain, need to be developed. Some are presently being studied (34); hopefully they will increase the validity of drug assessment.

THE THALAMUS AND CORTEX

Until recently, electrophysiological studies found few thalamic neurons responsive to noxious stimulation. Given the pronounced spinothalamic input to lateral and medial thalamus, these data were always disappointing. Early studies did report nociceptors in the centrum-median parafascicular complex of the medial thalamus (5), but the incidence of lateral thalamic nociceptors was rare. Most of the emphasis was placed on the nuclei of the posterior thalamus, located caudally to the ventroposterolateral (VPL) and ventroposteromedial (VPM) nuclei (54,55,75,99). More recently, however, several laboratories have recorded from cells within the ventrobasal thalamus that respond both to noxious as well as non-noxious stimulation (54,55,96). Some are driven by noxious heat. Most importantly, the nociceptors of the lateral thalamus can be distinguished from the population of neurons which conveys the traditional lemniscal, somatotopically organized inputs that arrive via the dorsal column nuclei. The nociceptors of VPL are not somatotopically organized. More recently, the cortical receiving area of VPL, namely the postcentral gyrus (SI), of the primate has also been shown to contain nociceptors (75).

Whether these populations of nociceptors contribute to pain sensation is, of course, unknown. It is of interest in this regard that large cortical ablations, that include SI, have been reported to only minimally effect pain sensation (77). Such clinical reports, in fact, led to the widely held view that the cortex is not necessary for pain sensation. It is likely, however, that large cortical removals, while not abolishing pain sensation completely, drastically affect the quality of the perception.

Do nociceptors of the lateral and medial thalamus convey information about acute and chronic pain, respectively, or do they both convey similar information? Given that most electrophysiological studies are performed in anesthetized animals, and use discrete noxious stimuli, it is particularly difficult to evaluate this question. Recent studies turned to an animal model of arthritis, which may be useful to model "chronic" pain. The results raised the interesting possibility that lateral thalamic neurons, normally concerned with acute noxious stimuli, change their responsiveness in the presence of chronic noxious inputs. For example, in the normal animal, most lateral thalamic neurons are selectively responsive to non-noxious stimulation, and have a very low spontaneous activity. In the "arthritic" rat, however, many lateral thalamic neurons become spontaneously active. More-over, nociceptors are more readily discovered (54). These data suggest that a given neuron's responsiveness to acute stimuli is a poor predictor of its potential contri-bution to chronic pain states. Thus, the lateral thalamic nuclei may be more relevant to chronic pain than is generally believed.

Given the cortical connections of the intralaminar nuclei, one might predict that it has a greater contribution to the motor response produced by a noxious stimulus, than to the perception of the stimulus. The central lateral nucleus, which receives dense spinothalamic tract fibers, projects heavily to the motor cortex (110). Con-ceivably, the medial thalamic-cortical connections are involved in the startle re-sponse that is generated by a noxious stimulus. Lesion studies of the thalamus are also equivocal. In animals, and in several cases in humans, large lesions of the medial thalamus have proven effective for pain relief (29). In numerous studies, however, medial ablations were very disappointing. What underlies the differential effectiveness of medial thalamic lesions is unknown.

The cortical location of the pain message is least understood. As described above, nociceptive responses have been recorded in the somatotopically organized SI region. Traditionally, however, emphasis was placed on the second somatosen-sory area, particularly its caudal aspect, which has nociceptive neurons. Other studies, however, argue differently. The location of cells with nociceptive inputs may be even more caudal, in the region of the retroinsular cortex. Obviously, the difficulty in recording from cortical nociceptors in anesthetized animals makes these studies particularly complicated. Since it has proven difficult to record from cortical nociceptors, the electrophysiological analysis of drug action on cortical nociceptors is limited. Perhaps an analysis of the metabolic changes introduced by noxious stimuli, and/or analgesics, in animals with the 2-deoxyglucose method, and in humans with PET scan methodology, will identify relevant cortical areas.

PAIN CONTROL MECHANISMS

It is clear that with the exception of the dorsal horn, our understanding of the mechanisms underlying the generation of pain is inadequate. On the other hand, the analysis of pain control mechanisms has moved rapidly. To some extent, the most dramatic advances resulted from the discovery of endogenous opiate systems, and their contribution to endogenous pain suppression systems. Perhaps what is most important is that the numerous anatomical and physiological studies of the endogenous opiates and endogenous pain suppression systems have greatly in-creased our understanding of the mechanisms through which *exogenous* opiates produce analgesia.

Discussions of pain control mechanisms often make reference to the Gate Control Theory of Melzack and Wall (89); therefore, it is appropriate to reevaluate this theory in light of recent evidence. Gate Control Theory was a response to two diametrically opposed theories as to how a peripheral stimulus is perceived as painful. One theory proposed that there is a specific pain transmission system; the other proposed that a particular pattern of activity in a variety of peripheral nerve fibers determines whether or not a stimulus is perceived as painful. Gate Control Theory took elements of both theories, and proposed that whether a given stimulus is perceived as painful depends not on the firing of any single element, but on the balance of activity in large and small diameter peripheral fibers. Through a complicated mechanism involving neurons of the SG, it was proposed that the large diameter fibers inhibit second order nociceptors of the dorsal horn. On the other hand, small diameter fibers were hypothesized to not only directly excite spinal nociceptors, but also to turn off the SG inhibitory neurons, thus "opening the gate," and producing pain. In effect, the SG was the key to the gate. Without doubt, Gate Control Theory was an impetus to numerous important studies of the spinal dorsal horn, and to the development of a variety of novel therapeutic approaches, for example, transcutaneous and dorsal column electrical stimulation.

Although it is clear that large diameter fibers exert an inhibitory action on spinal nociceptors, and that this may be generated through interactions in the SG, the analysis of the central effects of C fibers has produced a variety of contradictory results. Perhaps the most important legacy of the Gate Control Theory is that it focused attention on the SG, at a time when electrophysiological studies of the SG were nonexistent, and well before immunohistochemical techniques underscored its pharmacological complexity.

We know now that the SG contains a remarkably heterogenous group of neurons. Some almost certainly inhibit second order nociceptors. These include GABAergic and enkephalinergic cells. On the other hand, many SG neurons probably contribute to the firing of second order nociceptive projection neurons. For example, it has been proposed that some SG neurons are excitatory interneurons between primary afferent and second order, marginal nociceptors (100). As described above, one of the more surprising anatomical results is that large diameter fibers do not project directly into the SG. Thus, if their inhibitory action is mediated via the SG, then another population of neurons must also be involved, perhaps in lamina III. This is particularly true because few dendrites of SG neurons arborize beyond the SG.

The presence of enkephalin-containing neurons in the SG was, of course, consistent with the Gate Control Theory postulate of a local interneuron mediating an inhibitory control of nociceptors. More recently, it has been proposed that the pharmacological basis of acupuncture also reflects this anatomical organization. Acupuncture needling in the region where pain is perceived can apparently generate analgesia by at least two mechanisms. As Sjolund and Ericksson (109) demonstrated, the pharmacological basis of acupuncture analgesia depends on the parameters of needling. Low intensity, high frequency stimulation (which probably mimics a vibratory stimulus) generates analgesia in the area stimulated, but the analgesia is unaffected by the opiate antagonist, naloxone. On the other hand, analgesia can also be produced by high intensity, very low frequency stimulation, parameters that are more characteristic of traditional acupuncture needling. Naloxone abolished the analgesia produced with the latter parameters. It was hypothesized that the analgesia results from segmental activation of spinal enkephalin neurons, whose output can be blocked by naloxone. Clearly, one has to consider the central connections of afferent fibers which transmit the different parameters of stimulation. One can imagine, for example, that high intensity stimulation activates small diameter fibers, and that these excite dorsal horn enkephalin neurons. Gate Control Theory, in contrast, emphasized large fiber inhibition. The central connections of large fibers, and the pharmacological mechanism through which they generate analgesia are obviously different.

Gate Control Theory concentrated on the segmental control of nociceptive messages. Although a superspinal system was incorporated into the gate (the Central Control Trigger), the theory focused on the control exerted by large peripheral afferents. Recently, however, much attention has focused on the supraspinal control of spinal nociceptors and the relationship of endogenous opiate systems to that control. Reynolds (106), and Mayer and Liebeskind and Mayer and Price (86,87) demonstrated that profound analgesia can be produced by electrical stimulation of the midbrain periaqueductal gray. Many studies followed these early observations. Several studies demonstrated that the analgesic action of electrical brain stimulation involves descending systems, in part, through connections with the medullary serotonin-containing nucleus raphe magnus. A lesion of the dorsolateral funiculus of the spinal cord abolishes the analgesic affect of electrical brain stimulation (19); this apparently results from disruption of a raphe-spinal fiber system that terminates in laminae I, II, and V of the spinal dorsal horn, i.e., in those regions which contain spinal nociceptors (13,14,16,84). Electrical stimulation of either the periaqueductal gray (PAG) (93) or the raphe not only generates analgesia (94,95), but also inhibits spinal nociceptors (37,119). This is thought to be the basis of brain stimulation-produced analgesia (SPA).

The pharmacological basis of SPA has received considerable attention. Of particular importance are the striking similarities between the analgesic action of opiates and that produced by electrical brain stimulation. For example, the periaqueductal grey is the site most sensitive to intracranial opiate administration (127). Cross-tolerance between SPA and opiate analgesia has been demonstrated (85). Most importantly, the opiate antagonist naloxone not only reverses the analgesic action of systemic and intracerebrally administered opiates, but also that produced by electrical brain stimulation (4,66). It was thus proposed that electrical stimulation generates analgesia by activating an endogenous opiate system (15,36,87). The endorphin link in the system is the naloxone sensitive element.

Early hypotheses argued that there is an opiate receptor mediated event at the periaqueductal grey, and that exogenous opiates act at this site. On the other hand, the rostral ventromedial medulla is also exquisitely sensitive to opiate microinjection (2). In fact, nanogram doses elicit a potent analgesia; microgram doses are generally required in the PAG. Finally, it has been proposed that the opioid neuron in the cord is one of the final links in the descending neuronal chain, through which supraspinal control is exerted. Clearly multiple endogenous opioid components have been implicated in this endogenous pain suppression system; systemic naloxone could antagonize SPA by acting at superspinal sites or at the spinal opiate receptor.

LOCUS OF ACTION OF EXOGENOUS OPIATES

Given the model proposed above, it is likely that systemic opiates could produce analgesia by acting at the periaqueductal grey, in the medulla, or directly at the spinal cord; there is, in fact, evidence that all of these possibilities are true. Considerable discussion, however, has arisen concerning the predominant locus of action produced by systemic opiate injection. Those studies which demonstrated that the analgesic action of opiates is abolished by spinal cord transection (107), or by subtotal lesion (11,13,19), indicate that a supraspinal site of action predominates. On the other hand, Yaksh and Rudy (126) provide considerable evidence for a direct spinal action. Since the analgesic action of 10 mg/kg systemic morphine is abolished by spinal lesions and only reappears when the dose is increased to 15 mg/kg, it seems that at lower doses, the supraspinal site comes into play first (11). Yeung and Rudy (128), however, recently demonstrated that there is a multiplicative effect of morphine administered at supraspinal and spinal loci. These data indicate that neither the spinal nor the supraspinal site is activated independently; a systemic injection generates analgesia via interactions at both sites. From a practical point of view, of course, the effectiveness of local spinal opiate action is particularly important, and as described above, is the basis of important new analgesic therapies.

It is assumed that the mechanism of analgesia generated by supraspinal opiates is via activation of the descending control system that inhibits spinal nociceptors. On the other hand, the direct spinal action of morphine presumably generates analgesia by interaction with local binding sites, and consequent pre or postsynaptic inhibition of nociceptors (8,38,60,76). The presence of opiate binding sites on primary afferents is certainly consistent with a presynaptic action, despite the fact that enkephalin immunoreactive terminals presynaptic to primary afferents have not been unequivocally demonstrated. Still at issue, however, is whether the endogenous opiate neuron in the cord is part of a descending control system that is initiated in the periaqueductal grey (Fig. 5). Our early model proposed that 5HT axons from the medulla descend to the cord and synapse with enkephalin neurons (12,15). Behavioral studies of Yaksh (123), however, indicated that a 5HT-enkephalin connection was unlikely. He reported that the analgesic action of intracerebral morphine (injected into the periaqueductal grey) was not abolished by intrathecal naloxone. It was, however, antagonized by combined injection of the serotonin and norepinephrine antagonists, methysergide and phentolamine, respectively. He thus argued that an enkephalin link in the cord was not involved in the supraspinal control by the PAG. More recently, however, Zorman et al. (129,130), demonstrated that the suppression of the heat-evoked tail flick response by microstimulation in the medulla is abolished by intrathecal naloxone. Thus, their data implicate an enkephalin link in the spinal cord.

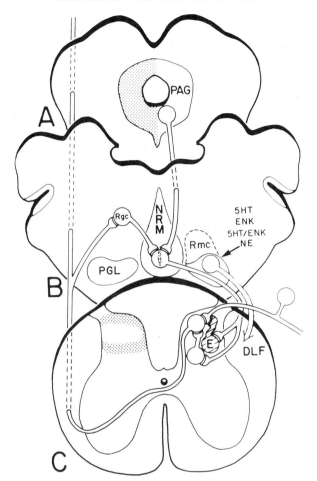

FIG. 5. Schematic diagram illustrating elements within a brainstem-spinal, endorphin, mediated pain suppression system. Enkephalin links are found in the periaqueductal grey, in the
medulla, and in the spinal dorsal horn. Enkephalin terminals are denoted by shading. Serotonergic
elements derive from the medullary nucleus raphe magnus (NRM) and from the adjacent nucleus
reticularis paragigantocellularis lateralis (PGL). In addition, the model indicates the possible contribution of norepinephrine-containing neurons, of neurons in which 5HT and enkephalin coexist,
and of neurons whose pharmacological identity has not been established (Rmc). Although a
presynaptic enkephalin action is indicated in the cord, postsynaptic actions are certain, and may,
in fact, predominate. Direct 5HT postsynaptic inhibition of spinal nociceptors is also likely. (Modified from Basbaum and Fields, ref. 15.)

Our laboratory directly evaluated this question using a combined ultrastructural,
immunocytochemical localization of enkephalin and autoradiographic localization
of serotonin (17). We demonstrated that there are, in fact, synaptic interactions
between descending serotonergic terminals and local spinal enkephalin neurons.
Obviously, the functional significance of this connection cannot be directly evaluated. Nevertheless, the connection clearly exists, and probably is involved in the

descending control. This, however, does not rule out a direct postsynaptic control of spinal nociceptors by descending serotonergic axons.

The issue of descending serotonergic-enkephalinergic interactions raises the more general question as to the mechanism by which the biogenic amines, their precursors, and a variety of specific uptake inhibitors either generate analgesia or enhance the analgesic action of a variety of compounds, including opiates. Tricyclic antidepressants, most commonly amitriptyline, are used for a variety of clinical pain syndromes, for example, postherpetic neuralgia (112). Admittedly, most chronic pain patients are depressed when they are seen by the neurologist; thus, any improvement in their psychological state will no doubt change their perception of the pain. Nevertheless, there is reason to believe that, in addition, to their antidepressant effect, the tricyclics exert a more direct antinociceptive action.

One possibility is that the antinociceptive action involves the descending serotonergic and noradrenergic terminals that play on spinal cord nociceptors. There is evidence, for example, that intrathecal application of either norepinephrine or serotonin exerts a potent analgesia, that is reversed by their appropriate blockers, but interestingly, not by naloxone (104,118). This, of course, suggests that either direct postsynaptic inhibitory effects are exerted by amines on spinal nociceptors, or that nonopioid interneuronal links are involved. Conceivably, any treatment that increases descending control exerted by the monoamines would facilitate or generate analgesia. A recent study indicated that intrathecal amitriptyline enhances opiate activity (25). Thus, uptake inhibitors would increase the concentration of serotonin and norepinephrine in the synaptic cleft, whereas precursor administration would increase the availability of the monoamine in the synaptic terminal. These treatments might enhance any analgesic therapy that uses these descending systems. Moreover, these drugs might minimize the "running down" of 5HT or norepinephrine with repeated analgesic therapy. This may explain how oral tryptophan can overcome some of the tolerance that occurs with repeated electrical brain stimulation (67,94).

Just as peripheral decarboxylase inhibitors significantly reduce the required dose of L-DOPA in the treatment of movement disorders, so a decarboxylase inhibitor coupled with tryptophan may be particularly helpful in the treatment of a variety of pain states. It should be emphasized, however, that tryptophan by itself is not an analgesic in humans. This suggests that the descending serotonergic control is not tonically active, but only comes into play when some analgesic treatment is initiated.

Although the association of serotonin with the antinociceptive properties of brain stimulation and morphine is quite strong, there is evidence that norepinephrine has contrasting spinal and supraspinal actions. At the spinal cord level, norepinephrine apparently synergizes with 5HT in inhibiting spinal nociceptors (57). In fact, norepinephrine may be more potent than 5HT. The origin of this noradrenergic control is certainly in the brainstem; however, the specific locus is unclear. Early studies pointed to the caudal medulla, e.g., in the A1 cell group, or in A6, i.e., the locus ceruleus; however, recent studies point to the midpontine, A5 group.

The spinal antinociceptive action of norepinephrine, however, is counterbalanced by an apparent antagonism of SPA and opiate analgesia at supraspinal sites. For example, microinjection of the α blocker phentolamine into the nucleus raphe magnus elicits a methysergide sensitive hypoalgesia (56), indicating that norepinephrine tonically *inhibits* descending, inhibitory raphe spinal axons. Earlier studies also reported antagonism of SPA by noradrenergic agonists (3). This dual noradrenergic action cautions against administering systemic norepinephrine agonists or antagonists. Complex agonist/antagonist effects will be generated. Clearly local application of the compound is necessary if a relatively undirectional effect, e.g., antinociception, is to be achieved. This point has general applicability. Not only can antagonistic actions be generated by systemic injections, but undesirable side effects also come into play. This is, of course, particularly true for the opiates; a major advantage of intrathecal opiate administration is that it offers a relatively selective analgesic treatment. The development of receptor specific opiate ligands may further narrow the biological effect produced.

If a drug has its analgesic effect by direct action on nociceptors, then the anatomy of "pain pathways" will dictate the best locus of administration. On the other hand, if the therapy activates a pain suppression system, then the best route and/or locus of drug therapy may differ significantly. There is evidence, for example, that endorphin-mediated endogenous pain suppression systems in part, underly the analgesic action of acupuncture (88), placebos (78), and a variety of "stress-producing" situations (79). If the pharmacology of those procedures which "tap into the endorphin" system can be identified, then new, specific avenues of analgesic therapy may be generated.

ACKNOWLEDGMENTS

I would like to thank the various authors who provided illustrations for this manuscript. I also thank Sandy Tsarnas and Alana Schilling for typing the manuscript. This work was supported by NS 14627, RCDA 00364, and the Sloan Foundation.

REFERENCES

1. Abols, I. A., and Basbaum, A. I. (1981): Afferent connections of the rostral medulla of the cat: A neural substrate for midbrain-medullary interactions in the modulation of pain. *J. Comp. Neurol.*, 201:285–297.
2. Akaike, A., Shibata, T., Satoh, M., and Takagi, H. (1978): Analgesia induced by microinjection of morphine into and electrical stimulation of the nucleus reticularis paragigantocellularis of rat medulla oblongata. *Neuropharmacology*, 17:775–778.
3. Akil, H., and Liebeskind, J. C. (1975): Monaminergic mechanisms of stimulation-produced analgesia. *Brain Res.*, 84:279–296.
4. Akil, H., Mayer, D. J., and Liebeskind, J. C. (1976): Antagonism of stimulation-produced analgesia by naloxone, a narcotic antagonist. *Science*, 191:961–962.
5. Albe-Fessard, D., and Besson, J. M. (1972): Convergent thalamic and cortical projections. The non-specific system. In: *Handbook of Sensory Physiology II: Somatosensory system*, edited by A. Iggo, pp. 489–560. Williams & Wilkins, Baltimore.
6. Applebaum, A. E., Leonard, R. B., Kenshalo, D. R., Martin, R. F., and Willis, W. D. (1979):

Nuclei in which functionally identified spinothalamic tract neurons terminate. *J. Comp. Neurol.*, 188:575–586.

7. Aronin, N., Difiglia, M., Liotta, A. S., and Martin, J. B. (1981): Ultrastructural localization and biochemical features of immunoreactive leu-enkephalin in monkey dorsal horn. *J. Neurosci.*, 1:561–578.

8. Atweh, S. E., and Kuhar, M. J. (1977): Autoradiographic localization of opiate-receptors in rat brain. I. Spinal cord and lower medulla. *Brain Res.*, 124:53–68.

9. Barber, R. P., Vaughn, J. E., Saito, K., McLaughlin, B. J., and Roberts, E. (1979): GABAergic terminals in the substantia gelatinosa of the rat spinal cord. *Brain Res.*, 141:35–55.

10. Barber, R. P., Vaughn, J. E., Slemmon, J. R., Salvaterra, P. M., Roberts, E., and Leeman, S. E. (1979): The origin distribution and synaptic relationships of substance P axons in rat spinal cord. *J. Comp. Neurol.*, 184:331–352.

11. Barton, C., Basbaum, A. I., and Fields, H. L. (1980): Dissociation of supraspinal and spinal actions of morphine: A quantitative evaluation. *Brain Res.*, 188:487–498.

12. Basbaum, A. I. (1981): Descending control of pain transmission: Possible serotonergic-enkephalinergic interactions. *Adv. Exp. Biol. Med.*, 133:177–189.

13. Basbaum, A. I., Clanton, C. H., and Fields, H. L. (1976): Opiate and stimulus-produced analgesia: Functional anatomy of a medullospinal pathway. *Proc. Natl. Acad. Sci. U.S.A.*, 73:4685–4688.

14. Basbaum, A. I., Clanton, C. H., Fields, H. L. (1978): Three bulbospinal pathways from the rostral medulla of the cat: An autoradiographic study of pain modulating systems. *J. Comp. Neurol.*, 178:209–224.

15. Basbaum, A. I., and Fields, H. L. (1978): Endogenous pain control mechanisms: Review and hypothesis. *Ann. Neurol.*, 4:451–462.

16. Basbaum, A. I., and Fields, H. L. (1979): The origin of descending pathways in the dorsolateral funiculus of the spinal cord of the cat and rat: Further studies on the anatomy of pain modulation. *J. Comp. Neurol.*, 187:513–522.

17. Basbaum, A. I., Glazer, E. J., and Lord, B. A. P. (1982): Simultaneous ultrastructural localization of tritiated serotonin and immunoreactive peptides. *J. Histochem. Cytochem.*, 30:780–784.

18. Basbaum, A. I., Glazer, E. J., and Oertel, W. (1981): A light and EM analysis of immunoreactive glutamic acid decarboxylase (GAD) in the spinal and trigeminal dorsal horn of the cat. *Neurosci. Abst.*, 7:528.

19. Basbaum, A. I., Marley, N. J. E., O'Keefe, J., and Clanton, C. H. (1977): Reversal of morphine and stimulus-produced analgesia by subtotal spinal cord lesions. *Pain*, 3:43–56.

20. Bennett, G. J., Abdelmoumene, M., Hayashi, H., and Dubner, R. (1980): Physiology and morphology of substantia gelatinosa neurons intracellulary stained with horseradish peroxidase. *J. Comp. Neurol.*, 194:809–828.

21. Bennett, G. J., Hayashi, H., Abdelmoumene, M., and Dubner, R. (1979): Physiological properties of stalked cells of the substantia gelatinosa intracellularly stained with horseradish peroxidase. *Brain Res.*, 164:285–289.

22. Bessou, P., and Perl, E. R. (1969): Response of cutaneous sensory units with unmyelinated fibers to noxious stimuli. *J. Neurophysiol.*, 32:1025–1043.

23. Boivie, J. (1979): An anatomical reinvestigation of the termination of the spinothalamic tract in the monkey. *J. Comp. Neurol.*, 186:343–370.

24. Boivie, J. (1971): The termination of the spinothalamic tract in the cat. An experimental study with silver impregnation methods. *Exp. Brain Res.*, 12:331–353.

25. Botney, M., and Fields, H. L. (1983): Amitryptyline potentiates morphine analgesia by a direct action on the central nervous system. *Ann. Neurol.*, 13:160–164.

26. Burgess, P. R., and Perl, E. R. (1967): Myelinated afferent fibers responding specifically to noxious stimulation of the skin. *J. Physiol.*, 190:541–562.

27. Carstens, E., and Trevino, D. L. (1978): Laminar origins of spinothalamic projections in the cat as determined by the retrograde transport of HRP. *J. Comp. Neurol.*, 182:151–166.

28. Casey, K. L. (1971): Somatosensory responses of bulboreticular units in awake cat: Relation to escape-producing stimuli. *Science*, 173:77–80.

29. Cassinari, V., and Pagni, C. A. (1969): *Central Pain*. Harvard University Press, Boston.

30. Cervero, F., and Iggo, A. (1980): The substantia gelatinosa of the spinal cord. A critical review. *Brain*, 103:717–772.

31. Cervero, F., Iggo, A., and Molony, V. (1979): An electrophysiological study of neurons in the substantia gelatinosa Rolandi of the cat's spinal cord. *Exp. Brain Res.*, 64:297–314.

32. Christensen, B. N., and Perl, E. R. (1970): Spinal neurons specifically excited by noxious or thermal stimuli: Marginal zone of the dorsal horn. *J. Neurol.*, 33:293–307.

33. Coggeshall, R. E., Applebaum, M. L., Fazen, M., Stubbs, T. B., and Stykes, M. (1975): Unmyelinated axons in human ventral roots: A possible explanation for the failure of dorsal rhizotomy to relieve pain. *Brain*, 98:157–166.

34. Dennis, S. G., and Melzack, R. (1980): Pain modulation by 5-hydroxytryptaminergic agents and morphine as measured by three pain tests. *Exp. Neurol.*, 69:260–270.

35. Duggan, A. W., Hall, J. G., and Headley, P. M. (1976): Morphine, enkephalin and the substantia gelatinosa. *Nature*, 264:456–458.

36. Fields, H. L., and Basbaum, A. I. (1978): Brainstem control of spinal pain transmission neurons. *Ann. Rev. Physiol.*, 40:193–221.

37. Fields, H. L., Basbaum, A. I., Clanton, C. H., and Anderson, S. D. (1977): Nucleus raphe magnus inhibition of spinal cord dorsal horn neurons. *Brain Res.*, 126:441–453.

38. Fields, H. L., Emson, P. C., Leigh, B. K., Gilbert, R. F. T., and Iverson, L. L. (1980): Multiple opiate receptor sites on primary afferent fibers. *Nature*, 284:351–353.

39. Fields, H. L., Wagner, G. M., and Anderson, S. D. (1975): Some properties of spinal neurons projecting to the medial brain stem reticular formation. *Exp. Neurol.*, 47:118–134.

40. Gamse, R., Holzer, P., and Lembeck, F. (1980): Decrease of substance P in primary afferent neurons and impairment of neurogenic plasma extravasation by capsaicin. *Br. J. Pharmacol.*, 68:207–214.

41. Giesler, G. J., Jr., Menetrey, D., and Basbaum, A. I. (1979): Differential origins of spinothalamic tract projections to medial and lateral thalamus in the rat. *J. Comp. Neurol.*, 194:107–126.

42. Giesler, G. J., Menetry, D., Guilbaud, G., and Besson, J. (1976): Lumbar cord neurons at the origin of the spinothalamic tract in the rat. *Brain Res.*, 118:320–324.

43. Giesler, G. J., Yezierski, R. P., Gerhart, K. D., and Willis, W. D. (1981): Spinothalamic tract neurons that project to medial and/or lateral thalamic nuclei: Evidence for a physiologically novel population of spinal cord neurons. *J. Neurophysiol.*, 46:1285–1308.

44. Glazer, E. J., and Basbaum, A. I. (1981): Immunohistochemical localization of leucine-enkephalin in the spinal cord of the cat: Enkephalin-containing marginal neurons and pain modulation. *J. Comp. Neurol.*, 196:377–390.

45. Glazer, E. J., and Basbaum, A. I. (1983): Opioid neurons and pain modulation: An ultrastructural analysis of enkephalin in cat superficial dorsal horn. *Neuroscience*, 10:357–376.

46. Glazer, E. J., Steinbusch, H., Verhofstad, A., and Basbaum, A. I. (1981): Serotonin and enkephalin coexist in neurons of the nucleus raphe dorsalis and paragigantocellularis of the cat. *J. Physiol. (Paris)*, 77:241–245.

47. Gobel, S. (1978): Golgi studies of the neurons in layer I of the dorsal horn of the medulla (trigeminal nucleus caudalis). *J. Comp. Neurol.*, 180:375–394.

48. Gobel, S. (1978): Golgi studies of the neurons in layer II of the dorsal horn of the medulla (trigeminal nucleus caudalis). *J. Comp. Neurol.*, 180:395–413.

49. Gobel, S., and Binck, J. M. (1977): Degenerative changes in primary trigeminal axons and in neurons in nucleus caudalis following tooth pulp extirpations in the cat. *Brain Res.*, 132:347–354.

50. Gobel, S., and Falls, W. M. (1979): Anatomical observations of horseradish peroxidase-filled terminal primary axonal arborizations in layer II of the substantia gelatinosa of Rolando. *Brain Res.*, 175:335–340.

51. Gobel, S., Falls, W. M., Bennett, G. J., Abdelmoumene, M., Hayashi, H., and Humphrey, E. (1980): An EM analysis of the synaptic connections of horseradish peroxidase filled stalked cells and islet cells in the substantia gelatinosa of adult cat spinal cord. *J. Comp. Neurol.*, 194:781–808.

52. Gobel, S., Falls, W. M., and Humphrey, E. (1981): A light and electron microscopical analysis of the morphology and synaptic connections of ultrafine primary axons which terminate in lamina I of the spinal dorsal horn. *Pain (Suppl.)*, 1:128.

53. Grant, G., and Arvidsson, J. (1975): Transganglionic degeneration in trigeminal primary neurons. *Brain Res.*, 95:265–279.

54. Guilbaud, G., Gautron, M., and Peschanski, M. (1981): Electrophysiological responses of neurons of the thalamic ventrobasal complex to cutaneous and articular stimulation in rats exhibiting inflammatory polyarthritis. *C.R. des Science*, 292:227–230.

55. Guilbaud, G., Peschanski, M., Gautron, M., and Binder, D. (1980): Neurons responding to

noxious stimulation in VB complex and caudal adjacent regions in the thalamus of the rat. *Pain*, 8:303–318.

56. Hammond, D. L., Levy, R. A., and Proudfit, H. K. (1980): Hypoalgesia induced by microinjection of a norepinephrine antagonist in the raphe magnus: Reversal by intrathecal administration of a serotonin antagonist. *Brain Res.*, 201:475–489.

57. Headly, P. M., Duggan, A. W., and Griersmith, B. T. (1978): Selective reduction by noradrenaline and 5HT of nociceptive responses of cat dorsal horn neurons. *Brain Res.*, 145:185–189.

58. Henry, J. L. (1976): Effects of substance P on functionally identified units in cat spinal cord. *Brain Res.*, 114:439–452.

59. Hentall, I. (1977): A novel class of unit in the substantia gelatinosa of the spinal cat. *Exp. Neurol.*, 53:792–806.

60. Hiller, J. M., Simon, E. J., Crain, S. M., and Peterson, E. R. (1978): Opiate receptors in cultures of fetal mouse dorsal root ganglia (DRG) and spinal cord: Predominance in DRG neurites. *Brain Res.*, 145:396–400.

61. Hokfelt, T., Elde, R., Johansson, O., Luft, R., Nilsson, G., and Arimura, A. (1976): Immuno-histochemical evidence for separate populations of somatostatin-containing and substance P-containing primary afferent neurons. *Neuroscience*, 1:131–136.

62. Hokfelt, T., Ljungdahl, A., Steinbusch, H., Verhofstad, A., Nilsson, G., Brodin, E., Pernow, B., and Goldstein, M. (1978): Immunohistochemical evidence of substance P-like immunoreactivity in some 5-HT-containing neurons in the rat central nervous system. *Neuroscience*, 3:517–538.

63. Hokfelt, T., Ljungdahl, A., Terenius, L., Elde, R., and Nilsson, G. (1977): Immunohistochemical analysis of peptide pathways possibly related to pain and analgesia: Enkephalin and substance P. *Proc. Natl. Acad. Sci. USA*, 74:3081–3085.

64. Hokfelt, T., Skirboll, L., Rehfeld, J. F., Goldstein, M., Markey, K., and Dann, O. (1980): A subpopulation of mesencephalic dopamine neurons projecting to limbic areas contains a chole-cytokinin-like peptide: Evidence from immunohistochemistry combined with retrograde tracing. *Neuroscience*, 5:2093–2124.

65. Hokfelt, T., Terenius, T., Kuypers, H. G. J. M., and Dann, O. (1979): Evidence for enkephalin immunoreactive neurons in the medulla oblongata projecting to the spinal cord. *Neurosci. Lett.*, 14:55–60.

66. Hosobuchi, Y., Adams, J. E., and Linchitz, R. (1977): Pain relief by electrical stimulation of the central gray matter in humans and its reversal by naloxone. *Science*, 197:183–186.

67. Hosobuchi, Y., Lamb, S., and Bascom, D. (1980): Tryptophan loading may reverse tolerance to opiate analgesics in humans: A preliminary report. *Pain*, 9:161–170.

68. Hunt, S. P., Kelly, J. S., and Emson, P. C. (1980): The electron microscopic localization of methionine-enkephalin within the superficial layers (I and II) of the spinal cord. *Neuroscience*, 5:1871–1890.

69. Hunt, S. P., Kelly, J. S., Emson, P. C., Kimmel, J. R., Miller, R. J., and Wu, J.-Y., (1981): An immunohistochemical study of neuronal populations containing neuropeptides or γ-aminobutyrate within the superficial layers of the rat dorsal horn. *Neuroscience*, 6:1883–1898.

70. Jancso, N. (1978): Desensitization with capsaicin and related acylamides as a tool for studying the function of pain receptors. In: *Pharmacology of Pain*, edited by R. K. S. Lin, pp. 33–55. Pergamon Press, New York.

71. Jancso, G., Kiraly, E., and Jansco-Gabor, A. (1977): Pharmacologically induced selective degeneration of chemosensitive primary afferent sensory neurons. *Nature*, 270:724–743.

72. Jessell, T. M., and Iversen, L. L. (1977): Opiate analgesics inhibit substance P release from rat trigeminal nucleus. *Nature*, 268:549–551.

73. Jessell, T. M., Iversen, L. L., and Cuello, A. C. (1978): Capsaicin-induced depletion of substance P from primary sensory neurons. *Brain Res.*, 152:183–188.

74. Jessell, T., Tsunoo, A., Kanazawa, I., and Otsuka, M. (1979): Substance P depletion in the dorsal horn of rat spinal cord after sections of the peripheral processes of primary sensory neurons. *Brain Res.*, 168:247–260.

75. Kenshalo, D. R., Jr., and Isensee, O. (1980): Response of primate SI cortical neurons to noxious stimuli. *Neurosci. Abstr.*, 6:245.

76. Lamotte, C., Pert, C. B., and Snyder, S. H. (1976): Opiate receptor binding in primate spinal cord: Distribution and changes after dorsal root section. *Brain Res.*, 112:407–412.

77. Lende, R. A., Kirsch, W. M., and Druckman, R. (1971): Relief of facial pain after combined removal of precentral and postcentral cortex. *J. Neurosurg.*, 34:537–543.

78. Levine, J. D., Gordon, N. C., and Fields, H. L. (1978): The mechanism of placebo analgesia. *Lancet*, 2:654–657.

79. Lewis, J. W., Cannon, J. T., and Liebeskind, J. C. (1980): Opioid and nonopioid mechanisms of stress analgesia. *Science*, 208:623–624.

80. Light, A. R., and Perl, E. R. (1979): Reexamination of the dorsal root projection to the spinal dorsal horn including observations on the differential termination of coarse and fine fibers. *J. Comp. Neurol.*, 186:117–132.

81. Light, A. R., and Perl, E. R. (1979): Spinal termination of functionally identified primary afferent neurons with slowly conducting myelinated fibers. *J. Comp. Neurol.*, 186:133–150.

82. Light, A. R., Trevino, D. L., and Perl, E. R. (1979): Morphological features of functionally defined neurons in the marginal zone and substantia gelatinosa of the spinal dorsal horn. *J. Comp. Neurol.*, 186:151–172.

83. Light, A. R., and Metz, C. B. (1978): The morphology of the spinal cord efferent and afferent neurons contributing to the ventral roots of the cat. *J. Comp. Neurol.*, 179:501–516.

84. Martin, R. F., Jordan, L. M., and Willis, W. D. (1978): Differential projections of cat medullary raphe neurons demonstrated by retrograde labelling following spinal cord lesions. *J. Comp. Neurol.*, 182:77–88.

85. Mayer, D., and Hayes, R. (1975): Stimulation-produced analgesia: Development of tolerance and cross-tolerance to morphine. *Science*, 188:941–943.

86. Mayer, D. J., and Liebeskind, J. C. (1974): Pain reduction by focal electrical stimulation of the brain: An anatomical and behavioral analysis. *Brain Res.*, 68:73–93.

87. Mayer, D. J., and Price, D. D. (1976): Central nervous system mechanisms of analgesia. *Pain*, 2:379–404.

88. Mayer, D. J., Price, D. D., and Rafii, A. (1977): Antagonism of acupuncture analgesia in man by the narcotic antagonist naloxone. *Brain Res.*, 121:368–372.

89. Melzack, R., and Wall, P. D. (1965): Pain mechanisms: A new theory. *Science*, 150:971–979.

90. Menetry, D., Chaouch, A., and Besson, J. M. (1980): Location and properties of dorsal horn neurons at origin of spinoreticular tract in lumbar enlargement of the rat. *J. Neurophysiol.*, 4:862–877.

91. Miletic, V., and Randic, M. (1979): Neurotensin excites cat spinal neurones located in laminae I–III. *Brain Res.*, 169:600–604.

92. Olgart, L., Hokfelt, T., Nilsson, G., and Pernow, B. (1977): Localization of substance P-like immunoreactivity in nerves in the tooth-pulp. *Pain*, 4:153–160.

93. Oliveras, J. L., Besson, J. M., Guilbaud, G., and Liebeskind, J. C. (1974): Behavioral and electophysiological evidence of pain inhibition from midbrain stimulation in the cat. *Exp. Brain Res.*, 20:32–44.

94. Oliveras, J. L., Hosobuchi, Y., Guilbaud, G., and Besson, J. M. (1978): Analgesic electrical stimulation of the feline nucleus raphe magnus: Development of tolerance and its reversal by 5-HTP. *Brain Res.*, 146:404–409.

95. Oliveras, J. L., Redjemi, F., Guilbaud, G., and Besson, J. M. (1975): Analgesia induced by electrical stimulation of the inferior central nucleus of the raphe in the cat. *Pain*, 2:139–146.

95a. Perl, E. R. The superficial dorsal horn: some ideas from the distant and not so distant past. In: *Spinal Cord Sensation*, edited by A. G. Brown and M. Rethelyi, pp. 59–77. Scottish Academic Press, Edinburgh.

96. Peschanski, M., Guilbaud, G., Gautron, M., and Besson, J. M. (1980): Encoding of noxious heat message in neurons of the ventrobasal thalamic complex of the rat. *Brain Res.*, 197:401–413.

97. Pepper, C. M., and Henderson, G. (1980): Opiates and opioid peptides hyperpolarize locus coeruleus neurons in vitro. *Science*, 209:394–396.

98. Piercey, M., Schroeder, L. A., (1981): Sensory and motor functions of spinal cord substance P. *Science*, 214:1361–1363.

99. Poggio, G. F., and Mountcastle, V. B. (1960): A study of the functional contributions of the lemniscal and spinothalamic systems to somatic sensibility. *Bull. Johns Hopkins Med. School*, 106:266–316.

100. Price, D. D., Hayashi, H., Dubner, R., and Ruda, M. A. (1979): Functional relationships between neurons of marginal and substantia gelatinosa layers of primate dorsal horn. *J. Neurophysiol.*, 42:1590–1608.

101. Proshansky, E., and Egger, M. D. (1977): Staining of the dorsal root projection to the cat's dorsal horn by anterograde movement of horseradish peroxidase. *Neurosci. Lett.*, 5:103–110.
102. Ralston, H. J., and Ralston, D. D. (1979): The distribution of dorsal root axons in laminae I, II and III of the macaque spinal cord: A quantitative electron microscopy study. *J. Comp. Neurol.*, 184:643–684.
103. Randic, M., and Miletic, V. (1978): Depressant actions of methionine-enkephalin and somatostatin in cat dorsal horn neurons activated by noxious stimuli. *Brain Res.*, 152:196–202.
104. Reddy, S. V. R., and Yaksh, T. L. (1980): Spinal noradrenergic terminal system mediates antinociception. *Brain Res.*, 189:391–402.
105. Rexed, B. (1952): The cytoarchitectonic organization of the spinal cord in the cat. *J. Comp. Neurol.*, 96:415–496.
106. Reynolds, D. V. (1969): Surgery in the rat during electrical analgesia induced by focal brain stimulation. *Science*, 164:444–445.
107. Satoh, M., and Takagi, H. (1971): Enhancement by morphine of the central descending inhibitory influence on spinal sensory transmission. *Eur. J. Pharmacol.*, 14:60–65.
108. Seybold, V., and Elde, R. (1982): Neurotensin immunoreactivity in the superficial laminae of the dorsal horn of the rat. I. Light microscopic studies of cell bodies and proximal dendrites. *J. Comp. Neurol.*, 205:89–100.
109. Sjolund, B. J., and Ericksson, M. B. E. (1979): The influence of naloxone and analgesia produced by peripheral conditioning stimulation. *Brain Res.*, 178:295–302.
110. Strick, P. L. (1975): Multiple sources of thalamic input to the primate motor cortex. *Brain Res.*, 88:372–377.
111. Swanson, L. W., and McKellar, S. (1979): The distribution of oxytocin- and neurophysin-stained fibers in the spinal cord of the rat and monkey. *J. Comp. Neurol.*, 188:87–106.
112. Taub, A. (1973): Relief of postherpetic neuralgia with psychotropic drugs. *Neurosurgery*, 39:235–239.
113. Theriault, E., Otsuka, M., and Jessell, T. (1979): Capsaicin-evoked release of substance P from primary sensory neurons. *Brain Res.*, 170:209–213.
114. Trevino, D. L., Coulter, J. D., and Willis, W. D. (1973): Location of cells of origin of spinothalamic tract in lumbar enlargement of the monkey. *J. Neurophysiol.*, 36:750–761.
115. Wall, P. D. (1967): The laminar organization of dorsal horn and effects of descending impulses. *J. Physiol.*, 188:403–423.
116. Wall, P. D., and Gutnick, M. (1974): Ongoing activity in peripheral nerves: The physiology and pharmacology of impulses orginating from a neuroma. *Exp. Neurol.*, 43:580–593.
117. Wall, P. D., Scadding, J. W., and Tomkiewica, M. M. (1979): The production and prevention of experimental anesthesia dolorosa. *Pain*, 6:175–182.
118. Wang, J. K. (1977): Antinociceptive effect of inthrathecally administered serotonin. *Anesthesiology*, 47:269–271.
119. Willis, W. D., Haber, L. H., and Martin, R. F. (1977): Inhibition of spinothalamic tract cells and interneurons by brainstem stimulation in the monkey. *J. Neurophysiol.*, 40:968–981.
120. Willis, W. D., Kenshalo, J. R., and Leonard, R. B. (1979): The cells of origin of the primate spinothalamic tract. *J. Comp. Neurol.*, 188:543–574.
121. Willis, W. D., Trevino, D. L., Coulter, J. D., and Maunz, R. A. (1974): Responses of primate spinothalamic tract neurons to natural stimulation of hindlimb. *J. Neurophysiol.*, 37:358–372.
122. Wilson, P. R., and Yaksh, T. L. (1978): Baclofen is antinociceptive in the spinal intrathecal space of animals. *Eur. J. Pharmacol.*, 51:323–330.
123. Yaksh, T. L. (1979): Direct evidence that spinal serotonin and noradrenaline terminals mediate the spinal antinociceptive effects of morphine in the periaqueductal gray. *Brain Res.*, 160:180–185.
124. Yaksh, T. L., Farb, D. H., Leeman, S. E., and Jessell, T. M. (1979): Intrathecal capsaicin depletes substance P in the rat spinal cord and produces prolonged thermal analgesia. *Science*, 206:481–483.
125. Yaksh, T. L., Jessell, T. M., Gamse, R., Mudge, A.W., and Leeman, S. E. (1980): Intrathecal morphine inhibits substance P release from mammalian spinal cord *in vivo*. *Nature*, 286:155–156.
126. Yaksh, T. L., and Rudy, T. A. (1976): Analgesia mediated by a direct spinal action of narcotics. *Science*, 192:1357–1358.
127. Yaksh, T. L., and Rudy, T. A. (1978): Narcotic analgesics: CNS sites and mechanisms of action as revealed by intracerebral injection techniques. *Pain*, 4:299–360.

128. Yeung, J. C., and Rudy, T. A. (1980): Multiplicative interaction between narcotic agonists expressed at spinal and supraspinal sites of antinociceptive action as revealed by concurrent intrathecal and intracerebroventricular injections of morphine. *J. Pharmacol. Exp. Ther.*, 215:633–642.
129. Zorman, G., Belcher, C., Adams, J. E., and Fields, H. L. (1982): Lumbar intrathecal naloxone blocks analgesia produced by microstimulation of the ventromedial medulla in the rat. *Brain Res.*, 236:77–84.
130. Zorman, G., Hentall, I. D., Adams, J. E., and Fields, H. L. (1981): Naloxone-reversible analgesia produced by microstimulation in the rat medulla. *Brain Res.*, 219:137–148.

Analgesics: Neurochemical, Behavioral, and Clinical Perspectives, edited by M. Kuhar and G. Pasternak. Raven Press, New York © 1984.

Chemistry of Opiate Analgesics and Antagonists

William F. Michne

Medicinal Chemistry Department, Sterling-Winthrop Research Institute, Rensselaer, New York 12144

The subject of pain and its relief is no doubt as old as the human race. Pain, of course, is an extremely important protective phenomenon; it tells the body that a health problem, either a disease or trauma, exists. On the other hand, pain from an injury may not be felt under extremely stressful conditions (the wounded soldier in battle is a frequently cited example). In such cases, the drive for survival preempts the perception of pain as a behavior determinant. Alleviation of the stressful condition is accompanied by an awareness of the pain, which may then be inordinately intense. Whatever the circumstances of its appearance, pain, after fulfilling its role as a warning signal, becomes a useless agony to be endured.

Throughout history, many techniques have been employed to alleviate the suffering of pain. Most were worthless, a few were dangerous, and some actually have been fatal. Opium, the dried exudate from lanced unripe seed capsules of *Papaver somniferum* was the most widely used effective remedy. The bad effects of opium such as respiratory depression, nausea and vomiting, constipation, and physical dependence, if recognized, were ascribed to the presence of noxious resins in the preparation. Early in the 19th century, pure morphine was isolated from opium, an event which allowed the developing science of pharmacology to clearly establish a causal relationship between the drug and its effects. During the 20th century, organic chemists deduced the structure of morphine, achieved its total synthesis, and prepared thousands of structurally similar compounds in an effort to minimize morphine's undesirable effects, while retaining its potent analgesic property. To some extent, that effort has been successful. Many agents are available, which exhibit some advantage over morphine. No single compound, however, has yet been identified which has advantages over morphine in all aspects of its pharmacologic profile. Thus, the search continues. The sheer immensity of the body of medicinal chemical knowledge which has been amassed, largely during this century, precludes all but a superficial treatment of the subject in this chapter. After a brief description of the most commonly used bioassay systems, attention will be focused on major developments in each of a number of important structural classes, including some new drugs in development. In addition, the recent and continuing discoveries of endogenous opioids have opened new fields of research on their functions in health and disease. The possibility of controlling aberrant opioid function through the use of pure opioid antagonists represents an exciting new challenge to the medicinal chemist. This aspect of opioid research will be briefly discussed.

Many in depth reviews of and monographs on various aspects of the medicinal chemistry of opioids have been published. The monograph edited by deStevens (30) is a good general treatment of the subject through the early sixties. The reviews by Casy (22,23) cover the period 1962 through 1977. The reviews by Archer and Harris (10) and by Archer and Michne (11) treat the subject of narcotic antagonists primarily as analgesics.

COMMON BIOASSAYS OF NEW COMPOUNDS

Some idea of the problem of devising an animal test system for the evaluation of a new compound's potential as an analgesic agent is evident from the great variety of approaches which have been described. The qualitative emotional aspects of the pain experience, and the variability of reactions to nociceptive stimuli of a given intensity among individual members of a species, make the development of meaningful bioassays a formidable task. Nevertheless, a few model systems have achieved a degree of importance because they possess, by accident or design, certain attributes. For example, these methods allow the threshold value of the nociceptive stimulus required to produce a reaction to be controlled and quantified. This is achieved either by graded stimulus intensity or by duration of a constant stimulus intensity. The stimulus and its intensity do not cause tissue damage, in the case of unmedicated preparations, as well as in preparations under the influence of active drugs where thresholds or durations are increased. The model systems are sufficiently sensitive to detect weak activity so that new lead compounds are not overlooked, but are not so sensitive as to give many false positive results. They are, for the most part, simple and inexpensive to conduct, highly reproducible, and give results that correlate well with the human data on standard drug substances. Described below are many of these test systems which are presently in common use throughout the opiate research community.

In Vivo Methods

The pioneering work of Hardy et al. (53), on the quantitative determination of pain threshold through the application of localized heat to elicit a response, resulted in the development of two thermal stimulus tests of importance. The first of these is the mouse hot-plate test first described by Woolfe and MacDonald (118). In this test, mice are placed on a plate, where the temperature can be controlled and varied, usually from 50 to 70°C. The time required for the mouse to kick with the hind paws or attempt to jump out of the apparatus is taken as the reaction time. The second test is the rat tail flick test first described by D'Armour and Smith (28). This test measures the time required for a rat to withdraw its tail on exposure to a radiant heat stimulus. Both of these tests are highly selective for pure narcotic agonist agents, and are reproducible in determining relative potencies of such compounds at doses approximately 10 times higher than those used in man. These tests and others may also be used to measure a new compound's antagonist activity by observing reversal of an agonist effect. For example, Harris and Pierson (54) reported a method for evaluating narcotic antagonist activity based on graded reaction times for the tail flick response of rats. Other assays for opioid antagonist activity include counteraction of oxymorphone induced narcosis in rats (17), prevention of the narcotic induced Straub tail phenomenon in mice (4), and reversal of respiratory depression produced in unanesthetized rabbits by morphine (84).

The hot-plate and tail flick tests have the disadvantage of not being able to predict the analgesic activity of mixed narcotic agonist/antagonist analgesics such as nalorphine and pentazocine. This led to a number of successful attempts to devise models which would be predictive of human analgesia for this very important class of compounds. One such group of tests is based on measuring the ability of a test compound to inhibit a characteristic abdominal response (writhe) of mice to intraperitoneal injections of chemical nociceptive agents. The most commonly used chemical agents are paraphenylquinone (PPQ) and acetylcholine (ACH). The PPQ test was first described by Siegmund et al. (106). Hendershot and Forsaith (58) reported that the technique gave too many "false positives," but Taber et al. (109) showed that narcotic antagonists, which were clinically active analgesics but gave negative reponses in the tail flick test, gave positive results in this assay. Furthermore, the order of potency was close to that observed clinically. Collier et al. (26) studied a variety of nociceptive agents and found that ACH produced a writhing response within 2 min. Although a number of false positives were observed, narcotic antagonist analgesics were active. A rank order correlation of 14 analgesics was made between the potencies in the ACH test with the potencies in man; a rho value of 0.908 was obtained.

An assay method using electrical stimulation of the tail of mice as first described by Nilsen (91), and modified by Helsley et al. (57), was suggested as being simple, economical, and predictive for the narcotic antagonists. Perrine et al. (94) reported what they believed to be improvements in instrumentation and methodology. They compared this method with the hot-plate procedure for several compounds including pure agonists, a pure antagonist, several mixed agonist/antagonists, and two compounds of relatively unknown pharmacology. The results obtained indicated the method's superior predictive value for man with those substances possessing antagonist properties. This method is now routinely used for compounds submitted for testing under the auspices of the Committee on Problems of Drug Dependence (CPDD).

The CPDD also sponsors a testing program in monkeys which addresses various aspects of the classical problem of physical dependence on opiates (2,117). The single dose suppression test (SDS) determines the ability of a drug to suppress the signs of abstinence in monkeys, which have been made physically dependent by the chronic administration of morphine. Compounds suspected of having morphine-antagonist properties are tested for their ability to precipitate the abstinence syndrome in nonwithdrawn (NW) morphine-dependent monkeys. Nondependent monkeys (normals) are used to determine whether the acute effects of the test drug are reversible by nalorphine or naloxone. In a primary addiction study (PAS), nondependent monkeys receive the test drug every 6 hr for 30 days to determine whether abstinence signs will appear when the animals are challenged with an antagonist, or when drug administration is discontinued. Some indication of a compound's euphorigenic properties, and hence, its potential for eliciting drug seeking behavior is obtained from self administration studies. Compounds are examined in animals which have been conditioned to self-inject codeine. Saline is used as a negative control. A number of doses of the test compound are administered until a maximum rate of responding is obtained or until, in the absence of evidence of a reinforcing effect, directly observable changes in behavior are elicited by the compound.

In Vitro Methods

In 1957, Paton (93) demonstrated that the contraction of the coaxially stimulated longitudinal muscle of the guinea pig ileum (GPI) was inhibited by opiates. Gyang and Kosterlitz (51) and Kosterlitz and Watt (72) exploited this observation and developed a very useful *in vitro* assay to evaluate the agonist and antagonist actions of narcotic antagonists. In this preparation, the ID_{50} is the concentration of drug needed to inhibit the twitch height by 50%, and is a measure of agonist potency. The Ke is an equilibrium constant and is that concentration of the antagonist which will shift the dose-response curve of the agonist to the right by a factor of 2; it is a measure of antagonist potency. A limitation of this assay is that it is impossible to evaluate the antagonist potencies of compounds which are also potent agonists. Henderson et al. (59) found that the mouse vas deferens (MVD) preparation behaved similarly to the GPI for pure agonists, but had an advantage, in that the dose-response curves for potent agonist/antagonists were flat or actually sloped downward. This allowed the evaluation of the antagonist activity of compounds with a potent agonist component.

Goldstein et al. (45) described a method for analyzing the association of the opiate narcotic levorphanol with brain tissue into three components: nonsaturable, saturable nonspecific, and saturable stereospecific. In mouse brain, the stereospecific binding of levorphanol represented only 2% of the total association of drug with tissue, but was found only in certain membrane fractions. They suggested that the material responsible for the stereospecific binding might be the opiate receptor. Pert and Snyder (95) and Simon et al. (107) used a modification of the Goldstein method, which consisted of using very low concentrations of labeled ligand, made possible by very high-specific radioactivity, and washing of the homogenates after incubation with a cold buffer to remove contaminating unbound and loosely bound radioactivity. The specific binding was of sufficient affinity to withstand the cold washes and constituted a major portion of the total residual binding. Pert and Snyder used [3H]naloxone and found binding unaffected by high ionic strength, whereas Simon et al. used [3H]etorphine, and found its binding effectively prevented by high ionic strength. Pert and Snyder (96) subsequently reported that receptor binding of antagonists is enhanced, and that receptor binding of agonists is diminished by sodium ions. This work resulted in the concept of the sodium index, the ratio of the compounds $ID_{50}s$ in the presence and absence of 100 mM sodium ion. Naloxone and other antagonists have low sodium indices, generally around 1.0 or less; pure agonists have indices in the 12 to 60 range; morphine's sodium index is 37. However, caution is advised in the interpretation of sodium index data, because some known agonists, notably the peptides, have lower than expected sodium indices (24).

MULTIPLE OPIATE RECEPTORS

The study of thousands of semisynthetic and synthetic opiates during this century led to speculations about the opiate receptor. One of the earliest and best known is that of Beckett and Casy (13) which essentially summarized the chemical structural requirements for analgesics based on structure-activity data. Portoghese (100) studied several discrepanices in such data, and was the first to speculate on the possible existence of multiple opiate receptors. Martin and co-workers (81), based on behavioral and neurophysiological observations on standard opiates in the chronic spinal dog model, postulated that there are at least three types of opiate receptors. Morphine is the prototype agonist for the μ-receptor, ketazocine for the κ-receptor, and SKF 10,047 for the σ-receptor. Lord et al. (79) studied both classical and peptide (*see* chapter by Fredrickson) opiates in the GPI and MVD assays, and found that some peptides were relatively more potent in the MVD. They proposed the existence in the MVD of a new type of receptor, the δ-receptor. Kosterlitz et al. (70) found that D-Ala^2-D-Leu^5-enkephalin (DADLE) was very selective for the δ-receptor. DADLE has become the prototype for this receptor. Recently, Gacel and co-workers (43) reported that the hexapeptide Tyr-D-Ser-Gly-Phe-Leu-Thr is a highly preferential ligand for the δ-receptor, about seven times more selective than DADLE. The pure antagonist naloxone is selective for the μ-receptor; no antagonists are known to be selective for either the κ- or δ-receptors. It is not at all clear what physiologic functions are subserved by each receptor population, if indeed there are any differences. Nevertheless, the identification of receptor subtypes represents an irresistable challenge to the medicinal chemist to attempt to synthesize agonists and antagonists with increased receptor selectivity.

CHEMISTRY AND STRUCTURE-ACTIVITY RELATIONSHIPS

Opium Alkaloids and Their Derivatives

Opium is the dried sap of the unripe seed capsule of *Papaver somniferum* or opium poppy, which is indigenous to Asia Minor. Its effects have been known since antiquity, the earliest medicinal uses being ascribed to the Sumerians ca. 4000 B.C. Throughout history, it has been used in the form of aqueous or alcoholic extracts, or consumed as the solid or suspensions for virtually every ill encountered by mankind. The harmful effects of these preparations were frequently blamed on the presence of impurities. In 1805, a pharmacist's assistant named Serturner described the isolation of a crystalline substance from opium, which he named morphine after Morpheus, the Greek god of sleep. Serturner observed that morphine was capable of neutralizing acids and he therefore referred to the material as "vegetable alkalai." That term later gave way to the term "alkaloid;" morphine was thus the first alkaloid to be isolated in the pure state. Sometime later, two other alkaloids, codeine and thebaine, were isolated and shown to be related structurally to morphine, although their precise structures were unknown. After years of chemical degradative work by generations of organic chemists, the correct structure of morphine (Fig. 1, **1a**) was proposed by Gulland and Robinson in 1925 (50), and the structures of codeine (**1b**), and thebaine (**2**) followed. These structures were firmly established by the report of the total syntheses of morphine by Gates and Tschudi (44) in 1952, and by Elad and Ginsburg (35) in 1954. The absolute

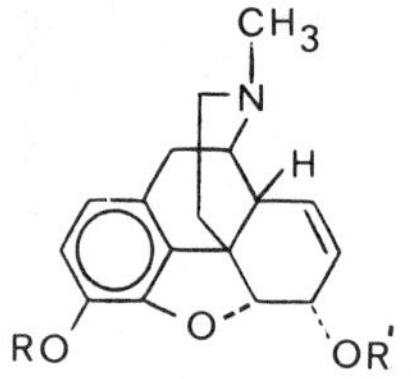

1a, R = R' = H
 b, R = CH₃, R' = H
 c, R = R' = CH₃CO

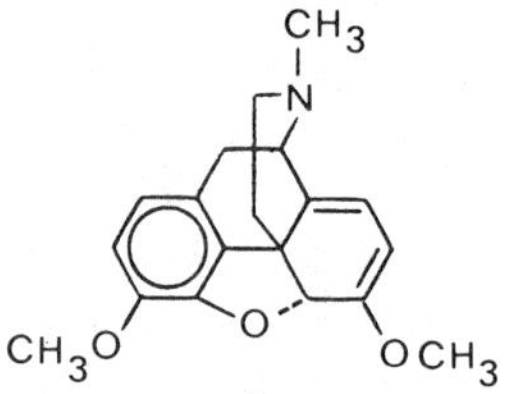

2

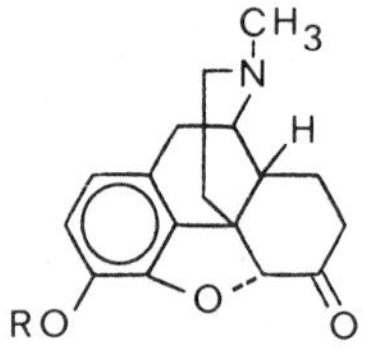

3a, R = H
 b, R = CH₃

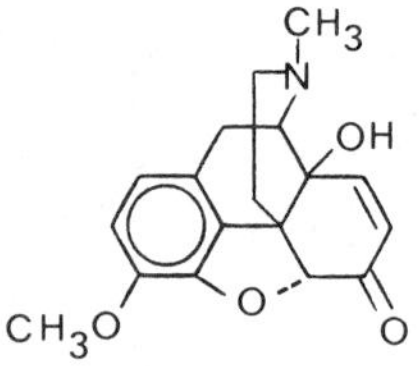

4

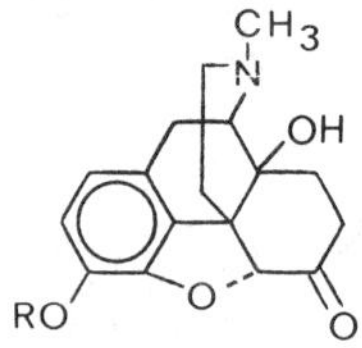

5a, R = CH₃
 b, R = H

FIG. 1. Alkaloids of opium and related compounds.

stereochemistry of morphine was established by X-ray crystallography in 1955 (80).

Pharmacologically, morphine is active in all the standard bioassays for analgesia. It is a potent analgesic in man, and is the standard against which all new analgesics are compared. It is indicated for the symptomatic relief of severe pain, and is usually administered intramuscularly. The onset of analgesia occurs within 1 hr, and lasts about 4 hr. The drug depresses the cough center; its principal side effects are nausea and vomiting, respiratory depression, and constipation. Continued use results in tolerance to its analgesic effect, leading to the need for increasing doses to obtain the same degree of pain relief. Continued use also leads to physical dependence on the drug, and abrupt withdrawal of the drug results in a characteristic withdrawal syndrome.

Codeine (**1b**) is the 3-O-methyl ether of morphine. In animal tests, it is less potent than morphine, and *in vitro* it is less potent still. The same is true for other 3-O-alkyl derivatives of morphine. It has been suggested (71) that the virtual inactivity of codeine *in vitro* is because it is not converted to morphine under these conditions. This conversion has been shown to be required for the activity of codeine *in vivo* (5). The compound is used orally for the relief of mild to moderate pain, and as an antitussive. It is frequently combined with mild analgesics such as acetaminophen. Because its action is much weaker than that of morphine (approximately one-sixth) it appears less likely to elicit nausea, vomiting, constipation, or respiratory depression. It also has a lower potential than morphine for development of tolerance and physical dependence.

Thebaine (**2**) is among the less abundant (0.3 to 1.5%) of the phenanthrene alkaloids of opium. It is of no value medicinally in that its actions are stimulatory to the point of causing seizures. Its real value lies in its use as a chemical-starting material for the preparation of a variety of semisynthetic opiates of considerable theoretical and practical significance. These uses will be discussed as they arise.

The clinical disadvantages of morphine have resulted in considerable synthetic activity which persists today. During the decade of the thirties, a large number of morphine derivatives were prepared and evaluated as analgesics under the auspices of the CPDD, and the results published in a monograph (108). These data allowed several general conclusions to be drawn. Among the more important are the following: (a) masking the phenolic hydroxyl with an alkyl group (e.g., morphine→codeine) decreases activity; (b) acylation of the phenolic hydroxyl (e.g., morphine→heroin, **1c**) increases activity; (c) if the C-6 hydroxyl is removed, or oxidized, or replaced by halogen, morphine-like activity is enhanced; (d) cleavage of the 4,5-oxygen bridge reduces activity; (e) reduction of the double bond has little effect. From this and related work, some compounds of interest emerged. For example, reduction of the 6,7-double bond of morphine and oxidation of the C-6 hydroxyl to a carbonyl gives hydromorphone, **3a** (101). The compound is readily absorbed, has a more rapid onset, and somewhat longer duration of analgesic action than does morphine. In addition, it is about twice as potent as morphine. Side effects are similar to those with morphine but are less frequently encountered and are less severe. The analogous codeine derivative **3b** is prepared from codeine in a similar fashion. This compound is somewhat more potent as an analgesic and antitussive than is codeine and is generally better tolerated; constipation and gastric upset are rarely seen.

Thebaine may be oxidized under a variety of conditions (e.g., H_2O_2/HOAc or chromic acid) to provide hydroxy codeinone **4** (42). Catalytic hydrogenation yields oxycodone **5a**. This compound is 5 to 6 times as potent an analgesic as codeine; its addiction potential is high. Its clinical value lies in its ready absorption after oral administration, rapid onset (15 min), and fairly long duration (up to 5 hr). Closely related structurally to oxycodone is oxymorphone **5b** obtained from **5a** by refluxing concentrated hydrobromic acid (115). Parenterally administered oxymorphone is about 10 times as potent as morphine, with rapid onset (as little as 5 min) and fairly long duration (up to 6 hr). This advantage of this drug is that it produces only mild sedation and little depression of the cough reflex.

The compounds discussed so far are all classical narcotic analgesics, i.e., to a greater or lesser extent they share with the parent morphine the same prominent agonist effects such as analgesia, sedation, respiratory depression, and miosis. In 1915, Pohl (98) reported the morphine antagonist properties of N-allylnorcodeine (Fig. 2, **6a**). About 10 years later, VonBraun and co-workers (113) reported the synthesis and antimorphine effects of a series of alkyl and cycloalkyl derivatives

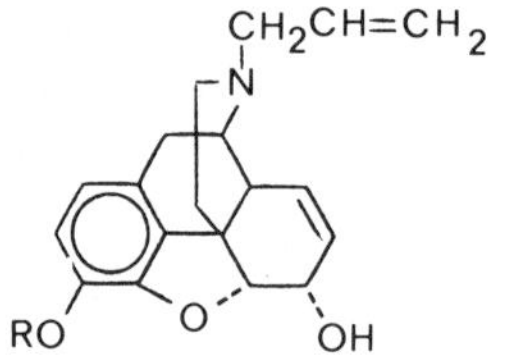

6a, R = CH$_3$
b, R = H

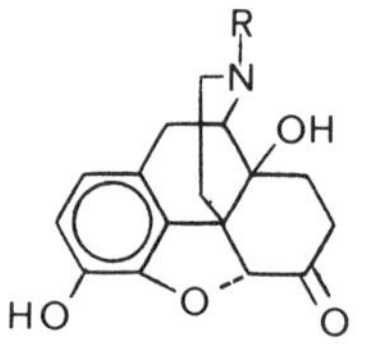

7a, R = CH$_2$CH = CH$_2$
b, R = CH$_2$◁

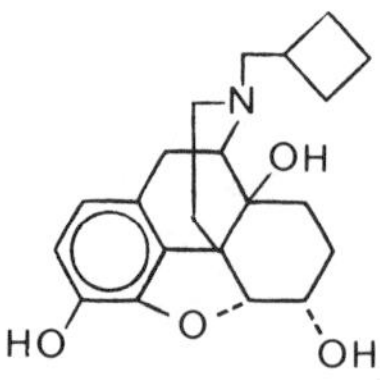

8

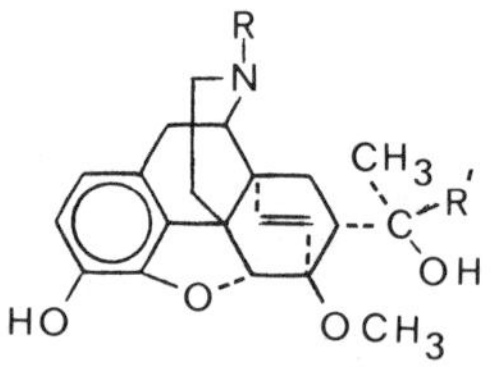

9a, R = CH$_3$, R' = C$_3$H$_7$
b, dihydro, R = CH$_2$◁,
R' = C(CH$_3$)$_3$

FIG. 2. Agonist/antagonists derived from opium alkaloids.

of norcodeine. These observations remained unnoticed until the early 1940s when the synthesis and pharmacological properties of N-allylnormorphine (nalorphrine, **6b**) were announced (55,114).

In the hope that a mixture of morphine and nalophine could be found which would not antagonize the analgesic properties of morphine and yet would abolish the respiratory depressant action, Lasagna and Beecher (74) undertook a controlled study of mixtures of these drugs using nalorphine alone as a control. In this way, the clinical analgesic effects of nalorphine were first observed. This observation was quickly confirmed and extended by Keats and Telford (68), who found that the antagonist was as effective as morphine in relieving postoperative pain. The psychotomimetic effects attending the use of nalorphine as an analgesic precluded its clinical acceptance, despite the fact that Isbell (65) found nalorphine nonaddicting.

These observations opened a period of intense research on narcotic antagonists. In a classic paper, Winter et al. (116) reported their studies of the effects on analgesic and antagonist activity of a variety of substituents on the nitrogen atom of morphine and related compounds. They found that in the morphine series, compounds with three carbon chains such as allyl, propyl, isobutyl, and methallyl have some degree of antimorphine activity. Lengthening the side chain beyond butyl resulted in a return to morphine-like activity. None of the morphine derivatives with aromatic side chains were antagonists; N-phenylethylnormorphine was an extraordinarily potent analgesic agent. Furthermore, N-allylnormeperidine was found not to be an antagonist. Thus, research focused on the attachment of short chains to the nitrogen atom of at least tricyclic ring systems (10). Because oxymorphone is a more potent agonist than morphine, it was speculated that the corresponding N-allyl derivative might be more potent than nalorphine, and perhaps show less of the latter's undesirable side effects, such as respiratory depression and psychotomimetic reactions. N-allylnoroxymorphone or naloxone **(7a)** was synthesized by Lewenstein and Fishman (75), was found by Blumberg et al. (18) to be 10 to 20 times more active than nalorphine when tested by prevention of Straub tail erection (s.c.) in mice, by counteraction of narcosis (s.c.) in rats, and by counteraction of narcotic depression of respiration (i.v.) in rabbits. Kosterlitz and Watt (72) found naloxone to be devoid of agonist effects in the guinea pig ileum. Naloxone was thus the first pure opioid antagonist to be identified. The closely related naltrexone, **7b**, is two to three times more active than naloxone as an antagonist, but shows some antinociceptive activity in the rat (16,19). Both drugs are essentially devoid of agonist effects in man (67,83). There is now considerable interest in the use of such compounds to prevent the resumption of drug seeking behavior in postaddicts (82). In addition, the implication of the recently discovered endogenous opioids as mediators in a variety of pathophysiological states suggests the use of pure opioid antagonists for the treatment of those states. For example, Holaday and Faden (60) reasoned that because the cardiovascular system is extremely sensitive to the effects of endogenous opiates, and the action of stressors seems to result in the release of β-endorphin, then it seems likely that β-endorphin is released during shock states, and that it might contribute to the hypotension. To test the hypothesis, they used an endotoxin shock model in the rat and found that naloxone pretreatment (10 mg/kg) blocked the effects of 4 mg of endotoxin on mean arterial blood pressure. Using a hypovolemic shock model in the rat, they showed (36) that 1 mg/kg naloxone significantly increased survival. Lightman and Jacobs (78), based on earlier reports that an enkephalin analog caused severe facial flushing and that naloxone inhibits the chlorpropamide induced alcoholic flushing of diabetics, investigated the effect of naloxone infusion on post menopausal flushing. Using only 4 patients, they found that the number of flushing episodes was significantly reduced during periods of naloxone infusion. Recently, Verebey et al. (112) reviewed the role of endorphins in psychiatry. The evidence presented in the review was compatible with a hypothesis that the level of functional endorphins may be related to psychological events, with a normal level needed for psychological homeostasis. A corollary of this hypothesis is that the level of opioids in the brains of the mentally ill may be disturbed; experiments with opiate antagonists have provided limited support for the hypothesis of endorphin excess and no support for the hypothesis of endorphine deficiency.

Efforts to find a useful mixed agonist/antagonist analgesic related to oxymorphone and naloxone resulted in the discovery of nalbuphine, **8**. In man, the compound is about equiactive with morphine. Houde et al. (61) found nalbuphine to be about three times more active than pentazocine and to produce less psychotomimetic effects.

A second major class of agonists and antagonists derived from thebaine are the result of Diels-Alder additions to thebaine's diene system followed by further transformations. The chemistry and biological activity of this group was described by Lewis and co-workers over several years (76,77). The complex structure-activity relationships depend largely on R, R' and the configuration of C-19 of structure **9**, and the effects of these changes are interrelated. For example, increasing the size of R' increases activity to a maximum at R'=propyl (etorphine, **9a**, is about 1,000 times as active as morphine), whereas in the C-19 epimer series activity is generally low and largely independent of the size of R'. Also, when R is an antagonist side chain such as cyclopropylmethyl, antagonist activity gives way to agonist activity as R' increases to propyl. A compound of major importance in the series is buprenorphine **9b**. Cowan et al. (27) studied the agonist and antagonist properties of buprenorphine. The compound is 25 to 40 times more active than morphine in the mouse writhing assay, and did not produce physical dependence in the monkey. They concluded that the compound represents a definite advance in the search for a narcotic antagonist analgesic of low physical dependence potential. However, this drug is not yet available in the United States.

Morphinans and Benzomorphans

Early reaction sequence modeling directed toward the total synthesis of morphine led Grewe (47) to the morphinan ring system **10** by the route shown in Fig. 3.

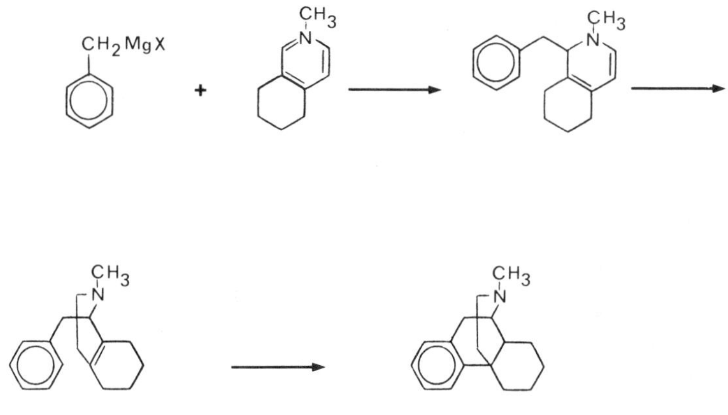

10

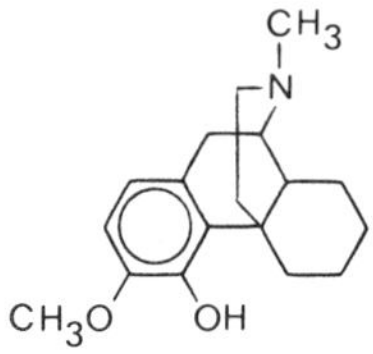

11

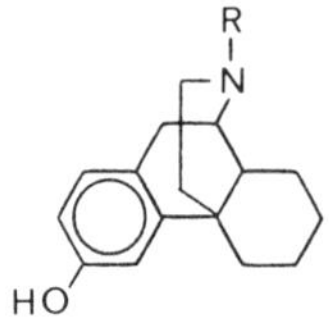

12a, (-), R = CH_3
b, (-), R = $CH_2CH{=}CH_2$

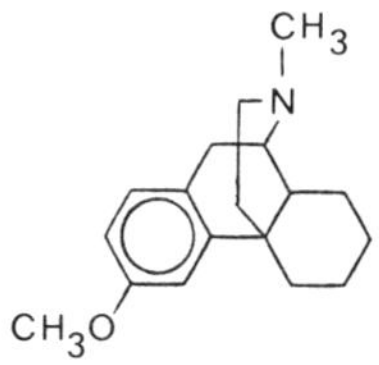

13, (+)-enantiomer

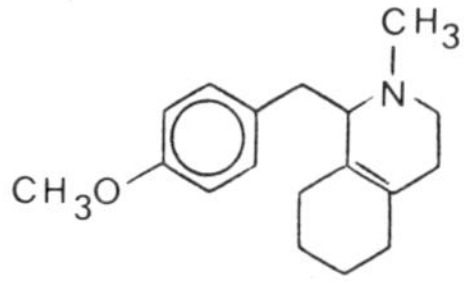

14

FIG. 3. Synthesis of morphinans.

Structure **10** contains the carbon/nitrogen framework of morphine and lacks the oxygen bridge and functionality in rings A and C; the compound is about one-fifth as active as morphine as an analgesic. Using a slightly different route, Grewe et al. (48) prepared tetrahydrodeoxycodeine **11** thereby establishing the gross structure and stereochemistry of the morphinans as being identical to those of the opium alkaloids. Using Grewe's original synthesis, Schnider and Grussner (104) prepared racemic **12a**. Resolution using L-(+)-tartaric acid gave **12a**, levorphanol, which contains virtually all of the activity of the racemate. Levorphanol in 2 mg doses either orally or parenterally provides analgesia equivalent to morphine for up to 8 hr. The N-allyl congener **12b**, levallorphan, was prepared (105) and found to be several times as potent as nalorphine as a narcotic antagonist. It was also found that most of the biological activity resides in the (-)-isomer (15). Finally, dextromethorphan **13** is analgetically inert. Its importance is as a nonaddictive antitussive. A procedure for its preparation has been developed, which involves resolution of the intermediate **14** (21). The unused portion of **14**, enriched in the undesired isomer, may be racemized, and the resolution step repeated.

A series of 14β-hydroxymorphinans (Fig. 4, **16**) has been described (90). These compounds are prepared, using as a key synthetic step, the rearrangement of the spirotetralin **14** to the phenanthrylethyl amine **15**. Several steps are required for ultimate transformation to **16**. More recently, a stereoselective total synthesis of 14β-hydroxymorphinans using a modified Grewe approach was reported (89). The appropriately substituted **17** is epoxidized with the oxiran hydrolyzed to the diol **18**. Cyclization of the borane complex of **18** with anhydrous phosphoric acid gives **19**, which can be readily converted to **16**. Use of optically active **17** as a starting material eliminates the costly last step resolution of the original synthesis. The undesired optical antipode of **17** may be recycled as in the dextromethorphan

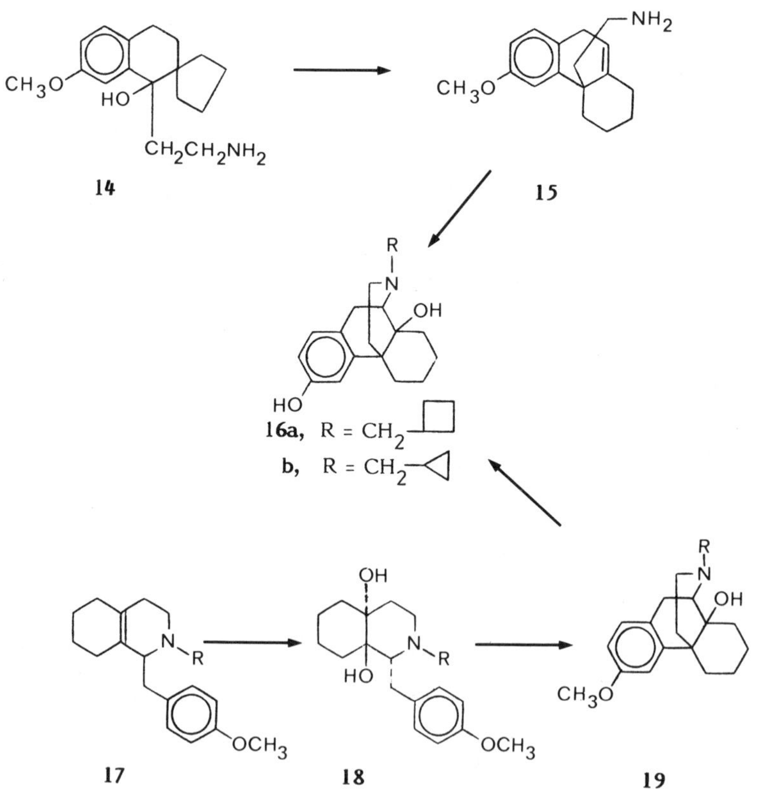

FIG. 4. Syntheses of 14-hydroxymorphinans.

synthesis *(vide supra)*. The most important compound to come out of this work is butorphanol, **16a**, which possesses both narcotic agonist and antagonist properties (56). As an analgesic, it is about five times as active as morphine and the effect lasts 3 to 4 hr. Its overall effect on respiration is similar to that seen with morphine, but unlike the latter drug, butorphanol's effect appears to reach a ceiling, beyond which higher doses do not produce a greater effect. The most frequently reported complaints are sedation, nausea, and diaphoresis. Another compound of importance in this series is the antagonist oxilorphan, **16b**. The compound is about equipotent with naloxone as an antagonist and has weak agonist properties in the PPQ test (97). It has been evaluated by Resnick et al. (102) for use in postaddicts. They found that a daily maintenance dose of 10 to 24 mg was required to block a 25 mg heroin challenge, and some side effects were noted during induction. The drug may be a promising candidate for this use.

Structurally simpler than the morphinans, the benzomorphans **22** (Fig. 5) have achieved considerable importance in the medicinal chemistry of analgesics. There are two major synthetic routes to this ring system. Historically, the first approach (12), now referred to as the tetralone approach, involves cyclization of an amino-ethyltetralone **20** via an intermediate α-bromoketone. The second approach involves a Grewe type synthesis using a tetrahydropyridine (or equivalent) **21**, first reported by May and Fry (85). The synthesis, stereochemistry, reactions, and spectroscopic characterizations of benzomorphans have been reviewed (92). Many theoretically important compounds have been discovered in this series. The first of these was phenazocine, **23a**, an effective analgesic with only marginal ability to substitute for morphine in the dependent monkey (33). This effect however was not totally carried over to man (40). The N-allyl derivative **23b** is a potent narcotic antagonist in animals (46). In man, the compound was found to be analgesic, but 15 mg was not equivalent to 10 mg of morphine. Higher doses could not be tested because of its psychotomimetic effects (69). Cyclazocine, **23c**, is one of the most potent antagonists in the series (8), and is an extremely potent analgesic in man, about 40 times stronger than morphine (29). It has also been studied for its ability to block heroin challenges in postaddicts (82); although effective, its dysphoric side effects required a long induction period to reach maintenance doses (41). Pentazocine, **23d**, was the result of a plan (9) to prepare a series of narcotic antagonists of varying potency and subject a few members to clinical evaluation as analgesics. Pentazocine became and remains the most important compound clinically in this series. It is firmly established as an analgesic of value in a wide range of pain situations. Parenterally, a 30-mg dose is equivalent to 10 mg of morphine, and orally, a 50-mg dose is equivalent to 60 mg of codeine. Onset of analgesic effect is 15 to 30 min, and lasts 3 to 4 hr.

Benzylic oxidation of the ring system (86) afforded a series of ketobenzomorphans, among which ketazocine (**24**, Fig. 6) was found to be active in the guinea pig ileum, but incapable of supporting morphine dependence in the monkey (64). In the chronic spinal dog model of Martin et al. (81), the compound was so unique that a subset of receptors, the so-called κ-receptors, were invoked to explain its

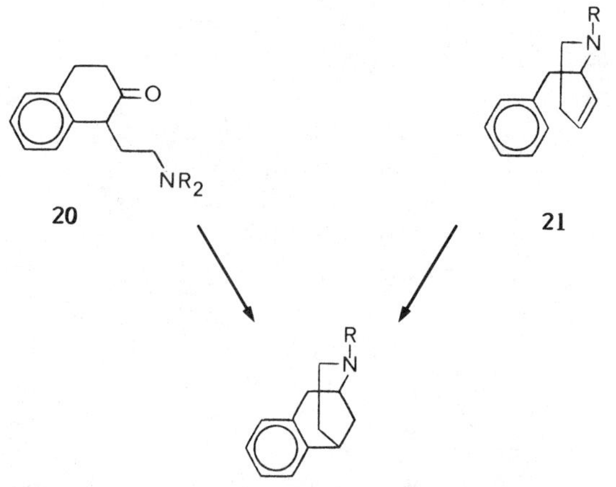

20 **21** **22**

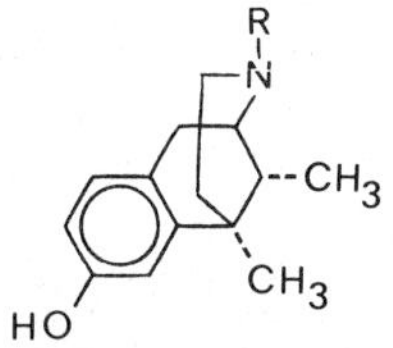

23a, R = $CH_2CH_2C_6H_5$
b, R = $CH_2CH{=}CH_2$
c, R = CH_2–cyclopropyl
d, R = $CH_2CH{=}C(CH_3)_2$

FIG. 5. Syntheses of benzomorphans.

action. Bremazocine, **25** (103), has been reported to be an agonist of the κ-type; in animals it is potent, long-acting, and free of physical and psychological dependence liability. A new series of benzomorphan derivatives (**26**), structurally analogous to the thebaine/Diels-Alder adduct series, has been reported by Michne et al. (87,88). The compounds are unusual in that potent antagonist activity is present among the N-CH_3 derivatives. For example, tonazocine (**26a**) is about equal to naloxone in antagonist potency (tail flick), and two times morphine in agonist potency. In the monkey (1,3), the drug promptly precipitated dose-related withdrawal signs; the duration of action was approximately twice that of naloxone. The compound did not produce a significant degree of morphine-like dependence, and little tolerance developed to its effects. At the doses used, the compound did not appear to be well tolerated, however. Nevertheless, no injection dose of this drug

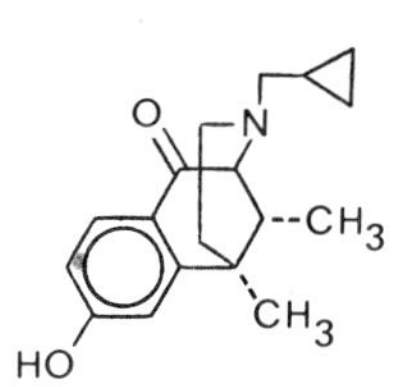

24

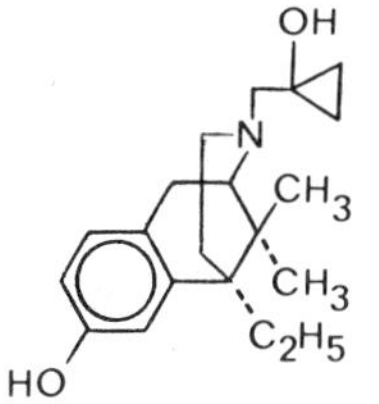

25

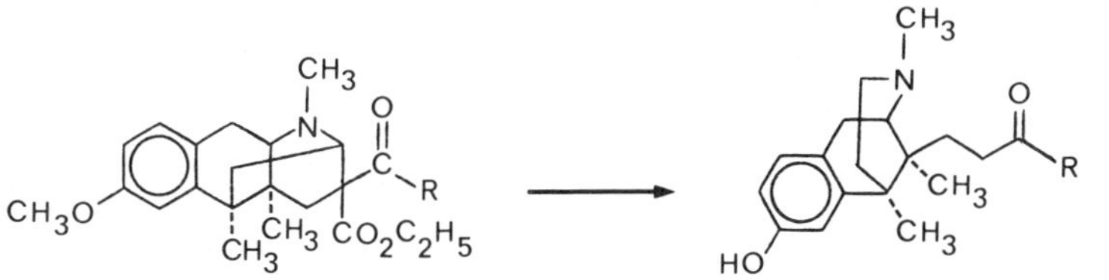

26a, R = $(CH_2)_4CH_3$
b, R = $(CH_2)_2CH(CH_3)_2$
c, R = CH_2CH_2–cyclopentyl

FIG. 6. Benzomorphans of theoretical significance.

maintained rates of self injection behavior higher than those maintained by saline. Win 42,964, **26b**, is less potent as an antagonist, but is about 10 times more potent than morphine as an agonist. Win 44,441, **26c**, is about equal to naloxone as an antagonist, and has very weak, if any, agonist properties.

Aryl-Piperidines and Related Compounds

In 1939, Eisleb and Schaumann (34) reported that in the course of routine pharmacologic screening of candidate antispasmodic compounds, **27** (meperidine, Fig. 7) was found to be an analgesic, and had other morphine-like properties as well. At first glance, the structure of **27** appears to have little in common with that of morphine **1a**. However, both compounds contain a 4-phenylpiperidine moiety, and in each case, the 4 position of the piperidine ring is quaternary. Meperidine was shown to be an effective analgesic clinically, and was quickly and widely accepted in clinical use. Parenteral doses of 60 to 80 mg are approximately equivalent to 10 mg of morphine; peak analgesia develops over about 45 min, and persists 2 to 4 hr. The potency of the drug is considerably less when administered orally.

The acceptance of meperidine stimulated considerable synthetic effort. Many analogs have been prepared more often than not using the general approach shown for meperidine itself. The resulting structure-activity relationships may be summarized as follows (14): (a) substitution of the phenyl ring generally reduces

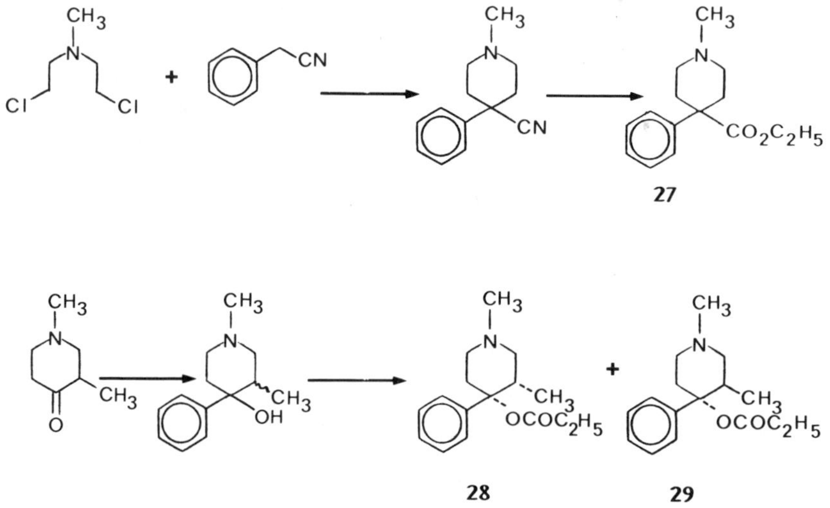

FIG. 7. Syntheses of 4-arylpiperidines.

activity; (b) methyl or phenethyl are the best substituents on nitrogen; (c) the carbethoxy group seems to be optimum.

Notwithstanding (c) above, the so-called reversed esters or prodines are active. Such compounds are usually prepared as shown for **28** and **29**, α- and β-prodine, respectively (119). The stereochemical assignments of **28** and **29** have been made unequivocally by X-ray crystallography (6,7). The α- or *trans*-phenyl/methyl form predominates, and is about equal to morphine as an analgesic; the less abundant β- or *cis*-phenyl/methyl form is about three times more potent than morphine. This is not generally true for substituents other than methyl; the corresponding ethyl compounds may have the opposite potency relationship. Clinically, α-prodine is a rapid acting analgesic with a short duration. Onset of analgesia is about 5 min, and lasts about 2 hr. It is particularly useful for short procedures such as encountered in obstetrics and urology.

Further explorations of the structure-activity relationships with this type of compound has resulted in a number of clinically useful products. Ethoheptazine **30** (Fig. 8) was prepared in several steps by Diamond et al. (31). The compound differs structurally from meperidine in that the piperidine ring of the latter has been replaced by a 7-membered hexamethyleneimine ring. It is a non-narcotic analgesic and is well absorbed orally. For the relief of mild to moderate pain, the drug may be used in place of or in combination with aspirin. On the other hand, fentanyl, **31**, is an extremely potent narcotic analgesic synthesized by Janssen and Gardocki (66). Its onset is rapid and its duration is short. The drug combined with droperidol is used in neuroleptanesthesia.

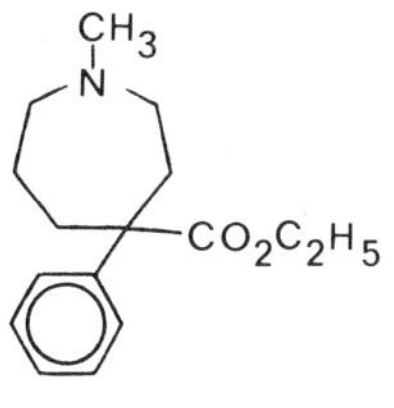

FIG. 8. Synthetic analgesics of diverse structure.

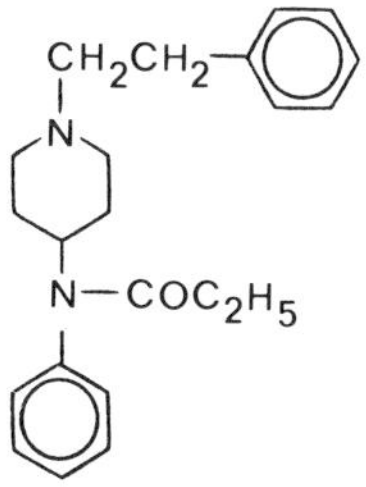

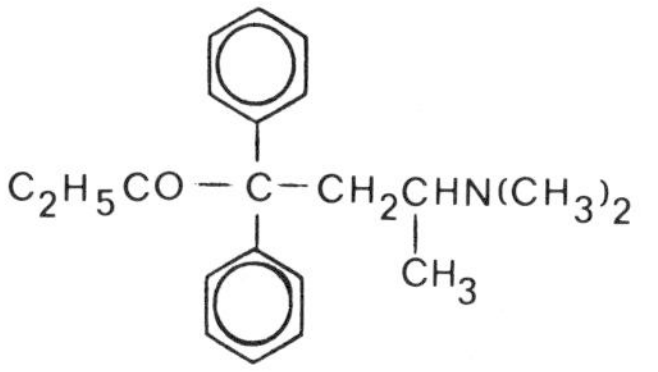

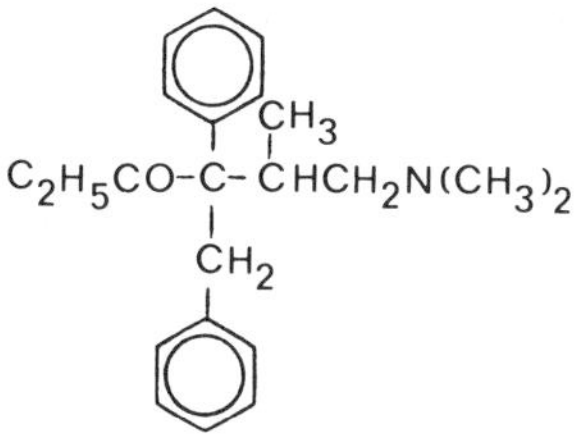

Somewhat more removed structurally are the acyclic aryl propyl amines methadone **32** and propoxyphene **33**. Methadone was discovered in Germany during World War II (20). The original synthesis produces both methadone and its C-methyl isomer isomethadone. Several unambiguous syntheses of these materials have since been reported (52). Methadone is about equal in potency to morphine as an analgesic, but has a much longer duration of action. It is fully effective orally at about twice the parenteral dose. The biological activity resides in the levorotatory enantiomorph (73,111). In addition to its use for analgesia, it is being studied for its ability to aid the rehabilitation of opiate addicts (32). Propoxyphene is a structural variation of methadone, which is about equivalent to codeine as an analgesic (49,99). In this case, the activity resides largely in the dextrorotatory enantiomorph. The napsylate salt is becoming a more frequently used form, because its low water solubility provides for more stable pharmaceutical formulations.

MISCELLANEOUS STRUCTURES

Occasionally, research directed toward areas other than analgesia has resulted in novel new structures with morphine-like activity. Some, like meperidine, achieve the level of wide acceptance in clinical practice. Others, for a variety of reasons, do not advance to such levels. Nevertheless, their pharmacology is undeniably opioid, and any theoretical concept of the molecular nature of the opiate receptor must take such structures into account. A few examples are presented here to emphasize the diversity of chemical structures which are recognized by the opiate receptor.

In 1957, Hunger et al. (62) reported a new class of analgesics containing a benzimidazole ring. Improvements in the original synthesis (63) allowed the expansion of the series and the establishment of the structure-activity relationships. The most potent compound found was etonitazene (**34**, Fig. 9), about 1,000 times as active as morphine. The nitro and ethoxy groups appear to be key functions, since the *des*-nitro compound (ethoxy present) is only 70 times as active, and the *des*-ethoxy compound (nitro present) is only twice as active as morphine. Clinical trials showed that members of the series were analgesics in man but were also respiratory depressants, and therefore offered no advantage over morphine. In addition, etonitazene's addiction potential was comparable to that of morphine (39). Feinberg et al. (37) proposed a model to explain structure-activity relationships of opiate agonists and antagonists. A key feature of their model is that potent agonists such as etonitazene contain an aromatic ring F as distinguished from the aromatic ring A of morphine. They suggested that the interaction of ring F with a specific site on the opiate receptor is crucial for the potent agonist activity of etonitazene. Clarke et al. (25) suggested that etonitazene's activity is owing to its nitro and ethoxy groups mimicking the carboxy and phenyl ring of phenylalanine, respectively, of the enkephalins.

A second unusual structure with morphine-like activity is the diazatwistane, **35** (38). Inspection of the molecule indicates identical nitrogens separated by four carbons through fused twist-boat rings. The molecule has a C_2 axis of symmetry making the 2 and 9 positions identical even in respect to absolute stereochemistry, although the molecule as a whole is resolvable. The activity resides largely in the (-)-isomer. Structure-activity relationships in this series do not correspond to those observed in the morphine series (110). Structural comparisons of **35** with probable conformations of enkephalins suggest that the primary binding sites for **35** may correspond to the basic nitrogen and the Phe of enkephalin, rather than the Tyr, as is thought to be the case with morphine.

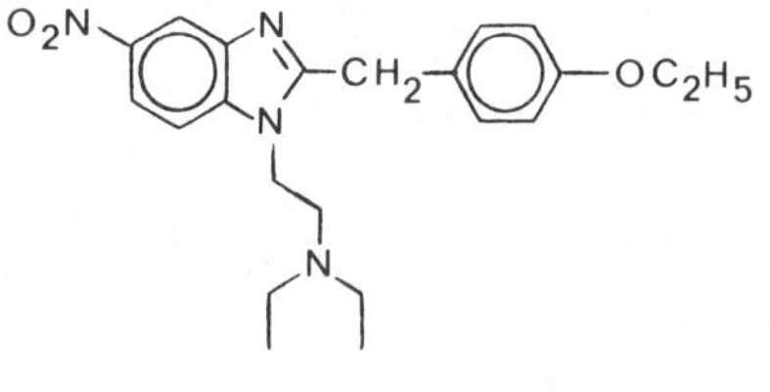

34 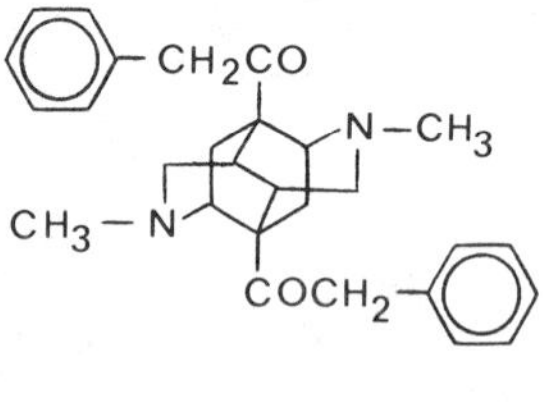   35

FIG. 9. Unusual analgesic structures.

FUTURE DIRECTIONS

To say that the discoveries of the opiate receptor and the endogenous opioids have changed the course of opiate research is an understatement. Our original concept of the opioid system as simply a processor of pain information has been expanded to one involving many aspects of the physiology of a variety of systems. It may eventually emerge that these discoveries are having more of an effect on how the medicinal chemist views the problem rather than on its ultimate solution. The multiplicity of opiate receptors is yet to be related to physiological effects. However, chemists are already synthesizing molecules which may have highly receptor-selective agonist or antagonist characteristics. When such highly selective agents are found, they will be used to define the physiologic effects of receptor events, and thereby, perhaps, define the characteristics of the ideal analgesic in terms of relative receptor agonist/antagonist selectivities. It is important to bear in mind that a great diversity of chemical structural types interact with opioid receptors, and that only a relatively few structural types have been studied in great detail. Thus, our knowledge of the structural requirements for agonist or antagonist activity at a particular receptor is limited. Further progress will be made as we base our thinking on, but not confine it to, those well-studied classes of compounds, and perhaps look for new compounds of theoretical and clinical significance among "novel" structural types.

REFERENCES

1. Aceto, M. D., Harris, L. S., Dewey, W. L., and May, E. L. (1979): Annual report: Dependence studies of new compounds in the rhesus monkey (1979): In: *Problems of Drug Dependence 1979*, edited by L. S. Harris, pp. 330–350. U.S. Government Printing Office, Washington, D.C.
2. Aceto, M. D., Harris, L. S., Dewey, W. L., and May, E. L. (1980): Annual report: Dependence studies of new compounds in the rhesus monkey. In: *Proceedings of the 42nd Annual Scientific Meeting, Committee on Problems of Drug Dependence*, pp. 297–326 (and references therein).
3. Aceto, M. D., Harris, L. S., Dewey, W. L., and May, E. L. (1981): Annual report: Dependence studies of new compounds in the rhesus monkey (1980): In: *Problems of Drug Dependence 1980*, edited by L. S. Harris, pp. 297–366. U.S. Government Printing Office, Washington, D.C.
4. Aceto, M. D., McKean, D. B., and Pearl, J. (1969): Effects of opiate antagonists on the Straub tail reaction in mice. *Br. J. Pharmacol.*, 36:225–239.
5. Adler, T. K. (1963): The comparative potencies of codeine and its demethylated metabolites after intraventricular injection in the mouse. *J. Pharmacol. Exp. Ther.*, 140:155–161.
6. Ahmed, F. R., Barnes, W. H., and Kartha, G. (1959): Configuration of the alpha-prodine molecule. *Chem. Ind.*, 485.
7. Ahmed, F. R., Barnes, W. H., and Masironi, L. A. (1962): Configuration of the beta-prodine molecule in *dl*-betaprodine hydrobromide. *Chem. Ind.*, 97.
8. Archer, S., Albertson, N. F., Harris, L. S., Pierson, A. K., and Bird, J. G. (1964): Pentazocine. Strong analgesics and analgesic antagonists in the benzomorphan series. *J. Med. Chem.*, 7:123–127.
9. Archer, S., Albertson, N. F., Harris, L. S., Pierson, A. K., Bird, J. G., Keats, A. S., Telford, J., and Papadopoulos, C. (1962): Narcotic antagonists as analgesics. *Science*, 137:541–543.
10. Archer, S., and Harris, L. S. (1965): Narcotic antagonists. In: *Progress in Drug Research, Vol. 8*, edited by E. Jucker, pp. 261–320. Birkhauser Verlag, Basel.
11. Archer, S., and Michne, W. F. (1976): Recent progress in research on narcotic antagonists. In: *Progress in Drug Research, Vol. 20*, edited by E. Jucker, pp. 45–100. Birkhauser Verlag, Basel.
12. Barltrop, J. A. (1947): Syntheses in the morphine series. Part I. Derivatives of bicyclo[3.3.1.]-2-azanonane. *J. Chem. Soc.*, 399–401.

13. Beckett, A. H., and Casy, A. F. (1954): Synthetic analgesics: Stereochemical considerations. *J. Pharm. Pharmacol.*, 6:986–1001.
14. Beckett, A. H., and Casy, A. F. (1962): The testing and development of analgesic drugs. In: *Progress in Medicinal Chemistry, Vol. 2*, edited by G. P. Ellis and G. B. West, pp. 43–87. Butterworth Ltd., London.
15. Benson, W. M., O'Gara, E., and VanWinkle, S. (1952): Respiratory and analgesic antagonism of dromoran by 3-hydroxy-N-allyl-morphinan. *J. Pharmacol. Exp. Ther.*, 106:373.
16. Blumberg, H., and Dayton, H. B. (1973): Naloxone and related compounds. In: *Agonist and Antagonist Actions of Narcotic Analgesic Drugs*, edited by H. W. Kosterlitz, H. O. J. Collier, and J. E. Villareal, pp. 110–119. University Park Press, Baltimore.
17. Blumberg, H., Dayton, H. B., George, M., and Rapaport, D. N. (1961): N-allynoroxymorphone: A potent narcotic antagonist. *Fed. Proc.*, 20:311.
18. Blumberg, H., Dayton, H. B., and Wolf, P. S. (1965): Narcotic antagonist activity of naloxone. *Fed. Proc.*, 24:676.
19. Blumberg, H., Dayton, H. B., and Wolf, P. S. (1967): Analgesic and narcotic antagonist properties of noroxymorphone derivatives. *Toxicol. Appl. Pharmacol.*, 10:406.
20. Bockmuhl, M., and Ehrhart, G. (1949): Uber eine neue Klasse von spasmolytisch und analgetisch wirkenden Verbindungen, I. *Ann. Chem.*, 561:52–85.
21. Brossi, A., and Schnider, O. (1956): 164. Hydroxymorphinane. Versuche zur racemisierung optisch aktiver 1-(p-hydroxybenzyl)-1,2,3,4,5,6,7,8-octahydroisochinoline. *Helv. Chim. Acta*, 39:1376–1386.
22. Casy, A. F. (1970): Analgesics and their antagonists: Recent developments. In: *Progress in Medicinal Chemistry*, edited by G. P. Ellis and G. B. West, pp. 229–284. Appleton Century Crofts, New York.
23. Casy, A. F. (1978): Analgesics and their antagonists. In: *Progress in Drug Research, Vol. 22*, edited by E. Jucker, pp. 149–227. Birkhauser Verlag, Basel.
24. Childers, S. R., Creese, I., Snowman, A. M., and Snyder, S. H. (1979): Opiate receptor binding affected differentially by opiates and opioid peptides. *Eur. J. Pharmacol.*, 55:11–18.
25. Clarke, F. H., Jaggi, H., and Lovell, R. A. (1978): Conformation of 2,9-dimethyl-3'-hydroxy-5-phenyl-6,7-benzomorphan and its relation to other analgetics and enkephalin. *J. Med. Chem.*, 21:600–606.
26. Collier, H. O. J., Dineen, L. C., Johnson, C. A., and Schneider, C. (1968): The abdominal constriction response and its suppression by analgesic drugs in the mouse. *Br. J. Pharmacol.*, 32:295–310.
27. Cowan, A., Lewis, J. W., and Macfarlane, I. R. (1977): Agonist and antagonist properties of buprenorphine, a new antinociceptive agent. *Br. J. Pharmacol.*, 60:537–545.
28. D'Armour, F. E., and Smith, D. L. (1941): A method for determining loss of pain sensation. *J. Pharmacol. Exp. Ther.*, 72:74–79.
29. DeKornfeld, T. J., and Lasagna, L. (1963): Win 20740, a potent new analgesic agent. *Fed. Proc.*, 22:248.
30. deStevens, G., editor (1965): *Analgetics*. Academic Press, Inc., New York.
31. Diamond, J., Bruce, W. F., and Tyson, F. T. (1957): Synthesis of azacycloheptane derivatives related to piperidine analgesics. *J. Org. Chem.*, 22:399–405.
32. Dole, V. P., and Nyswander, M. (1965): A medical treatment for diacetylmorphine (heroin) addiction. *J.A.M.A.*, 193:646–650.
33. Eddy, N. B., and May, E. L. (1966): *Synthetic Analgesics, Part 2(B)*. Pergamon Press, London.
34. Eisleb, O., and Schaumann, O. (1939): Dolantin, a new antispasmodic and analgesic. *Dtsch. Med. Wochenschr.*, 65:967–968.
35. Elad, D., and Ginsburg, D. (1954): Syntheses in the morphine series. Part VI. The synthesis of morphine. *J. Chem. Soc.*, 3052–3056.
36. Faden, A. I., and Holaday, J. W. (1979): Opiate antagonists: A role in the treatment of hypovolemic shock. *Science*, 205:317–318.
37. Feinberg, A. P., Creese, I., and Snyder, S. H. (1976): The opiate receptor: A model explaining structure-activity relationships of opiate agonists and antagonists. *Proc. Natl. Acad. Sci. U.S.A.*, 73:4215–4219.
38. Fisher, M. H., Grabowski, E. J. J., Patchett, A. A., ten Broeke, J., Flataker, L. M., Lotti, V. J., and Robinson, F. M. (1977): 5,11-Dimethyl-2,9-bis(phenylacetyl)-5,11-diazatetracy-

clo[6.2.2.0^{2,7}.0^{4,9}]dodecane, a potent, novel analgesic. *J. Med. Chem.*, 20:63–66.

39. Fraser, H. F., Isbell, H., and Wolback, R. (1960): *Bull. Drug Addiction and Narcotics, Addendum 2*, p. 35.
40. Fraser, H. F., and Isbell, H. (1960): Human pharmacology and addiction liabilities of phenazocine and levophenacylmorphan. *Bull. Narc., U.N., Dept. Social Affairs*, 12:15–23.
41. Freedman, A., Fink, M., Sharoff, R., and Zaks, A. (1968): Clinical studies of cyclazocine in the treatment of narcotic addiction. *Am. J. Psychiatry*, 124:1499–1504.
42. Freund, M., and Speyer, E. (1916): Uber die Umwandlung von thebain in oxycodeinon und dessen derivate. *J. Prakt. Chem.*, 94:135–178.
43. Gacel, G., Fournie-Zaluski, M. C., and Roques, B. P. (1980): Tyr-D-Ser-Gly-Phe-Leu-Thr, a highly preferential ligand for δ-opiate receptors. *FEBS Lett.*, 118:245–247.
44. Gates, M., and Tschudi, G. (1952): The synthesis of morphine. *J. Am. Chem. Soc.*, 74:1109–1110.
45. Goldstein, A., Lowney, L. I., and Pal, B. K. (1971): Stereospecific and nonspecific interactions of the morphine congener levorphanol in subcellular fractions of mouse brain. *Proc. Natl. Acad. Sci. U.S.A.*, 68:1742–1747.
46. Gordon, M., Lafferty, J. J., Tedeschi, D. H., Eddy, N. B., and May, E. L. (1961): A new potent analgetic antagonist. *Nature*, 192:1089.
47. Grewe, R. (1947): Synthetische Arzneimittel mit Morphin-Wirkung. *Angew. Chem.*, 59:194–199.
48. Grewe, R., Mondon, A., and Nolte, E. (1949): Die Totalsynthese des tetrahydrodesoxycodeins. *Ann. Chem.*, 564:161–198.
49. Gruber, C. M. (1955): The analgesic activity of Lilly compound 16298, acetylsalicyclic acid, and codeine in humans with chronic pain. *J. Pharmacol. Exp. Ther.*, 113:25–26.
50. Gulland, J. M., and Robinson, R. (1925): Constitution of codeine and thebaine. *Mem. Proc. Manchester Lit. Phil. Soc.*, 69:79–86.
51. Gyang, E. A., and Kosterlitz, H. W. (1966): Agonist and antagonist actions of morphine-like drugs on the guinea pig isolated ileum. *Br. J. Pharmacol.*, 27:514–527.
52. Hardy, R. A., and Howell, M. G. (1965): Synthetic analgetics. In: *Analgetics*, edited by G. deStevens, pp. 179–279. Academic Press Inc., New York.
53. Hardy, J. D., Wolff, H. G., and Goodell, H. (1940): Studies on pain. A new method for measuring pain threshold: Observations on spatial summation of pain. *J. Clin. Invest.*, 19:649–657.
54. Harris, L. S., and Pierson, A. K. (1964): Some narcotic antagonists in the benzomorphan series. *J. Pharmacol. Exp. Ther.*, 143:141–148.
55. Hart, E. R. (1941): N-Allylnorcodeine and N-allylnormorphine, two antagonists to morphine. *J. Pharmacol. Exp. Ther.*, 72:19.
56. Heel, R. C., Brogden, R. N., Speight, T. M., and Avery, G. S. (1978): Butorphanol: A review of its pharmacological properties and therapeutic efficacy. *Drugs*, 16:473–505.
57. Helsley, G. C., Richman, J. A., Lunsford, C. D., Jenkins, H., Mays, R. P., Funderberk, W. H., and Johnson, D. N. (1968): Analgetics. Esters of 3-pyrrolidinemethanols. *J. Med. Chem.*, 11:472–475.
58. Hendershot, L. C., and Forsaith, J. (1959): Antagonism of the frequency of phenylquinone-induced writhing in the mouse by weak analgesics and nonanalgesics. *J. Pharmacol. Exp. Ther.*, 125:237–240.
59. Henderson, G., Hughes, J., and Kosterlitz, H. W. (1972): A new example of a morphine-sensitive neuro-effector junction: Adrenergic transmission in the mouse vas deferens. *Br. J. Pharmacol.*, 46:764–766.
60. Holaday, J. W., and Faden, A. I. (1978): Naloxone reversal of endotoxin hypotension suggests role of endorphins in shock. *Nature*, 275:450–451.
61. Houde, R. W., Wallenstein, S. L., and Rogers, A. (1975): Analgesic studies in cancer patients: SU-19713B, nalbuphine, propiram, and butorphanol. In: *Proceedings of the 37th Annual Scientific Meeting, Committee on Problems of Drug Dependence*, pp. 162–177. National Academy of Sciences, Washington, D.C.
62. Hunger, A., Kebrle, J., Rossi, A., and Hoffmann, K. (1957): Synthese basisch substituierter, analgetisch wirksamer benzimidazol-derivate. *Experientia*, 13:400–401.
63. Hunger, A., Kebrle, J., Rossi, A., and Hoffmann, K. (1960): Benzimidazol-Derivate und verwandte heterocyclen III. Synthese von 1-aminoalkyl-2-benzyl-nitrobenzimidazolen. *Helv. Chim. Acta*, 43:1032–1046.
64. Hutchinson, M., Kosterlitz, H. W., Leslie, F. M., Waterfield, A. A., and Terenius, L. (1975):

Assessment in the guinea pig ileum and mouse vas deferens of benzomorphans which have strong antinociceptive activity but do not substitute for morphine in the dependent monkey. *Br. J. Pharmacol.*, 55:541–546.

65. Isbell, H. (1956): Attempted addiction to nalorphine. *Fed. Proc.*, 15:442.

66. Janssen, P. A. J., and Gardocki, J. F. (1964): Method for producing analgesia. *U.S. Patent*, 3,141,823.

67. Jasinski, D. R., Martin, W. R., and Haertzen, C. A. (1967): The human pharmacology and abuse potential of N-allylnoroxymorphone (naloxone). *J. Pharmacol. Exp. Ther.*, 157:420–426.

68. Keats, A. S., and Telford, J. (1956): Nalorphine, a potent analgesic in man. *J. Pharmacol. Exp. Ther.*, 117:190–196.

69. Keats, A. S., and Telford, J. (1964): Studies of analgesic drugs. VIII. A narcotic antagonist analgesic without psychotomimetic effects. *J. Pharmacol. Exp. Ther.*, 143:157–164.

70. Kosterlitz, H. W., Lord, J. A. H., Paterson, S. J., and Waterfield, A. A. (1980): Effects of changes in the structure of enkephalins and of narcotic analgesic drugs on their interactions with μ- and δ-receptors. *Br. J. Pharmacol.*, 68:333–342.

71. Kosterlitz, H. W., and Waterfield, A. A. (1975): In vitro models in the study of structure-activity relationships of narcotic analgesics. In: *Annual Review of Pharmacology, Vol. 15*, edited by H. W. Eliot, R. George, and R. Okun, pp. 29–47. Annual Reviews, Inc., Palo Alto.

72. Kosterlitz, H. W., and Watt, A. J. (1968): Kinetic parameters of narcotic agonists and antagonists, with particular reference to N-allylnoroxymorphone (naloxone). *Br. J. Pharmacol.*, 33:266–276.

73. Larsen, A. A., Tullar, B. F., Elpern, B., and Buck, J. S. (1948): The resolution of methadone and related compounds. *J. Am. Chem. Soc.*, 70:4194–4197.

74. Lasagna, L., and Beecher, H. K. (1954): The analgesic effectiveness of nalorphine and nalorphine-morphine combination in man. *J. Pharmacol. Exp. Ther.*, 112:356–363.

75. Lewenstein, M. J., and Fishman, J. (1966): Morphine derivative. *U.S. Patent* 3,254,088.

76. Lewis, J. W. (1973): Ring C-bridged Derivatives of thebaine and oripavine. In: *Advances in Biochemical Psychopharmacology, Vol. 8: Narcotic Antagonists*, edited by M. C. Braude, L. S. Harris, E. L. May, J. P. Smith, and J. E. Villareal. Raven Press, New York.

77. Lewis, J. W., Bentley, K. W., and Cowan, A. (1971): Narcotic analgesics and antagonists. In: *Annual Review of Pharmacology, Vol. 11*, edited by H. W. Eliot, R. Okun, and R. H. Dreisbach, pp. 241–270. Annual Reviews, Inc., Palo Alto.

78. Lightman, S. L., and Jacobs, H. S. (1979): Naloxone: Non-steroidal treatment for postmenopausal flushing? *Lancet*, 2:1071.

79. Lord, J. A. H., Waterfield, A. A., Hughes, J., and Kosterlitz, H. W. (1977): Endogenous opioid peptides: Multiple agonists and receptors. *Nature*, 267:495–499.

80. Mackay, M., and Hodgkin, D. (1955): A crystallographic examination of the structure of morphine. *J. Chem. Soc.*, 3261–3267.

81. Martin, W. R., Eades, C. G., Thompson, J. A., Huppler, R. E., and Gilbert, P. E. (1976): The effects of morphine and nalorphine-like drugs in the nondependent and morphine dependent chronic spinal dog. *J. Pharmacol. Exp. Ther.*, 197:517–532.

82. Martin, W. R., Gorodetzky, C. W., and McLane, T. M. (1966): An experimental study in the treatment of narcotic addicts with cyclazocine. *Clin. Pharmacol. Ther.*, 7:455–465.

83. Martin, W. R., Jasinski, D. R., and Mansky, P. A. (1973): Naltrexone, an antagonist for the treatment of heroin dependence. *Arch. Gen. Psychiatry*, 28:784–791.

84. Matsumoto, S., Oka, T., Takemori, A. E., and Hosoya, E. (1972): Comparative studies on the antagonism of naloxone and nalorphine to the morphine-induced respiratory depression in rabbits. *Jpn. J. Pharmacol.*, 22: Suppl., 89.

85. May, E. L., and Fry, E. M. (1957): Structures related to morphine. VIII. Further syntheses in the benzomorphan series. *J. Org. Chem.*, 22:1366–1369.

86. Michne, W. F., and Albertson, N. F. (1972): Analgetic 1-oxidized-2,6-methano-3-benzazocines. *J. Med. Chem.*, 15:1278–1281.

87. Michne, W. F., Lewis, T. R., Michalec, S. J., Pierson, A. K., Gillan, M. G. C., Paterson, S. J., Robson, L. E., and Kosterlitz, H. W. (1978): Novel developments of N-methylbenzomorphan narcotic antagonists. In: *Characteristics and Function of Opioids*, edited by J. M. vanRee and L. Terenius, pp. 197–206. Elsevier North-Holland, Amsterdam.

88. Michne, W. F., Lewis, T. R., Michalec, S. J., Pierson, A. K., and Rosenberg, F. J. (1979): (2,6-Methano-3-benzazocin-11β-yl)-alkanones. 1. Alkylalkanones: A new series of N-methyl derivatives with novel opiate activity profiles. *J. Med. Chem.*, 22:1158–1163.

89. Monkovic, I., Bachand, C., and Wong, H. (1978): A stereoselective total synthesis of 14-hydroxymorphinans. Grewe Approach. *J. Am. Chem. Soc.*, 100:4609–4610.

90. Monkovic, I., Conway, J. J., Wong, H., Perron, Y. G., Pachter, I. J., and Belleau, B. (1973): Total synthesis and pharmacological activities of N-substituted-3,14-dihydroxymorphinans. I. *J. Am. Chem. Soc.*, 95:7910–7912.

91. Nilsen, P. L. (1961): Studies on algesimetry by electrical stimulation of the mouse tail. *Acta Pharmacol. Toxicol.*, 18:10–22.

92. Palmer, D. C., and Strauss, M. J. (1977): Benzomorphans: Synthesis, stereochemistry, reactions, and spectroscopic characterizations. *Chem. Rev.*, 77:1–36.

93. Paton, W. D. M. (1957): The action of morphine and related substances on contraction and on acetylcholine output of coaxially stimulated guinea pig ileum. *Br. J. Pharmacol.*, 12:119–127.

94. Perrine, T. D., Atwell, L., Tice, I. B., Jacobson, A. E., and May, E. L. (1972): Analgesic activity as determined by the Nilsen method. *J. Pharm. Sci.*, 61:86–88.

95. Pert, C. B., and Snyder, S. H. (1973): Opiate receptor: Demonstration in nervous tissue. *Science*, 179:1011–1013.

96. Pert, C. B., and Snyder, S. H. (1974): Opiate receptor binding of agonists and antagonists affected differentially by sodium. *Mol. Pharmacol.*, 10:868–879.

97. Pircio, A. W., and Gylys, J. A. (1975): Oxilorphan (1-N-cyclopropylmethyl-3,14-dihydroxymorphinan): A new synthetic narcotic antagonist. *J. Pharmacol. Exp. Ther.*, 193:23–34.

98. Pohl, J. (1915): N-allylnorcodenine, an inhibitor of morphine. *Z. Exp. Path. Ther.*, 17:370–382.

99. Pohland, A., and Sullivan, H. R. (1953): Analgesics: Esters of 4-dialkylamino-1,2-diphenyl-2-butanols. *J. Am. Chem. Soc.*, 75:4458–4461.

100. Portoghese, P. S. (1965): A new concept on the mode of interaction of narcotic analgesics with receptors. *J. Med. Chem.*, 8:609–616.

101. Rapoport, H., Naumann, R., Bissell, E. R., and Bonner, R. M. (1950): The preparation of some dihydroketones in the morphine series by Oppenauer oxidation. *J. Org. Chem.*, 15:1103–1107.

102. Resnick, R. B., Schwartz, L. K., Kestenbaum, R. S., and Amerling, R. (1975): Oral oxilorphan in man. In: *Proceedings of the 37th Annual Scientific Meeting, Committee on Problems of Drug Dependence*, pp. 391–400. National Academy of Sciences, Washington, D.C.

103. Romer, D., Buscher, H., Hill, R. C., Mauer, R., Petcher, T. J., Welle, H. B. A., Bakel, H. C. C. K., and Akkerman, A. M. (1980): Bremazocine: A potent, long acting opiate kappa-agonist. *Life Sci.*, 27:971–978.

104. Schnider, O., and Grussner, A. (1949): Synthese von oxy-morphinanen. *Helv. Chim. Acta.*, 32:821–828.

105. Schnider, O., and Hellerbach, J. (1950): Synthese von morphinanen. *Helv. Chim. Acta.*, 33:1437–1448.

106. Siegmund, E., Cadmus, R., and Lu, G. (1957): A method for evaluating both non-narcotic and narcotic analgesics. *Proc. Soc. Exp. Biol. Med.*, 95:729–731.

107. Simon, E. J., Hiller, J. M., and Edelman, I. (1973): Stereospecific binding of the potent narcotic analgesic [³H]-etorphine to rat brain homogenate. *Proc. Natl. Acad. Sci. U.S.A.*, 70:1947–1949.

108. Small, L. F., Eddy, N. B., Mosettig, E., and Himmelsbach, C. K. (1938): *Studies on Drug Addiction, Suppl. No. 138 to the Public Health Reports*, U.S. Government Printing Office, Washington, D.C.

109. Taber, R. I., Greenhouse, D. D., and Irwin, S. (1964): Inhibition of phenylquinone-induced writhing by narcotic antagonists. *Nature*, 204:189–190.

110. TenBroeke, J., Hudgin, R. L., Patchett, A. A., Rackham, A., Robinson, F. M., and Williams, M. (1978): Some structure activity relationships in the diazatwistane series. In: *Characteristics and function of opioids*, edited by J. M. vanRee, and L. Terenius, pp. 241–242. Elsevier North-Holland, Amsterdam.

111. Thorp, R. H., Walton, E., and Ofner, P. (1947): Optical isomers of amidone, with a note on isoamidone. *Nature*, 160:605–606.

112. Verebey, K., Volavka, J., and Clouet, D. (1978): Endorphins in psychiatry: An overview and a hypothesis. *Arch. Gen. Psychiatry*, 35:877–888.

113. VonBraun, J., Kuhn, M., and Siddiqui, S. (1926): Ungesattigte reste in chemischer und pharmakologischer Beziehung. *Ber. Dtsch. Chem. Ges.*, 59:1081–1090.

114. Weijlard, T., and Erickson, A. E. (1942): N-allylnormorphine. *J. Am. Chem. Soc.*, 64:869–870.

115. Weiss, U. (1955): Derivatives of morphine. I. 14-Hydroxydihydromorphinone. *J. Am. Chem. Soc.*, 77:5891–5892.

116. Winter, C. A., Orahovits, P. D., and Lehman, E. G. (1957): Analgesic activity and morphine antagonism of compounds related to nalorphine. *Arch. Int. Pharmacodyn. Ther.*, 150:186–202.

117. Woods, J. H., Medzihradsky, F., Smith, C. B., Young, A. M., and Swain, H. H. (1980): Annual Report: Evaluation of new compounds for opioid activity. *Proceedings of the 42nd Annual Scientific Meeting, Committee on Problems of Drug Dependence*, pp. 327–366 (and references therein). U.S. Government Printing Office, Washington, D.C.

118. Woolfe, G., and MacDonald, A. D. (1944): The evaluation of the analgesic action of pethidine hydrochloride (Demerol). *J. Pharmacol. Exp. Ther.*, 80:300–307.

119. Ziering, A., and Lee, J. (1947): Piperidine derivatives. V. 1,3-Dialkyl-4-aryl-4-acyloxypiperidines. *J. Org. Chem.*, 12:911–914.

Analgesics: Neurochemical, Behavioral, and Clinical Perspectives, edited by M. Kuhar and G. Pasternak. Raven Press, New York © 1984.

Nonopioid Analgesics

K. Brune and R. Lanz

Institute of Pharmacology and Toxicology, University of Erlangen-Nürnberg, D-8520 Erlangen, West Germany

Non-narcotic analgesics exerting their effects in the periphery (65, Fig. 1) belong to the most widely distributed and most frequently used drugs worldwide. Relative to the quantity of packages, they make up about 10% of the drugstore turnover (32a). Of all analgesics, only 5% of the packages sold contain drugs acting on the central nervous system (CNS). The remainder are represented by peripherally-acting analgesics. In combination with various admixtures, they are marketed not only as analgesics, but also as antirheumatics, remedies for the common cold, menstrual discomfort, sensitivity to changes in the weather, hang-overs, and many other disorders.

The peripherally-acting analgesics can be divided into two pharmacologically and physicochemically different subclasses. The first one comprises the anti-inflammatory, antipyretic analgesics, which all show acidic properties, and are effective mainly against inflammatory pain. They influence partial aspects of the complex inflammatory process, mainly pain and oedema. On the other hand, some nonacidic drugs are classified as peripherally-acting antipyretic analgesics. Since these drugs show almost no anti-inflammatory activity at therapeutic doses, the distinction of these two subclasses is of therapeutic relevance.

ANTI-INFLAMMATORY, ANTIPYRETIC ANALGESICS (ACIDS)

Characteristics

The apparently considerable structural differences within this subclass often veil the pharmacological and physicochemical similarities. In principle, these substances consist of a hydrophilic and a lipophilic part of the molecule. The structural differences and physicochemical similarities of some acidic anti-inflammatory analgesics are presented in Table 1. All these drugs show a marked hydrophilic/lipophilic polarity and comparable acidity with pKa values around 4 to 5 (40,60, 103). At therapeutic doses they are bound, to a high degree, to human blood plasma proteins (37). These properties seem to be essential with regard to the anti-inflammatory activity, because in contrast to most other drugs, the analgesic and anti-inflammatory potency of acidic analgesics appears to be directly correlated

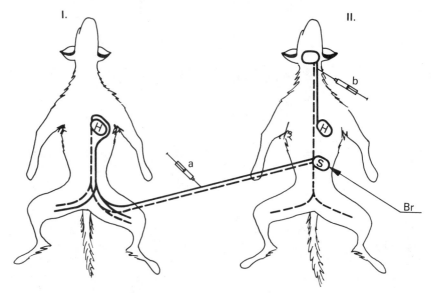

FIG. 1. Arrangement of a test to define the therapeutic site of action of analgesics. Two anaesthetised dogs (I and II) are positioned side by side. The femoral artery and vein of I are cannulated and connected to the cannulated splenic artery and vein of the exposed spleen (S) of II, i.e., the spleen of II is supplied by the blood circulation of I. The splenic nerves of II are, however, intact and connected to the CNS of II. By injecting bradykinin (Br) into the spleen, a nociceptive reaction ("pain") can be produced in II. This reaction is suppressed when analgesics are administered. Depending on whether the application causes an analgesic effect ($+$) or is ineffective ($-$) in *a* or *b*, one can assume either a peripheral or a central site of action (65).

	Efficacy after injection into:	
Drug	**a** *(Splenic artery)*	**b** *(Brachiocephalic artery)*
Morphine	$-$	$+$
Acetylsalicylic acid	$+$	$-$
Salicylic acid	$+$	$-$
Acetaminophen	$+$	$-$
Dimethylaminophenazone	$+$	$-$

with the degree of albumin binding (41). Further, molecular modifications leading to a distinct increase or decrease of the pKa value, as well as the introduction of a hydrophilic group into the lipophilic part of the molecule, cause a large or total loss of activity (Fig. 2). Of course, the characteristics mentioned here also determine the pharmacokinetic behaviour of these drugs (*see* below).

Pharmacodynamics

In contrast to the opioids, the mode of action of peripherally-acting anti-inflammatory analgesics remains unclear, even today, after decades of research in this field. At present, there are two theories that cannot be rejected on the basis of

TABLE 1. *Characteristics of anti-inflammatory, analgesic acids*

Drug name (trademark®)	Structure — Lipophilic part	Structure — Hydrophilic part	(a) pKa value (b) Binding to plasma proteins (c) Absorption	Refs.
Salicylates Acetylsalicylic acid (Aspirin)			(a) 3.5 (b) >75% (c) rapid complete	61 70 73
Diflunisal (Dolobid)			(a) 3–4 (b) ~99% (c) complete	102
Profens (arylpropionic acids) Ibuprofen (Brufen)			(a) ~5 (b) ~99% (c) complete	114
Naproxen (Naprosyn)			(a) 4–5 (b) ~99% (c) rapid complete	4
Aryl- and heteroarylacetic acids Tolmetin (Tolectin)			(a) 4–5 (b) ~99% (c) complete	30
Zomepirac (Zomax)			(a) 4–5 (b) ~99% (c) rapid complete	78
Diclofenac (Voltaren)			(a) 4–5 (b) ~99% (c) rapid complete	98
Indomethacin (Indocin)			(a) 4–5 (b) ~99% (c) rapid complete	44
Acidic ketoenols Piroxicam (Felden)			(a) ~5 (b) ~99% (c) complete	47
Phenylbutazone (Butazolidin)			(a) 4–5 (b) ~99% (c) complete	1 28

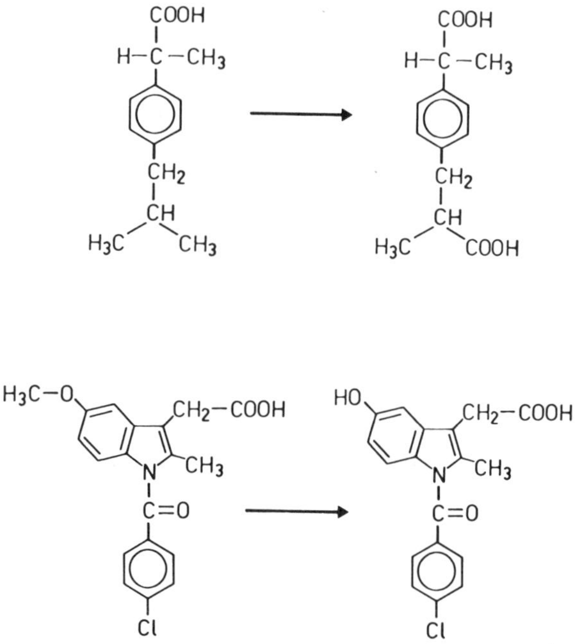

FIG. 2. Metabolic transformations *(left to right)* of active drugs ibuprofen *(top, left)* (2), and indomethacin *(bottom, left)* (95) leading to their total *(top, right)* or partial *(bottom, right)* inactivation by introduction of a second polar group.

current knowledge. The first one postulates that the analgesic acids act by inhibiting the synthesis of prostaglandins and other metabolites of unsaturated fatty acids of the cellular membrane, mainly arachidonic acid (Fig. 3). This very popular concept (36,37,97) is based on the pioneering observations of Vane and Willis et al. They found that the anti-inflammatory analgesics inhibit the biosynthesis of prostaglandins *in vitro* (106). Slightly later it was discovered that they have the same effect *in vivo* (116). Prostaglandins and their partly very unstable precursors formed in the inflamed tissue are able to elicit and/or intensify the symptoms of inflammation, namely, pain, erythema, and oedema (58,111). Thus, inhibition of prostaglandin synthesis in the inflamed tissue might well cause an analgesic/anti-inflammatory effect. The correlation between analgesic and prostaglandin inhibitory relative

FIG. 3. Recent concepts of the biological effects of arachidonic acid metabolites and the actions of analgesic acids. The so-called "slow-reacting substances" (SRSs), now identified as leukotrienes (LTs) (64,84,94) and the thromboxanes are known to be formed from arachidonic acid in addition to prostaglandins (PGs, synthesis inhibited by, e.g., indomethacin (Ind)). The formation of thromboxane A can be inhibited by imidazole derivatives (Imid) (80), and the formation of LTs by experimental drugs like BW 755 c (46). Further, leukotactic hydroxy acids are synthesized, the formation of which is inhibited by salicylic acid (Sal) and other acidic analgesics (96). Besides reactive oxygen, ($\cdot O_2^-$; $\langle O \rangle$; $\cdot OH$) is formed, which is able to oxidize macromolecules of possible functional importance in the development of inflammation (58,71). Reactive oxygen is inactivated in part by the enzyme superoxide dismutase (SOD) (50). SOD of bovine origin is on the market as an anti-inflammatory drug (Orgotein).

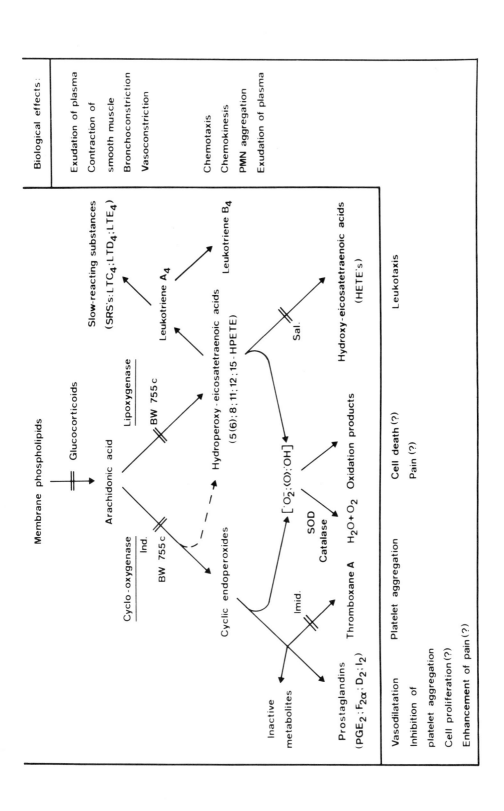

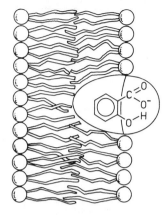

FIG. 4. Incorporation of the ionised form of salicylic acid in the lipid bilayer of a cell membrane (hypothetically) (13).

potencies of the analgesic acids emphasises the relationship (37). However, prostaglandins are formed, not only in the inflamed tissue, but by almost all cells throughout the human body. As so called tissue hormones, they are assumed to modulate the functions of most cells, except liver and skeletal muscle cells (Table 2). The regulation of gastrointestinal (7,8) and kidney (59,72) functions, and also of platelet aggregation (75) by prostaglandins, might be particularly important, because all anti-inflammatory analgesic acids have side effects in these systems (18,76,99). However, the prostaglandin hypothesis is not quite satisfactory, because the analgesic acids are effective even in animals unable to synthesize the known inflammagenic prostaglandins because of essential fatty acid deficient feed (9). Nevertheless, this concept has become accepted, and the basis of many screening systems in search of new anti-inflammatory analgesics.

An alternative but less popular hypothesis assumes that analgesic acids, similar to local anaesthetics or inhalation narcotics, are attached to cellular membranes (Fig. 4) where they inhibit, at sufficiently high concentrations, many cell functions, including the metabolic conversion of unsaturated fatty acids to prostaglandins (14). By these multiple actions (112), the analgesic acids might exert their manifold effects and side effects (Table 3). This concept has not yet been proved.

Whether the analgesic acids act by inhibition of the ubiquitous prostaglandin synthesis, or other processes occurring in all cells, at equal distribution throughout the body they should exert effects everywhere in the living organism. As far as these compounds show a certain organ selectivity in their actions, it must be because of an unequal distribution, i.e., these drugs have to distribute unequally in order to act selectively. Therefore, the pharmacokinetic behaviour of these drugs is an important factor for the understanding of their effects and side effects (13,16). In this respect, they differ from the opioids, which interact with specific pharmacological receptors, and thus are effective only in structures endowed with these receptors. How the simultaneous lowering of raised body temperature by anti-inflammatory analgesics occurs remains unclear (22,35). This effect is relevant only in the therapy of pain, owing to infections which are accompanied by fever.

TABLE 2. *Biological effects of prostaglandins (PGs) and thromboxane A (TXA)*

Body system	Type of prostaglandin	Effects	Indomethacin causes (37,95)	Refs.
CNS	E	Behavioural changes	Psychoses (very rare)	21
		Fever	Lowering of fever	35
Autonomous nervous system	E	Inhibition of NA release	?	43
	F	Increase of NA release	?	43
Endocrine system	E,F	Release of ACTH STH Prolactin Gonadotropins LH TH Insulin	?	49
Heart	$F_{2\alpha}$	Lysis of corpus luteum		32
	E,F	Contractility increased	?	7
Smooth musculature	all PGs + TXA	Contraction or relaxation depending on muscle type, localization, hormonal status (uterus), and species		
Intestine			Prolongation of labour	53
Urogenital tract			Bronchial asthma	24
Respiratory system			Closure of the ductus arteriosus Botalli	32,39,45
Vessel wall			Shock (very rare)?	
Exocrine glands (gastrointestinal tract)	E,F,I	Inhibition of H+ secretion but augmented production of mucus and digestive enzymes	Stomach ulcers	8
			Inhibition of some forms of diarrhea	51
Kidney	E,I	Diuresis (H_2O, K^+, Na^+)	Retention of H_2O and salts	72
Blood cells	I,D,E	Inhibition of platelet aggregation	Impaired blood clotting (only in cases of pre-existing deficiencies of blood coagulation)	75
	TXA	Platelet aggregation		75

This table is not exhaustive. The biological relevance of most observations remains undefined (?) or controversial.

TABLE 3. *Anti-inflammatory analgesic acids*

Effects, mode of actions, and therapeutic uses	Side effects (approximate frequency (%))

Effects
Inhibition of pain and inflammation
Lowering of fever
 	
Mode of action
Inhibition of prostaglandin synthesis
Alternatively: inhibition of the production and action of many inflammatory mediators
 	
Therapeutic use
Pain related to inflammation
Acute
  Toothache
  Sunburn
  Muscle stiffness
  Posttraumatic pain
  Dysmenorrhea (pain relief)
  Headache (some types)
  → Short-acting anti-inflammatory acids
Chronic
  Rheumatoid arthritis
  Osteoarthrosis, etc.
  → Long-acting anti-inflammatory acids or short-acting compounds adequately dosed
	Gastrointestinal tract
	Nausea, pain, diarrhea, obstipation (10)
	Blood loss, ulcers (particularly with aspirin) (2)
	
	Kidney
	H_2O and salt retention (particularly with phenylbutazone and piroxicam) (5)
	Papillary necrosis and interstitial nephritis (very rare)
	
	Blood
	Inhibition of platelet aggregation (particularly pronounced and lasting with aspirin) (100)
	
	Bone marrow and liver
	Damage (particularly with phenylbutazone but altogether very rare)
	
	CNS
	Chronic administration (particularly with indomethacin) (50)
	Nausea, somnolence, headache, psychosis
	Overdosage (particularly with aspirin)
	Auditory and visual disturbances
	Fever, alkalosis, acidosis, coma (salicylism)
	
	Additional side effects
	Drug allergy (anaphylactoid and anaphylactic) (5)
	Drug interactions with
	  Antacids
	  Vitamin K-antagonists
	  Oral antidiabetic drugs
	  Cardiac glycosides
	  Diuretics (well-documented for aspirin, indomethacin, and phenylbutazone)
	All side effects have also been observed in some cases with more modern anti-inflammatory analgesic acids

All known analgesic acids cause considerable side effects in the upper gastrointestinal tract. Particularly, ulcerations of the stomach comprise a major problem of the treatment with these drugs (27,87). It is assumed that gastric irritation is caused by two processes. On one hand, inhibition of prostaglandin synthesis in the stomach

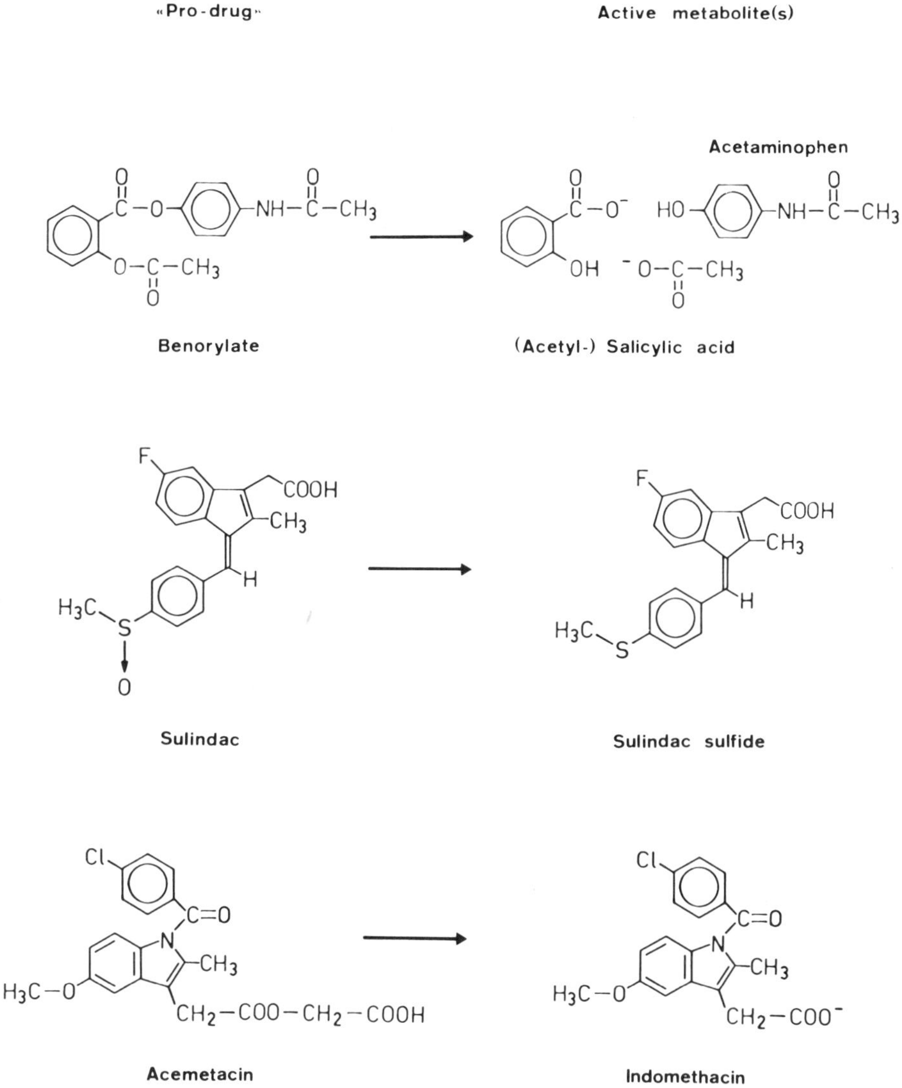

"Pro-drug"   Active metabolite(s)

Benorylate   (Acetyl-) Salicylic acid

Sulindac   Sulindac sulfide

Acemetacin   Indomethacin

FIG. 5. "Pro-drugs" of analgesic acids: Benorylate (91), sulindac (95), and acemetacin (25).

wall may deprive the stomach of a protective factor (7). In addition, high concentrations of these acidic drugs in cells of the stomach wall may lead to local damage (*see* below). Many attempts have been made to find compounds devoid of gastric irritating effects (88). Thus, new drugs with novel chemical structure have been developed. They are reported to be less ulcerogenic than acetylsalicylic acid (aspirin) at equianalgesic doses (11). The justification of the claim that these new compounds are superior with regard to this side effect is questionable, although many double-blind studies show a lower incidence of gastrotoxic side effects with these new compounds. The question, however, often remains if equianalgesic doses were applied in these studies. Another method of reducing the gastrotoxicity of analgesic acids is to apply "pro-drugs," which are metabolized to active forms after absorption, perhaps not before they have reached their site of action (25,54,91,95). Three examples of such "pro-drugs" are shown in Fig. 5. Their superiority in analgesic/anti-inflammatory therapy is not yet definitely proved, but the claim that they are less ulcerogenic is based on the theory that less absorption is to be expected in the stomach. Finally, it is possible to provide the active drugs with coatings resistant to gastric fluid. Indeed, the rapid decay of these preparations in the small intestine may lead to very high concentrations and to ulcerations in this area. Therefore, this pharmaceutical variety shows no clear advantage. Recently, devices for controlled intestinal release and absorption of substances such as indomethacin have been developed (5). The clinical advantage of these systems has to be documented.

Pharmacokinetics

After oral administration, acidic anti-inflammatory analgesics are absorbed at different rates in the upper gastrointestinal tract (19,89, Fig. 6). Extensive transformation during the primary liver passage (first pass effect) has been reported for fenbufen (54). Aspirin too is metabolized esterolytically in the stomach, the cells of the intestinal tract, and the blood plasma during or shortly after absorption (70). In both cases, acids are formed again, which conform to the structural requirements defined at the beginning of the chapter. All acidic analgesics distribute unequally throughout the body (16,19,89). Particularly high concentrations are present in the stomach wall (after oral administration, exceptions: *see* "pro-drugs"), in the kidney, liver, bone marrow, and the inflamed tissue (Figs. 6 and 7; 30,56,68,74,114). Relatively low concentrations are observed in the not inflamed muscular, adipose, and connective tissue but also, after a single therapeutic dose, in the CNS. In all organs where the acidic analgesics reach high concentrations, they exert typical effects and side effects (Table 3). The latter include hypersensitivity reactions ("aspirin asthma") (101,113) because the high degree of protein binding presumably

---

FIG. 6. Autoradiographs of the whole body distribution of ^{14}C-labelled aspirin (a) and diflunisal (b) in rats. Rats were given a single oral dose of [^{14}C-acetyl]-labelled aspirin (100 μCi in 10 mg/kg body weight) or [^{14}C-carboxyl]-labelled diflunisal (100 μCi in 100 mg/kg), respectively. At 1 hr (aspirin) and 3 hr (diflunisal) after drug administration, the animals were sacrificed and sections prepared for autoradiography (89,90). High concentrations of radioactivity *(dark)* are observed in organs with high blood content like liver (L) and kidney (K). High specific accumulation of aspirin **(a)** is evident in the stomach (S) wall and the bone marrow (BM). This high labelling, stemming from the acetyl moiety of aspirin lasts up to more than 5 hr after drug administration as a consequence of acetylation of macromolecules in these organs (90). In contrast, high concentrations of diflunisal **(b)** are present in the stomach lumen even 3 hr after administration, whereas the mucosa remains practically unstained by radioactivity. The apparent low rate of penetration of this compound into the cells of the stomach mucosa compared to aspirin may explain why diflunisal causes less gastric irritation than other salicylates (11).

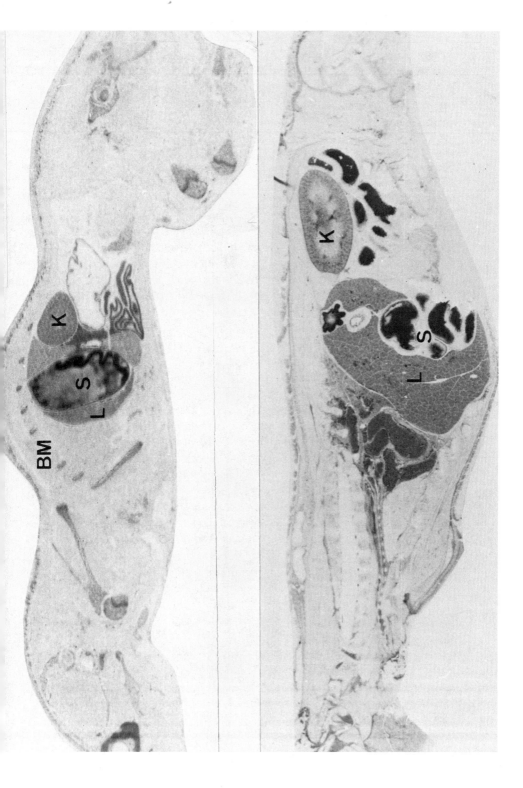

favours sensitization. However, the so-called "aspirin asthma" is not always caused by a true allergic reaction. Apparently the blockade of prostaglandin synthesis by inhibition of the enzyme cyclo-oxygenase (Fig. 3) enhances the formation of lipoxygenase products like slow-reacting substance A (SRS-A, leukotrienes) (34,42,52,84,109) which may cause bronchoconstriction (77,82,83). This reaction may thus be provoked by any analgesic acid applied. Also, the most frequent drug interactions, displacement of other drugs from plasma proteins by overloading the binding capacity (100), are essentially a consequence of the high plasma concentrations reached by all acidic analgesics (30,33,56,68,74,104,114). The observed unequal distribution of these drugs in the body is owing to the already mentioned physicochemical properties of the drugs (Table 1) as well as to the physiology and anatomy of the involved tissues. The following appear to be responsible for the accumulation of acidic analgesics in certain body regions. First, high drug concentrations are present in the gastric mucosa after oral administration because of intensive absorption of acidic compounds in the stomach (48,69). It appears noteworthy that some other acidic drugs, e.g., furosemide, probenecid, and valproic acid also cause stomach irritation, although they do not inhibit prostaglandin synthesis. Second, inflammation causes capillary damage and extravasation of plasma proteins together with protein-bound drugs (115). Because protein binding is reversible, a redistribution of acidic analgesics into the intracellular space may take place (*see* below). Further, high drug concentrations are found in the kidney because of active secretion of organic cations in the proximal tubules followed by passive back diffusion in the distal tubules at acidic pH-values of the urine (110). Finally, a direct cellular contact with the high drug concentrations in plasma is expected in the liver, spleen, and bone marrow. In these organs, the cells are not well protected by tight capillary walls as in the CNS, where closed layers of endothelial cells plus glia cells prevent this direct contact.

However, these findings and considerations are not sufficient to explain the effects and side effects of acidic analgesics, because other drugs are also orally administered, renally eliminated, and show a high degree of binding to plasma proteins. An additional reason for the unequal distribution of acidic analgesics is the acidic pH values found in the gastric fluid, the distal tubules of the kidney (acidic urine), and also in the inflamed tissue (23). According to the principle of nonionic diffusion, acidic pH values in the extracellular space together with alkaline values in the

--->

FIG. 7. Cross-section **(a)** and whole body autoradiograph **(b)** of a rat treated with ^{14}C-labelled phenylbutazone. A young rat (30 g body weight) was given a single dose of ^{14}C-labelled phenylbutazone (100 μCi in 10 mg/kg) by a stomach tube. At the same time, an inflammatory reaction was induced in the neck by subcutaneous injection of an irritant agent (carrageenan). At 5 hr after drug administration, the animal was exsanguinated, frozen, and sectioned in slices of about 100 μm by a cryomicrotome. Sections were freeze-dried and subsequently exposed by direct contact for 8 days to x-ray film (18). *Dark regions* correspond to areas of high activity. Particularly high concentrations are found in the inflamed tissue (IT), kidney (K) and liver (L). It is noteworthy that the stomach (S) lumen is free of activity, whereas the stomach wall is markedly stained. Opposite conditions are observed in the intestine (I), probably because of excretion of metabolites with the bile.

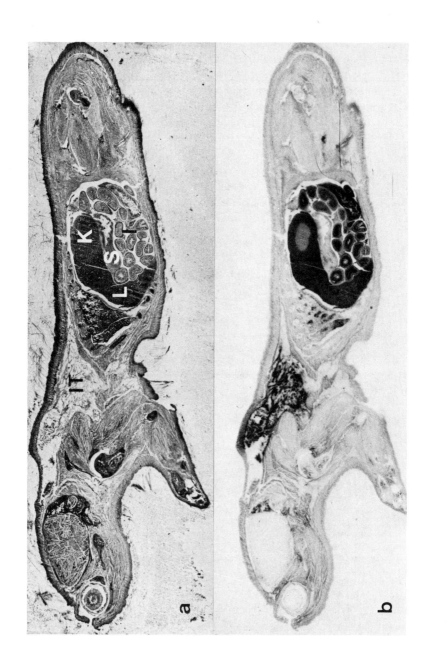

cell interior (108) cause a considerable shift of acidic compounds into the intra-cellular space (17). Thus, the acidic analgesics already accumulated in the extra-cellular space by the mechanisms mentioned above, reach the sites of possible pharmacodynamic actions in relatively high concentrations.

The characteristic distribution pattern of acidic anti-inflammatory analgesics is important not only for the understanding of their typical side effects. It also explains why the duration of action is generally (systematic investigations are lacking) longer than expected from their plasma half-life (29, Table 4). The inflamed tissue, which is the site of action of these drugs, presumably behaves as a deep compartment retaining high drug concentrations at the site of action, long after blood concen-trations have begun to decline (30,33,56,68,74,93,104,114). Conversely, central nervous side effects increase after prolonged high-dose therapy or acute overdosage, especially with aspirin at acidotic conditions (salicylism) (20). In the CNS, distri-bution of the drug into the intracellular space leads to coma, which can sometimes be overcome instantaneously by infusion of bicarbonate (81).

Applications

All acidic analgesics are indicated, particularly in inflammatory pain, indepen-dent of the inflammagen which may consist, e.g., in urate crystals in gout, UV-

TABLE 4. *Analgesic acids: dosage and duration of action*

Drug name (trademark®)	Usual adult dose (g/day)	Duration of action (plasma half-life)
Acetylsalicylic acid (Aspirin)	3	Hours (2–8 hr depending on dose; salicylic acid)
Diflunisal (Dolobid)	1.5	Hours (12 hr)
Ibuprofen (Brufen)	1	Hours (3 hr)
Tolmetin (Tolectin)	1	Hours (3 hr)
Zomepirac (Zomax)	0.3	Hours (4 hr)
Diclofenac (Voltaren)	0.2	Hours (2 hr)
Indomethacin (Indocin)	0.1	Hours (2 hr)
Naproxen (Naprosyn)	0.5	1 day (13 hr)
Piroxicam (Felden)	20 mg/day	Days (40 hr)
Phenylbutazone (Butazolidin)	Initial dose: e.g., 0.4 g/day over a 5-day period Maintenance dose: 0.2 g/day	Days (70 hr)

For complete references, see Table 1.

radiation in sunburn, or bacteria in toothache. Carcinoma metastases are also often accompanied by an inflammatory reaction. Injuries of any kind (fractures, surgery) represent inflamed areas according to pathophysiological criteria. Finally, some headaches seem to have an inflammatory component (exudation of plasma into the perivascular tissue). Thus, acidic analgesics may be therapeutically successful in such cases as well. Under all painful conditions mentioned, the analgesic and the anti-inflammatory effects cannot be separated because they are causally related. The characteristic side effects of several acidic analgesics are listed in Table 3. They often limit the use of those drugs that are to be administered therapeutically for a long period of time. Thus, indomethacin, with its high incidence of central nervous side effects such as dizziness, headaches, and daze is obviously not suitable for the therapy of headaches. The long-lasting inhibitory effect of aspirin on platelet aggregation excludes this drug from pain relief in every case of impaired blood coagulation (6,92). The new compounds introduced into therapy during the last few years appear to have these side effects to a lesser extent than the older ones. It remains to be seen whether the apparent superiority is real. The duration of action is another essential factor in the choice of an acidic analgesic drug for the therapy of a certain type of pain. Although the analgesic effect of the short-acting analgesic acids uniformly lasts for about 6 to 8 hr, and is apparently independent of the plasma half-life of the drug (Table 4), the duration of action of piroxicam (47) or even phenylbutazone (66) is very much longer (days!). Because these drugs may cumulate, they are to be used at adequate doses in chronic inflammatory pain only. Corresponding caution, e.g., of bone marrow function, must be exercised.

NONACIDIC, ANTIPYRETIC ANALGESICS

Characteristics

In contrast to the acidic analgesics, the pharmacological and physicochemical properties of the peripherally-acting nonacidic antipyretic analgesics are much less homogenous. Essentially, they belong to two classes of compounds, namely, the p-aminophenol derivatives (Table 5) and the nonacidic pyrazoles (Table 6). Common structural characteristics or physicochemical properties are not evident.

Pharmacodynamics

p-Aminophenol Derivatives

The p-aminophenol derivatives have antipyretic and analgesic effects, the mode of action being unclear for both effects. Often, inhibition of prostaglandin synthesis in the CNS is argued to be responsible for the actions of these drugs (38), but the experimental data are unsatisfactory, because a significant inhibition of prostaglandin biosynthesis occurs only at doses or concentrations hardly reached in therapy (12).

TABLE 5. *Antipyretic analgesics: p-aminophenol derivatives*

Drug name:	Phenacetin	Acetaminophen (paracetamol)
Structure:	(phenacetin structure: benzene ring with NH–C(=O)–CH₃ and O–CH₂–CH₃) → (acetaminophen structure: benzene ring with NH–C(=O)–CH₃ and OH)	
	↓ (benzene ring with NH₂ and O–CH₂–CH₃)	↓ (quinone-imine structure with N=C(=O)–CH₃ and =O)

Toxic metabolites:	p-Phenetidin (→methemoglobinemia)	N-Acetyl-p-benzoquinone-imine (→liver cell necrosis)
Absorption:	Complete	Complete
Duration of action ($t_{50\%}$ of acetaminophen) (67):	2–4 hr	2–4 hr
		(~2 hr)
Dosage:	0.5–1.0 g	0.5–1.0 g
Effects:	Analgesic, antipyretic effect	Analgesic, antipyretic effect
Mode of action:	Undefined (15)	Undefined (15)
Therapeutic use:	Occasional pain and virus infection related fever (pediatrics)	Occasional pain and virus infection related fever (pediatrics)
Side effects:	Methemoglobinemia (105) Probably important in small children only Chronic use Interstitial nephritis, cancer (31,85)	Overdosage (10–40 g) Severe hepatic centrolobular necrosis resulting in death (3) Chronic ingestion Kidney damage not excluded so far

For details see (refs.).

Phenacetin (acetophenetidin) is hardly in clinical use any more because of the risk of methemoglobin formation and kidney damage (interstitial nephritis). Methemoglobin formation comprises a considerable risk in children, especially newborns, because they lack the enzyme NAD-methemoglobin reductase which reactivates methemoglobin. Acetaminophen does not lead to methemoglobin formation. It causes liver cell necrosis in high doses. High doses lead to the metabolic formation of reactive N-acetyl-p-benzoquinone-imine. If given within 15 hr after ingestion of acetaminophen, acetylcysteine can prevent liver cell necrosis (86, Fig. 8).

Nonacidic Pyrazoles

The analgesic and antipyretic efficacy of some pyrazoles is higher than those of the p-aminophenol derivatives. The actions are explained by an inhibitory effect on prostaglandin synthesis (26), although the pyrazoles are hardly administered at doses sufficient to clearly inhibit prostaglandin synthesis in the organism (15). Therefore, the mode of action of these drugs is unknown at present.

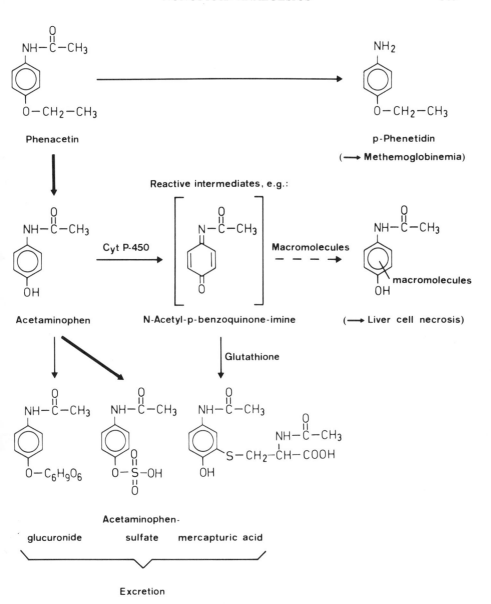

FIG. 8. Biotransformation of phenacetin and acetaminophen (for details see text).

Pharmacokinetics

Both types of nonacidic analgesics are metabolized rapidly and extensively in the human organism. The distribution of the primary compounds and their major metabolites throughout the body and the contribution to the analgesic effectiveness and the essential side effects are still unknown. No remarkable accumulation of

TABLE 6. *Antipyretic analgesics: nonacidic pyrazoles*

Drug name:	4-Dimethylaminophenazone	Isopyrine	Dipyrone	Propyphenazone
Structure:				
Major metabolite (107):			4-Aminophenazone	—

Absorption: Complete
Duration of action: 2–4 hr
   ($t_{50\%}$ of 4-
   aminophenazone) (~1 hr)

Effects: Analgesic, antipyretic effects
Slightly spasmolytic effects
Anti-inflammatory effect (in very high
   doses)

Mode of action: Undefined (15)
Therapeutic use: Fever-related pain (e.g. headache
   during virus infections)
Colic pain (e.g., stones of the gall
   bladder or urinary tract)

Side effects: Anaphylactic and anaphylactoid
   reactions (101)
Pruritus, urticaria, shock (particularly
   following i.v. administration)
Bone marrow damage (incidence is
   probably much lower than suspected)
   (10, 63)
Aminophenazone:
   Formation of nitrosamines
    (carcinogenic effects are
    postulated) (57)

For details, see refs.

acetaminophen and aminophenazone or their metabolites in certain body regions has been observed (19). The biotransformation of phenacetin (and acetaminophen) strikingly shows how relative (genetically determined) or absolute (overdosage) overload of metabolic pathways may lead to the formation of toxic metabolites and side effects (Fig. 8).

If the dealkylation of phenacetin to acetaminophen is limited (for unknown reasons), phenacetin is metabolized to a major extent to p-phenetidin and its oxidation products, which may be responsible for methemoglobin formation (105). Phenacetin treatment may thus cause methemoglobinemia and symptoms of poisoning, particularly in the newborn, for lack of the enzyme methemoglobin reductase.

In addition, overdosage of acetaminophen not only leads to conjugation but also oxidation reactions. In the presence of reactive SH-groups (glutathione) the supposed unstable N-acetyl-p-benzoquinone-imine is conjugated to a nontoxic mercapturic acid (79). If this conjugation system is overloaded, e.g., owing to overdosage but possibly also by drugs like salicylamide (62) or others, the unstable intermediate is bound covalently to cellular macromolecules (DNA, proteins). Liver cell necrosis may be the consequence (3).

Finally, the lack of reduced glutathione in erythrocytes of individuals deficient in the enzyme glucose-6-phosphate dehydrogenase may be increased by acetaminophen and lead to acute hemolysis (55). The incidence of bone marrow damage caused by pyrazoles and the contribution of their metabolites to this side effect is still unknown.

Applications

For decades, the p-aminophenol derivatives and nonacidic pyrazoles were considered exceptionally harmless and useful (in Europe). However, during the last few years, they were exposed to vehement criticism because physicians and patients have shown that these drugs have potential dangers (Tables 5 and 6). Nevertheless, most of the side effects reported are owing to improper use. It is not surprising that dangerous toxic reactions like shock may occur if pyrazoles, e.g., dipyrone, are administered intravenously at doses of more than 2 g as 20% solutions. On the other hand, it is a small wonder that high doses of phenacetin, taken over decades, cause kidney damage (interstitial nephritis), and that doses of 10 to 40 g of acetaminophen lead to liver cell necrosis.

REFERENCES

1. Aarbakke, J. (1978): Clinical pharmacokinetics of phenylbutazone. *Clin. Pharmacokinet.*, 3:369–380.
2. Adams, S. S., McCullough, K. F., and Nicholson, J. S. (1969): The pharmacological properties of ibuprofen, an anti-inflammatory, analgesic and antipyretic agent. *Arch. Int. Pharmacodyn. Ther.*, 178:115–129.
3. Ameer, B., and Greenblatt, D. J. (1977): Acetaminophen. *Ann. Intern. Med.*, 87:202–209.
4. Anttila, M., Haataja, M., and Kasanen, A. (1980): Pharmacokinetics of naproxen in subjects with normal and impaired renal function. *Eur. J. Clin. Pharmacol.*, 18:263–268.

5. Bayne, W., Place, V., Theeuwes, F., Rogers, J. D., Lee, R. B., Davies, R. O., and Kwan, K. C. (1982): Kinetics of osmotically controlled indomethacin delivery systems after repeated dosing. *Clin. Pharmacol. Ther.*, 32:270–276.

6. Beaver, W. T. (1965 and 1966): Mild analgesics: A review of their clinical pharmacology. *Am. J. Med. Sci.*, 250:577–604, and 251:576–599.

7. Bennett, A. (1977): The role of prostaglandins in gastrointestinal tone and motility. In: *Prostaglandins and Thromboxanes*, edited by F. Berti, B. Samuelsson, and G. P. Velo, pp. 275–285. Plenum Press, New York.

8. Bennett, A., Stamford, I. F., and Unger, W. A. (1973): Prostaglandin E_2 and gastric acid secretion in man. *J. Physiol. (Lond.)*, 229:349–360.

9. Bonta, I. L., Bult, H., v.d. Ven, L. L. M., and Noordhoek, J. (1976): Essential fatty acid deficiency: A condition to discriminate prostaglandin and non-prostaglandin mediated components of inflammation. *Agents Actions*, 6:154–158.

10. Böttiger, L. E., Furhoff, A. K., and Holmberg, L. (1979): Drug-induced blood dyscrasias. *Acta Med. Scand.*, 205:457–461.

11. Brogden, R. N., Heel, R. C., Pakes, G. E., Speight, T. M., and Avery, G. S. (1980): Diflunisal: A review of its pharmacological properties and therapeutic use in pain and musculoskeletal strains and sprains and pain in osteoarthritis. *Drugs*, 19:84–106.

12. Bruchhausen, F., and Baumann, J. (1982): Inhibitory actions of desacetylation products of phenacetin and paracetamol on prostaglandin synthetases in neuronal and glial cell lines and rat renal medulla. *Life Sci.*, 30:1783–1791.

13. Brune, K. (1974): How aspirin might work: A pharmacokinetic approach. *Agents Actions*, 4:230–232.

14. Brune, K. (1982): Prostaglandins, inflammation and anti-inflammatory drugs. *Eur. J. Rheumatol. Inflammation*, 5:335–349.

15. Brune, K. (1983): Prostaglandins and the mode of action of antipyretic analgesic drugs. *Am. J. Med.*, 75(5a):19–23.

16. Brune, K., Graf, P., and Rainsford, K. D. (1977): A pharmacokinetic approach to the understanding of therapeutic effects and side-effects of salicylates. In: *Aspirin and Related Drugs: Their Actions and Uses*, edited by K. D. Rainsford, K. Brune, and M. W. Whitehouse. *Agents Actions (Suppl.)*, 1:9–26.

17. Brune, K., and Graf, P. (1978): Non-steroid anti-inflammatory drugs: Influence of extra-cellular pH on biodistribution and pharmacological effects. *Biochem. Pharmacol.*, 27:525–530.

18. Brune, K., Gubler, H., and Schweitzer, A. (1979): Autoradiographic methods for the evaluation of ulcerogenic effects of anti-inflammatory drugs. *Pharmacol. Ther.*, 5:199–207.

19. Brune, K., Rainsford, K. D., and Schweitzer, A. (1980): Biodistribution of mild analgesics. *Br. J. Clin. Pharmacol.*, 10:279S–284S.

20. Buchanan, N., and Rabinowitz, L. (1974): Infantile salicylism—a reappraisal. *J. Pediatr.*, 84:391–395.

21. Coceani, F. (1974): Prostaglandins and the central nervous system. *Arch. Intern. Med.*, 133:119–129.

22. Cranston, W. I. (1979): Central mechanisms of fever. *Fed. Proc.*, 38:49–51.

23. Cummings, N. A., and Nordby, G. L. (1966): Measurement of synovial fluid pH in normal and arthritic knees. *Arthritis Rheum.*, 9:47–56.

24. Cuthbert, M. F. (1973): Prostaglandins and respiratory smooth muscle. In: *The Prostaglandins: Pharmacological and Therapeutic Advances*, edited by M. F. Cuthbert, pp. 253–286. J. B. Lippincott Co., Philadelphia.

25. Dell, H.-D., Doersing, M., Fischer, W., Jacobi, H., Kamp, R., Köhler, G., and Schöllnhammer, G. (1980): Metabolism and pharmacokinetics of acemetacin in man. *Drug. Res.*, 30:1391–1398.

26. Dembińska-Kieć, A.,Żmuda, A., and Krupińska, J. (1976): Inhibition of prostaglandin synthetase by aspirin-like drugs in different microsomal preparations. In: *Advances in Prostaglandin and Thromboxane Research, Vol. 1*, edited by B. Samuelsson, and R. Paoletti, pp. 99–103. Raven Press, New York.

27. Desbaillets, L. G. (1974): Side-effects of anti-inflammatory agents. *Adv. Clin. Pharmacol.*, 6:23–30.

28. Dieterle, W., Faigle, J. W., Früh, F., Mory, H., Theobald, W., Alt, K. O., and Richter, W. J. (1976): Metabolism of phenylbutazone in man. *Drug. Res.*, 26:572–577.

29. Doménech, J., Lauroba, J., Moreno, J., and Plá-Delfina, J. M. (1981): A relationship between

biological half-life and effective half-life according to pharmacological response in non-steroid antiinflammatory drugs. *Drug. Res.*, 31:445–452.

30. Dromgoole, S. H., Furst, D. E., Desiraju, R. K., Nayak, R. K., Kirschenbaum, M. A., and Paulus, H. E. (1982): Tolmetin kinetics and synovial fluid prostaglandin E levels in rheumatoid arthritis. *Clin. Pharmacol. Ther.*, 32:371–377.

31. Duggin, G. G. (1980): Mechanisms in the development of analgesic nephropathy. *Kidney Int.*, 18:553–561.

32. Dusting, G. J., Moncada, S., and Vane, J. R. (1979): Prostaglandins, their intermediates and precursors, their cardiovascular actions and regulatory roles in normal and abnormal circulatory systems. *Prog. Cardiovasc. Dis.*, 21:405–430.

32a. Editorial (1982): Mehr Nutzen und weniger Kosten durch die richtige Auswahl von Arzeimitteln. *Arznei-Telegramm*, 4:33–41.

33. Emori, H. W., Champion, G. S., Bluestone, R. S., and Paulus, H. E. (1973): Simultaneous pharmacokinetics of indomethacin in serum and synovial fluids. *Ann. Rheum. Dis.*, 32:433–435.

34. Engineer, D. M., Niederhauser, U., Piper, P. J., and Sirois, P. (1978): Release of mediators of anaphylaxis: Inhibition of prostaglandin synthesis and the modification of release of slow-reacting substance of anaphylaxis and histamine. *Br. J. Pharmacol.*, 62:61–66.

35. Feldberg, W. (1974): Fever, prostaglandins and antipyretics. In: *Prostaglandin Synthetase Inhibitors*, edited by H. J. Robinson, and J. R. Vane, pp. 197–203. Raven Press, New York.

36. Ferreira, S. H., and Vane, J. R. (1974): New aspects of the mode of action of nonsteroid antiinflammatory drugs. *Annu. Rev. Pharmacol.*, 14:57–73.

37. Flower, R. J. (1974): Drugs which inhibit prostaglandin biosynthesis. *Pharmacol. Rev.*, 26:33–67.

38. Flower, R. J., and Vane, J. R. (1972): Inhibition of prostaglandin synthetase in brain explains the anti-pyretic activity of paracetamol (4-acetamidophenol). *Nature*, 240:410–411.

39. Friedman, W. F., Printz, M. P., and Kirkpatric, S. E. (1978): Blocker of prostaglandin synthesis. A novel therapy in the management of the premature human infant with patent ductus arteriosus. In: *Advances in Prostaglandin and Thromboxane Research, Vol. 4*, edited by F. Coceani, and P. M. Olley, pp. 373–381. Raven Press, New York.

40. Goldstein, A., Aronow, L., and Kalman, S. M. (1969): The absorption, distribution, and elimination of drugs. In: *Principles of Drug Action*, edited by A. Goldstein et al., pp. 106–205. Harper & Row, New York.

41. Grant, N. H., Alburn, H. E., and Singer, C. A. (1971): Correlation between *in vitro* and *in vivo* models in anti-inflammatory drug studies. *Biochem. Pharmacol.*, 20:2137–2140.

42. Hamberg, M. (1976): On the formation of thromboxane B_2 and 12-L-hydroxy-5,8,10,14-eicosatetraenoic acid (12 ho-20:4) in tissues from the guinea pig. *Biochim. Biophys. Acta*, 431:651–654.

43. Hedqvist, P. (1976): Prostaglandin action on transmitter release at adrenergic neuroeffector junctions. In: *Advances in Prostaglandin and Thromboxane Research, Vol. 1*, edited by B. Samuelsson and R. Paoletti, pp. 357–363. Raven Press, New York.

44. Helleberg, L. (1981): Clinical pharmacokinetics of indomethacin. *Clin. Pharmacokinet.*, 6:245–258.

45. Heymann, M. A., and Rudolph, A. M. (1978): Effects of prostaglandins and blockers of prostaglandin synthesis on the ductus arteriosus: Animal and human studies. In: *Advances in Prostaglandin and Thromboxane Research, Vol. 4*, edited by F. Coceani and P. M. Olley, pp. 363–371. Raven Press, New York.

46. Higgs, G. A., Flower, R. J., and Vane, J. R. (1979): A new approach to anti-inflammatory drugs. *Biochem. Pharmacol.*, 28:1959–1961.

47. Hobbs, D. C., and Twomey, T. M. (1979): Piroxicam pharmacokinetics in man: Aspirin and antacid interaction studies. *J. Clin. Pharmacol.*, 19:270–281.

48. Hogben, C. A. M., Tocco, D. J., Brodie, B. B., and Schanker, L. S. (1959): On the mechanism of intestinal absorption of drugs. *J. Pharmacol. Exp. Ther.*, 125:275–282.

49. Horton, E. W. (1972): *Prostaglandins. Monographs on Endocrinology, Vol. 7.* Springer-Verlag, Berlin.

50. Huber, W. (1980): Future trends in free radical studies. In: *Inflammation: Mechanisms and Treatment*, edited by D. A. Willoughby and J. P. Giroud, pp. 27–42. MTP Press Limited, Lancaster.

51. Jaffe, B. M. (1978): Prostaglandins and serotonin in diarrheogenic syndromes. *Adv. Exp. Biol. Med.*, 106:285–295.
52. Jakschik, B. A., Falkenhein, S., and Parker, C. W. (1977): Precursor role of arachidonic acid in release of slow reacting substance from rat basophil leukaemia cells. *Proc. Natl. Acad. Sci. U.S.A.*, 74:4577–4581.
53. Karim, S. M. M. (1972): Prostaglandins and human reproduction: Physiological roles and clinical uses of prostaglandins in relation to human reproduction. In: *The Prostaglandins: Progress in Research*, edited by S. M. M. Karim, pp. 71–164. John Wiley & Sons, Inc., New York.
54. Kerwan, S. S., and Sloboda, A. E. (1982): Pharmacological properties of fenbufen. *Pharmacology, (Suppl. 1)*, 25:12–20.
55. Kirkman, H. N. (1968): Glucose-6-phosphate dehydrogenase variants and drug-induced hemolysis. *Ann. NY Acad. Sci.*, 151:753–764.
56. Köhler, G., and Mohing, W. (1980): Zur Kinetik von Diclofenac-NA in Plasma und Synovialflüssigkeit. *Akt. Rheumatol.*, 5:151–155.
57. Kramer, M. (1980): Chronic toxicity of pyrazolones: The problem of nitrosation. *Br. J. Clin. Pharmacol.*, 10:313S–317S.
58. Kuehl, F. A., Humes, J. L., Egan, R. W., Ham, E. A., Beveridge, G. C., and Van Arman, C. G. (1977): Role of prostaglandin endoperoxide in inflammatory processes. *Nature*, 265:170–173.
59. Lee, J. B. (1972): The antihypertensive and natriuretic endocrine function of the kidney: Vascular and metabolic mechanisms of the renal prostaglandins. In: *Prostaglandins in Cellular Biology, Vol. 1*, edited by P. W. Ramwell and B. B. Pharriss, pp. 399–450. Plenum Press, New York.
60. Levitan, H., and Barker, J. L. (1972): Salicylate: A structure activity study of its effects on membrane permeability. *Science*, 176:1423–1425.
61. Levy, G. (1980): Clinical pharmacokinetics of salicylates: A re-assessment. *Br. J. Clin. Pharmacol.*, 10:285S–290S.
62. Levy, G., and Yamada, H. (1971): Drug biotransformation interactions in man III: Acetaminophen and salicylamide. *J. Pharmacol. Sci.*, 60:215–221.
63. Levy, M. (1980): Epidemiological evaluation of rare side-effects of mild analgetics. *Br. J. Clin. Pharmacol.*, 10:395S–399S.
64. Lewis, R. A., Drazen, J. M., Figueiredo, J. C., Corey, E. J., and Austen, K. F. (1982): A review of recent contributions on biologically active products of arachidonate conversion. *Int. J. Immunopharmacol.*, 4:85–90.
65. Lim, R. K. S. (1970): Pain. *Annu. Rev. Physiol.*, 32:269–288.
66. Lombardino, J. G. (1974): Enolic acids with anti-inflammatory activity. In: *Anti-inflammatory Agents, Vol. 1*, edited by R. A. Scherrer and M. W. Whitehouse, pp. 130–158. Academic Press, Inc., New York.
67. Lowenthal, D. T.,Øie, S., Van Stone, J. C., Briggs, W. A., and Levy, G. (1976): Pharmacokinetics of acetaminophen elimination by anephric patients. *J. Pharmacol. Exp. Ther.*, 196:570–578.
68. Mäkelä, A.-L., Lempiäinen, M., and Ylijoki, M. (1981): Ibuprofen levels in serum and synovial fluid. *Scand. J. Rheumatol. Suppl.*, 39:15–17.
69. Martin, B. K. (1963): Accumulation of drug anions in gastric mucosal cells. *Nature*, 198:896–897.
70. Mason, W. D., and Winer, N. (1981): Kinetics of aspirin, salicylic acid, and salicyluric acid following oral administration of aspirin as a tablet and two buffered solutions. *J. Pharmacol. Sci.*, 70:262–265.
71. McCord, J. M. (1974): Free radicals and inflammation: Protection of synovial fluid by superoxide dismutase. *Science*, 185:529–531.
72. McGiff, J. C., Crowshaw, K., and Itskovitz, H. D. (1974): Prostaglandins and renal function. *Fed. Proc.*, 33:39–47.
73. Miaskiewicz, S. L., Shively, C. A., and Vesell, E. S. (1982): Sex differences in absorption kinetics of sodium salicylate. *Clin. Pharmacol. Ther.*, 31:30–37.
74. Mitchell, W. B., Scott, P., Kennedy, A. C., Brooks, P. M., Templeton, R. S., and Jefferies, M. G. (1975): Clinico-pharmacological studies on ketoprofen (Orudis). *Curr. Med. Res. Opin.*, 3:423–430.
75. Moncada, S., and Vane, J. R. (1978): Unstable metabolites of arachidonic acid and their role in haemostasis and thrombosis. *Br. Med. Bull.*, 34:129–136.
76. Morales, A., and Steyn, J. (1971): Papillary necrosis following phenylbutazone ingestion. *Arch. Surg.*, 103:420–421.

77. Murphy, R. C., Hammarström, S., and Samuelsson, B. (1979): Leukotriene C: A slow-reacting substance from murine mastocytoma cells. *Proc. Natl. Acad. Sci. U.S.A.*, 76:4275–4279.

78. Muschek, L. D., and Grindel, J. M. (1980): Review of the pharmacokinetics and metabolism of zomepirac in man and animals. *J. Clin. Pharmacol.*, 20:223–229.

79. Nelson, S. D., Forte, A. J., Vaishnav, Y., Mitchell, J. R., Gillette, J. R., and Hinson, J. A. (1981): The formation of arylating and alkylating metabolites of phenacetin in hamsters and hamster liver microsomes. *Mol. Pharmacol.*, 19:140–145.

80. Nijkamp, F. P., Moncada, S., White, H. L., and Vane, J. R. (1977): Diversion of prostaglandin endoperoxide metabolism by selective inhibition of thromboxane A_2 biosynthesis in lung, spleen or platelets. *Eur. J. Pharmacol.*, 44:179–186.

81. Oliver, T. K., and Dyer, M. E. (1963): The prompt treatment of salicylism with sodium bicarbonate. *Am. J. Dis. Child.*, 99:553–565.

82. Orange, R. P., and Austen, K. F. (1969): Slow reacting substance of anaphylaxis. In: *Advances in Immunology, Vol. 10*, edited by F. J. Dixon, and H. G. Hunkel, pp. 106–139. Academic Press, New York.

83. Parker, C. W., Jakschik, B. A., Huber, M. G., and Falkenhein, S. F. (1979): Characterisation of slow reacting substance as a family of thiolipids derived from arachidonic acid. *Biochem. Biophys. Res. Commun.*, 89:1186–1192.

84. Piper, P. J. (1983): Leukotrienes. *Trends Pharmacol. Sci.*, 4:75–77.

85. Porpáczy, P., and Schramek, P. (1981): Analgesic nephropathy and phenacetin-induced transitional cell carcinoma-analysis of 300 patients with long-term consumption of phenacetin-containing drugs. *Eur. Urol.*, 7:349–354.

86. Prescott, L. F., Illingworth, R. N., Critchley, J. A. J. H., Stewart, M. J., Adam, R. D., and Proudfoot, A. T. (1979): Intravenous N-acetylcysteine: The treatment of choice for paracetamol poisoning. *Br. Med. J.*, 2:1097–1100.

87. Rainsford, K. D. (1975): The biochemical pathology of aspirin-induced gastric damage. *Agents Actions*, 5:326–344.

88. Rainsford, K. D., and Whitehouse, M. W. (1976): Gastric irritancy of aspirin and its analogues: Anti-inflammatory effects without this side-effect. *J. Pharm. Pharmacol.*, 28:599–601.

89. Rainsford, K. D., Schweitzer, A., and Brune, K. (1981): Autoradiographic and biochemical observations on the distribution of non-steroid anti-inflammatory drugs. *Arch. Int. Pharmacodyn. Ther.*, 250:180–194.

90. Rainsford, K. D., Schweitzer, A., and Brune, K. (1983): Distribution of the acetyl compared with the salicyl moiety of acetylsalicylic acid: Acetylation of macromolecules in organs wherein side-effects are manifest. *Biochem. Pharmacol.*, 32:1301–1308.

91. Robertson, A. (1973): Benorylate—the rationale. *Rheumatol. Rehabil. Suppl.:* 7–16.

92. Roth, G. J., Stanford, N., and Majerus, P. W. (1975): Acetylation of prostaglandin synthetase by aspirin. *Proc. Natl. Acad. Sci. U.S.A.*, 72:3073–3076.

93. Saccetti, G., Ferrati, G. C., Parrinello, L., and Salami, A. (1978): Kinetics of analgesic response in man; an example with two non-steroidal anti-inflammatory analgesic drugs. *J. Int. Med. Res.*, 6:312–316.

94. Samuelsson, B. (1981): Leukotrienes: Mediators of allergic reactions and inflammation. *Int. Arch. Allergy Appl. Immunol., (Suppl. 1)*66:98–106.

95. Shen, T.-Y., and Winter, C. A. (1977): Chemical and biological studies on indomethacin, sulindac and their analogs. In: *Advances in Drug Research*, edited by N. J. Harper, and A. B. Simmons, pp. 89–245. Academic Press, Inc., New York.

96. Siegel, M. I., McConnell, R. T., Porter, N. A., and Cuatrecasas, P. (1980): Arachidonate metabolism via lipoxygenase and 12-L-hydroperoxy-5,8,10,14-icosatetraenoic acid peroxidase sensitive antiinflammatory drugs. *Proc. Natl. Acad. Sci. U.S.A.*, 77:308–312.

97. Simon, L. S., and Mills, J. A. (1980): Nonsteroidal antiinflammatory drugs. *N. Engl. J. Med.*, 302:1179–1185.

98. Sioufi, A., Stierlin, H., Schweizer, A., Botta, L., Degen, P. H., Theobald, W., and Brechbühler, S. (1982): Neuere Befunde zur klinisch relevanten Pharmakokinetik von Diclofenac Na. In: *Voltaren®, neue Ergebnisse*, edited by E. Kåss. Verlag Hans Huber, Bern.

99. Smith, J. B., and Willis, A. L. (1971): Aspirin selectively inhibits prostaglandin production in human platelets. *Nature New Biol.*, 231:235–237.

100. Svihovec, J. (1980): Anti-inflammatory analgesics and drugs used in gout. In: *Meyler's Side*

Effects of Drugs, 9th edition, edited by M. N. G. Dukes, pp. 141–164. Excerpta Medica, Amsterdam.

101. Szczeklik, A., Gryglewski, R. J., and Czerniawska-Mysik, G. (1977): Clinical patterns of hypersensitivity to nonsteroidal anti-inflammatory drugs and their pathogenesis. *J. Allergy Clin. Immunol.*, 60:276–284.

102. Tempero, K. F., Cirillo, V. J., and Steelman, S. L. (1977): Diflunisal: A review of pharmacokinetic and pharmacodynamic properties, drug interactions, and special tolerability studies in humans. *Br. J. Clin. Pharmacol.*, 4:31S–36S.

103. Terada, H., Muraoka, S., and Fujita, T. (1974): Structure-activity relationships of fenamic acids. *J. Med. Chem.*, 17:330–334.

104. Thomas, G. M., Rees, P., Dippy, J. E. S., and Maddock, J. (1975): Simultaneous pharmacokinetics of alclofenac in plasma and synovial fluid in patients with rheumatoid arthritis. *Curr. Med. Res. Opin.*, 3:264–267.

105. Uehleke, H. (1973): Biochemical pharmacology and toxicology of phenacetin. In: *International Symposium on Problems of Phenacetin Abuse*, edited by H. Haschek, pp. 31–44. Facta Publication, Wien.

106. Vane, J. R. (1971): Inhibition of prostaglandin-synthesis as a mechanism of action of aspirin-like drugs. *Nature New Biol.*, 231:232–235.

107. Volz, M., and Kellner, H.-M. (1980): Kinetics and metabolism of pyrazolones (propyphenazone, aminopyrine and dipyrone). *Br. J. Clin. Pharmacol.*, 10:299S–308S.

108. Waddell, W. J., and Bates, R. G. (1969): Intracellular pH. *Physiol. Rev.*, 49:285–329.

109. Walker, J. L. (1973): The regulatory role of prostaglandins in the release of histamine and SRS-A from passively sensitized human lung tissue. In: *Advances in the Biosciences, Vol. 9*, edited by S. Bergström, and S. Bernhard, pp. 235–239. Pergamon Press, New York.

110. Weiner, J. M., and Mudge, G. H. (1964): Renal tubular mechanisms for excretion of organic acids and bases. *Am. J. Med.*, 36:743–762.

111. Weissmann, G., Smolen, J. E., and Korchak, H. (1980): Prostaglandins and inflammation: Receptor/cyclase coupling as an explanation of why PGEs and PGI_2 inhibit functions of inflammatory cells. In: *Advances in Prostaglandin and Thromboxane Research, Vol. 8*, edited by B. Samuelsson, P. W. Ramwell, and R. Paoletti, pp. 1637–1653. Raven Press, New York.

112. Whitehouse, M. W. (1968): The molecular pharmacology of anti-inflammatory drugs: Some possible mechanisms of action at the biochemical level. *Biochem. Pharmacol. (Suppl.)*:293–307.

113. Whitehouse, M. W., and Rainsford, K. D. (1977): Side-effects of anti-inflammatory drugs. Are they essential or can they be circumvented? In: *Inflammation Mechanisms and their Impact on Therapy*, edited by I. L. Bonta, J. Thompson, and K. Brune. *Agents Actions (Suppl.)*, 3:171–187.

114. Whitlam, J.B., Brown, K. F., Crooks, M. J., and Room, G. F. W. (1981): Transsynovial distribution of ibuprofen in arthritic patients. *Clin. Pharmacol. Ther.*, 29:487–492.

115. Williams, T. J., and Morley, J. (1974): Measurement of rate of extravasation of plasma protein in inflammatory responses in guinea-pig skin using a continuous recording method. *Br. J. Exp. Pathol.*, 55:1–12.

116. Willis, A. L., Davison, P., Ramwell, P. W., Brocklehurst, W. E., and Smith, B. (1972): Release and actions of protaglandins in inflammation and fever: Inhibition by anti-inflammatory and antipyretic drugs. In: *Prostaglandins in Cellular Biology, Vol. 1*, edited by P. W. Ramwell and B. B. Pharriss, pp. 227–259. Plenum Press, New York.

Analgesics: Neurochemical, Behavioral, and
Clinical Perspectives, edited by M. Kuhar and
G. Pasternak. Raven Press, New York © 1984.

Animal Models in Analgesic Testing

Paul L. Wood

Douglas Hospital Research Centre, Verdun, Quebec, Canada H4H 1R3

Despite the vast amount of research in the area of analgesics, a potent nonaddicting analgesic is still needed. The complexity involved in solving this problem has only recently begun to be fully appreciated.

The demonstration of stereospecific CNS opiate receptors (71), the identification of endogenous opiate ligands (41), and the evolution of the concept of multiple opiate receptors (61) all form major advances in this area. Such advances have clearly demonstrated that specific but multiple opiate receptors are present in the CNS, and that activation of specific subsets of these populations can elicit analgesia independent of classical opiate side effects. Therefore, the design of a safer analgesic will depend on definition of the structural attributes which contribute to selective high affinity for opiate receptor subpopulations.

A tentative classification scheme (115) for the agonists of these receptor populations is presented in Table 1. This scheme includes the classical mu or alkaloid agonists, the partial mu agonists which bind to the mu receptor but dissociate very slowly (18,78), the delta or enkephalin agonists, the epsilon agonist β-endorphin, the sigma or dysphoric agonist SKF 10,047, and the kappa agonists (ketazocines and N-furyl benzomorphans). An additional drug class is also presently available for clinical use. These are the agonist/antagonist (Ag/Ant) agents which possess multiple receptor affinities (61) including kappa angonism, mu antagonism, and partial sigma agonism.

This classification scheme is based on many behavioral and neurochemical studies which are only briefly summarized in Table 2. However with these listed parameters, one can delineate the receptor characteristics of experimental narcotics. In regard to analgesia, it has become clear that sigma receptor activation is responsible for the dysphoric activity of Ag/Ant analgesics but that this receptor is not involved in analgesia (64,118). This contrasts with the analgesia elicited by mu, epsilon, and kappa receptor activation. The role of delta receptors in analgesia is still not clearly defined because the enkephalin analogs presently available all possess mu and delta receptor affinities. However, peptides with a high degree of delta receptor affinity exhibit much weaker analgesia than mu-preferring peptides (3,81,91). Further answers to this problem will inevitably come with studies of the apparent delta-selective peptide Tyr-D-Ser-Gly-Phe-Leu-Thr (29).

TABLE 1. *Narcotic classification scheme*

(A)	Mu agonists:	Morphine
		Methadone
		Dihydromorphine
		FK33 824[a]
(B)	Partial mu agonists:	Buprenorphine
		Profadol
		Propiram
(C)	Delta agonists:	DADLE [b]
		DSLET[c]
(D)	Epsilon agonists:	β-endorphin
(E)	Sigma agonists:	SKF 10,047 (N-allylnorphenazocine)
(F)	Kappa agonists:	Ethylketazocine[d]
		MR-2034[e]
(G)	Ag/Ant:	Nalorphine
		Nalbuphine
		Pentazocine
		Cyclazocine
		Butorphanol[f]

[a]D-Ala²-MePhe⁴-Met-O-OH enkephalin (*Drugs of the Future*, [1978]: 3:511).

[b]D-Ala²-D-Leu⁵-enkephalin; BW-180C (*Drugs of the Future*, [1980]: 8:395).

[c]D-Ser²-Leu⁵-enkephalin-Thr⁶; (29).

[d](73).

[e](-)-α-(1R, 5R, 9R)-5,9-dimethyl-2-(L-tetrahydrofurfuryl-2'-hydroxy-6, 7-benzomorphan (*Drugs of the Future*, [1980]: 5:303).

[f](75).

Of the active analgesic drug classes, it has become clear that mu agonists characteristically possess dependence potential and varying degrees of autonomic side effects. Although the partial mu agonists do not exhibit a marked withdrawal syndrome in man (46,47), they do act via mu receptors and therefore produce dependence and classical opiate side effects. Dependence is also a problem with enkephalin analogs which possess mu and delta receptor affinities. For example, FK33 824, which is a potent mu analgesic in animals and man (96,115), also elicits dependence on chronic administration in rats (110), and is self-injected by monkeys (122). In contrast, kappa agonists and Ag/Ant agents elicit analgesia with a much reduced dependence potential. Kappa agonists are unique in that they are not self-injected by rats or monkeys (121,123), nor do these agents express cross-tolerance with morphine (123). However, only two kappa agonists are presently available as clinical candidates: (a) EKC, which is an analgesic in man (123), unfortunately has a very short half-life, and (b) the N-furyl benzomorphan MR-2034 awaits clinical testing.

Ag/Ant are also potent analgesics in man (39,43). However, these agents vary considerably in their relative affinities for opiate receptor subpopulations and therefore express variable side effects. Characteristically, acute dysphoric and psycho-

TABLE 2. *Behavioral and neurochemical actions of narcotics*

Parameter	Drug class				
	Mu	Kappa	Sigma	Delta	Ag/Ant
Pulse rate (D)	−	0	+	−	
Skin twitch reflex (D)	−	−	0	−	−
Suppress morphine abstinence (D)	Y	N	N	Y	N
Suppress cyclazocine abstinence (D)	Y	Y	N	Y	Y
Analgesia (M)	Y	Y	N	Y	Y
Locomotor stimulation (M)	Y	N	Y	Y	N
Straub tail (M)	Y	N	N	Y	N
Striatal DOPAC (R)	+	0	+ [a]	+	+ [b]
Cortical TR$_{ACh}$ (R)	−	0	0	−	−
Hippocampal TR$_{ACh}$ (R)	−	0	0	−	0

(D), dog, (61).
(M), mouse, (64).
(R), rat, (114, 117, 118).
Y, yes.
N, no.
DOPAC, Dihydroxyphenylacetic acid.
[a], not reversed by naloxone.
[b], reversal at high drug doses.
−, decrease.
+, increase.
0, no effect.

tomimetic effects limit the clinical utility of Ag/Ant. This action was originally thought to involve a sigma narcotic receptor (61), but more recent behavioral and receptor binding studies suggest this may involve a phencyclidine receptor (115). Separation of the analgesic and dysphoric action of Ag/Ant is therefore a key goal of future drug development for this drug class. In this regard, several research data indicate that Ag/Ant analgesia may be independent of mu or kappa receptor activation. These data include the inability of Ag/Ant to elicit analgesia after local injections into the periaqueductal gray and the spinal cord (126). In marked contrast, mu, delta, and epsilon agonists are active at both sites (70,115,126), whereas kappa agonists are most active at the spinal level (119). These data suggest that Ag/Ant analgesia involves a unique receptor population and/or receptor distribution.

Other potential approaches to analgesia include anti-inflammatory agents and novel non-narcotic agents (e.g., α_2 agonists, GABAergics, and cholinergics); however, in both cases potent analgesia has not been achieved.

STATEMENT OF THE PROBLEM

A modern analgesic testing progam must have a defined goal in terms of the type of desired analgesic, and must utilize a battery of tests to define whether this goal has been achieved. The test battery, by definition, must include receptor

TABLE 3. *Test battery used to characterize kappa agonists*

A. Primary tests
   1. Opiate receptor binding (116): Displacement of ^{3}H-naloxone binding (Na$^+$ ratio).
   2. Potent analgesic activity (118): RTF (naloxone reversible).
   3. Mouse behavioral parameters (103): No Straub tail or locomotor stimulation.
   4. Lack of antagonist activity (72): No antagonism of morphine analgesia in the RTF
B. Secondary tests
   1. Striatal dopamine metabolites (117): No change in striatal DOPAC or HVA.
   2. Hippocampal acetylcholine turnover (114,118): No change in ACh turnover.
   3. Selective receptor protection (120): Pretreatment with the cold ligand should
      provide selective protection of the ^{3}H-EKC binding site, but not the ^{3}H-
      dihydromorphine or ^{3}H-D-Ala^2-D-Leu^5 enkephalin sites from inactivation by N-
      ethylmaleimide.

binding, behavioral, and neurochemical assays of narcotic activities. Such a test battery and the order of operations utilized in our laboratory to characterize kappa receptor agonists is presented in Table 3. This protocol is useful for characterizing kappa and Ag/Ant analgesics, both of which are key targets for the pharmaceutical industry today. In the case of Ag/Ant, auxillary procedures are required to delineate relative receptor affinities and the potential for dysphoric and psychotomimetic effects.

This chapter will concentrate on the animal models available to detect analgesics and to define the putative receptor populations involved. Other assay techniques essential to a successful screening battery should be consulted: (a) receptor binding (chapter 3 and refs. 116 and 120), (b) neurochemical parameters (114,117,118), and (c) *in vitro* smooth muscle preparations (51).

ANALGESIA TESTING

Pain is a subjective parameter which expresses a large variability among individuals. However, in animal tests, only behavioral responses subsequent to a painful stimulus are monitored. Therefore, it is inherent in all of the animal testing procedures that false negatives may be encountered with stringent protocols (e.g., rat tail flick assay) and false positives with less stringent tests (e.g., writhing assays). When considering data from such animal screening tests, the following points should be considered:

1. *Test validity:* Is the test predictive of the clinical utility of known analgesics?
2. *Test Reliability:* Is the test response reproducible throughout an experimental day and from day-to-day?
3. *Test Simplicity:* Does the procedure use a standard defined noxious stimulus, measure a well-defined animal response, and is the test easily utilized?
   Stimulus strength must be clearly defined because this parameter affects the results dramatically. For example, in the hot-plate (124) and the Haffner assay (99), only weak algesic stimuli enable detection of Ag/Ant agents and non-narcotic analgesics. A problem of increased variability in the animal

response, however, occurs with these weaker stimuli as compared to stronger algesic stimuli.

4. *Test Sensitivity:* Can different analgesic doses be discriminated and can the procedure detect weak and Ag/Ant analgesics?

5. *Data Analysis:* Analgesic ED_{50}s for representative narcotics assayed in our laboratories are presented in Table 4. These ED_{50}s are defined as a 100% increase in reaction times in 50% of the tested animals; however, in some studies ED_{50}s have been defined by various workers as a 50% increase in reaction time in 50% of the tested animals. These ED_{50} values are determined from linear regression analysis of log reaction time versus log dose or probit analysis using log dose. For probit analysis, the probit of percent responders, of percent inhibition of writhing (phenylquinone writhing assay), or of percent maximum possible effect[1] can be used. These methods of data analysis all yield reproducible ED_{50} values with defined confidence limits.

Using these criteria, Taber (98) has rated various analgesiometric procedures and given the highest ratings to the rat tail flick (RTF) or D'Amour and Smith test (19), the mouse phenylquinone writhing protocol (6,68), and the yeast-induced hyperalgesia (31,79) or Randall and Selitto procedure (79). These assays and others, which utilize chemical, thermal, electrical, and pressure as algesic stimuli will be considered (Table 4).

CHEMICAL STIMULI

Writhing Assays

The i.p. administration of noxious chemical agents to rats and mice results in peritoneal irritation which elicits a writhing response consisting of abdominal constriction, turning of the trunk, and extension of the hind legs. Blockade of these behavioral responses serves as a rapid and sensitive screen for analgesic activity. Many chemical irritants have been utilized, and include phenylquinone (35,93), acetylcholine (5,60), bradykinin (5,8,25,86,87), acetic acid (50), benzoquinone (44), serotonin (13,60), alloxan (11), and hypertonic saline (30).

These tests have the advantages of simplicity and sensitivity to all known clinically useful analgesics. For example, Ag/Ant agents are readily detected by this assay (6,98). Periaqueductal gray stimulation also inhibits visceral pain in response to hypertonic saline (30). The major disadvantage of writhing tests, however, is their lack of specificity with depressants and stimulants generating false positives. These false positives include muscle relaxants, antihistamines, MAO inhibitors, neuroleptics, cholinomimetics, and adrenergic blockers (12,35,60). Auxillary tests can be utilized to maintain false positives to a minimum. For example, although Ag/Ant analgesics are more active in the mouse phenylquinone writhing (MPQW)

---

[1]Maximum possible effect = [(Postdrug latency minus predrug latency)/(cut-off time minus predrug latency)] 100.

TABLE 4. Actions of analgesics in standard screening procedures

Drug (Straub tail)[a]	Dose in man (mg)[b]	^{3}H-naloxone[c]		MPQW[d]	RTF[e]	MHP[f]	RYPP[g]	
		−Na	+Na/−Na				Normal	Hyperalgesic
A. Mu								
Morphine (+)	10	3.5	30	0.5	2.0	4.0	3.0	1.0
Methadone (+)	10	7.3	97	—	0.8	0.5	1.5	0.5
Etorphine (+)	0.03	0.2	7	0.002	0.002	0.003	—	—
B. Delta/Mu								
DADLE (+)	—	5.7	131	—	5.0	—	—	—
FK33 824 (+)	1.0	1.0	36	0.02	0.4	0.8	0.8	0.1
C. Kappa								
EKC (−)	—	7.5	7.5	0.10	2.0	1.5	1.5	1.0
MR-2034 (−)	—	0.2	16.9	0.05	0.5	0.05	—	—
D. Partial Mu								
Buprenorphine (+)	0.4	1.6	1.3	0.02	0.06	—	—	—
E. Ag/Ant								
Butorphanol (−)	3	0.3	5.1	0.1	0.6	0.06	0.5	0.06
Cyclazocine (−)	30	0.2	2.1	0.4	IA	3.0	0.75	0.2
Nalbuphine (−)	10	2.4	6.2	—	4	4.0	0.5	0.25
Pentazocine (−)	40	13.5	12	2.0	40	32.0	8.0	8.0
Nalorphine (−)	15	3.7	2.1	1.0	IA	IA	IA	2.0
F. Anti-inflammatory								
Aspirin (−)	600	IA	—	4.0	IA	IA	IA	225
Zomepirac (−)	100	IA	—	1.0	IA	IA	IA	16

[a] +, present; −, absent.
[b] (43).
[c] IC_{50} (nM).
[d] Mouse phenylquinone writhing (ED_{50}, mg/kg, ip).
[e] Rat tail flick (ED_{50}, mg/kg, ip).
[f] Mouse hot-plate (ED_{50}, mg/kg, ip).
[g] Rat yeast paw pressure (ED_{50}, mg/kg, ip).

procedure than in the rotorod test, depressants and stimulants tend to be equiactive in both tests (68). Using these tests in parallel, drug-induced motor changes can therefore be distinguished from analgesia.

Discrimination between narcotic and anti-inflammatory agents has also been described for the benzoquinone writhing assay. In this procedure, PGE_2 and arachidonic acid potentiation of benzoquinone writhing are blocked by morphine, whereas only arachidonate potentiation is blocked by ASA (44).

More sophisticated analyses can also be performed in anesthetized animals but are not applicable for routine screening. For example, recording of dorsal horn interneurons (5) and quantitation of flexor reflex activity (86,87) in response to i.v. bradykinin have been investigated. The flexor reflex procedure has the advantage of insensitivity to muscle relaxants, contrasting with the writhing assays.

Hyperesthesia

Yeast-Induced

Hyperesthesia can be induced in the rat hindpaw by subplantar injection of an aqueous suspension of yeast, and the sensitivity to pressure measured 1 hr later (79). A vocalization response to the applied pressure is best quantitated by transducer measurements of the cylinder pressure applied to the foot at the time of vocalization (112). When the protocol was originally developed, it was proposed that the test could discriminate between narcotic and anti-inflammatory analgesics. This has generally proven to be the case for potent narcotics; however, Ag/Ant agents are an exception, because in some cases, they only possess analgesic activity in the inflamed paw (31).

Adjuvant-Induced

Intradermal injection of *Mycobacterium butyricum* with Freund's adjuvant into the tail of rats has been used as a model of polyarthritis (74,113). Hypersensitivity to pain develops within a few hours and is stable for testing at 18 to 24 hr (113). At 7 to 14 days, the paws also become hyperalgesic. This pain model demonstrates sensitivity to narcotic and nonsteroidal anti-inflammatory drugs (15,38,53), but not to CNS depressants or anti-inflammatory steroids (38,53).

Because of the chronic nature of this model, the painful stimuli are tonic and not phasic in nature. These polyarthritic rats have therefore been utilized as a model of chronic pain in addition to acute narcotic testing protocols. Of interest, a recent study (14) of this model has indicated that morphine analgesia, as measured with the tail withdrawal assay (55°C), does not express the same degree of tolerance as in the naive rat. These data suggest that under chronic pain conditions, tolerance to opiate agonists may not be a major problem for clinical treatment.

Neurochemically, 5-HT metabolites have been found to be elevated in the spinal cords of these animals (108).

Intra-Articular Inflammation

Intra-articular inflammation of the rat or dog knee joint can be obtained by local injections of *M. butyricum* (9,42) or chemicals such as carrageenan, sodium urate, and ellagic acid (67,104). In this case, the inflammation is restricted to the injected joint and does not spread.

Formalin Test

In this procedure, 50 μliters of a 5%-formalin solution are injected s.c. in the forepaws of the rat (1,21,23). An acute inflammatory response develops and yields a paw which is hypersensitive to pain for up to 2 hr. The inflammation is followed by a blister and then scar tissue. As with other inflammatory stimuli, this procedure results in continuous algesic input rather than periodic input.

NOXIOUS HEAT STIMULI

RTF

The tail flick procedure of D'Amour and Smith (19) has become a standard screening procedure for testing analgesics in both rats and mice. In this procedure, the time required for the test animal to remove its tail from a radiant heat source is recorded. Generally, two predrug reaction times are determined 30 min apart. The stimulus intensity is set to obtain a base-line reaction time of 2 to 4 sec. Drugs are then administered and the tail flick latency measured at 30-min intervals, with a stimulus cutoff time of 10 to 20 sec set to eliminate potential tissue damage.

The intensity of the stimulus can also be varied according to the desired stringency of the testing protocol. At low settings, methotrimeprazine (32), chlorpromazine (32), and most Ag/Ant analgesics (32) can be detected. Ag/Ant with marked antagonist potency (e.g., cyclazocine), however, are not detected (32).

Tail Withdrawal Assay

The rodent tail withdrawal reflex can be consistently elicited by immersion of the tail in hot water (45 to 65°C). This behavioral response is stable throughout the day and sensitive to strong narcotics (45). However, at low stimulus intensities (45°C), pentazocine and other Ag/Ant analgesics can also be detected (16,33,90).

CO$_2$ Laser

A new advance (10) in analgesic testing appears to be laser-induced heat stimulation which can be performed with unrestrained rats in their home cage. With this procedure, no tissue damage occurs, and the threshold to stimulation is stable with repeated testing. Consistent behavioral responses can be elicited by focusing the heat on the ear, tail, or paw. Clear dose-response data have been described for morphine (10). However, the actions of Ag/Ant and anti-inflammatory agents remain to be reported with this procedure.

Mouse Hot-Plate

The mouse hot-plate test (124) has also found extensive use as a screening procedure, mainly because of its simplicity and sensitivity. Briefly, the mouse is placed on a heated plate at 50 to 60°C, and the reaction time for reflex responses recorded. The key responses include paw-licking, limb withdrawal, and escape attempts.

The major limitation of this procedure is the sensitivity to sedatives and muscle relaxants (124).

ELECTRICAL STIMULATION

Stimulation of the Tail

Both the rat (11) and mouse (63,65) have been utilized for electrical stimulation of the tail. The end response is tail movement and vocalization. Electrical stimulation at the base of the tail has been found to yield the most consistent response. The procedure is sensitive to classical opiate agonists and anti-inflammatory agents (65). The predrug threshold is determined via a stepwise increase in the stimulation voltage with two tests at each step. Drugs are next administered and animals tested with four shocks at the predrug threshold; analgesia is defined as no behavioral response under these conditions.

A simpler and less innocuous variant of this procedure has been introduced (127) in which ultrasonic stimulation replaces electrical stimulation.

Trigeminal Stimulation

Modulation of facial nociceptive input to the trigeminal complex has been investigated extensively in the rat and dog. In the rat, direct stimulation of the ophthalmic division of the trigeminal nerve can be used to test analgesics (83), with the current required to elicit a vocal response being measured. More refined measurements of neuronal activity in the trigeminal nucleus can also be undertaken. Biochemical measurements of substance P release from trigeminal slices *in vitro* (48) and electrophysiological studies (2) have also demonstrated that nociceptive afferents to this nucleus possess presynaptic opiate receptors.

Recently, a facial mask has been devised for trigeminal stimulation in the unanesthetized rat (84). This device is fixed to the skull and applies radiant heat to the facial skin. The end response consists of a facial rub which may represent a behavior high in the hierarchy of potential responses to heat (84). In the dog, stimulation of the dental pulp has also been utilized (105) to test narcotics.

Flinch-Jump Assay

In the flinch-jump protocol (7,26,27), an electrical shock is applied to the grid floor of a rat cage, and the subsequent flinch (crouch, startle, or twitch), jump, and vocalization responses monitored.

Shock-Titration

The shock-titration (ST) procedure has been used successfully both with rodents (125) and primates (24). In this behavioral pardigm, the test animal has operant control over the magnitude of the maximum intensity of an applied nociceptive stimulus, with the shock intensity increasing in a stepwise manner unless suppressed by a bar press. The test animal therefore determines the level of shock that it will tolerate, thereby eliminating problems with drug-induced sedation or incapacitation. An additional advantage to this procedure is the sensitivity to Ag/Ant analgesics (24). Of interest, this Ag/Ant-induced analgesia requires 100 times more naloxone for reversal than morphine analgesia (24).

PRESSURE STIMULI

Mechanical pressure applied to the rat or mouse tail with artery clips (Haffner assay) has also been used as an algesic stimulus which can be applied at different pressures (99). This assay is insensitive to anti-inflammatory agents (77) but does detect mild analgesics like nefopam (54).

CHRONIC PAIN

Many technical and ethical problems have hampered the development of chronic pain models. At the present time, two models have attained significant use. Deafferentation hypersensitivity, in response to dorsal rhizotomy or peripheral neurectomy, consists of excessive responsiveness to touch, scratching, and self-mutilation (20,59,97,109). The polyarthritic rat (*see* Hyperesthesia, Yeast-Induced) also may represent a chronic pain model.

NARCOTIC PROPERTIES

In addition to analgesic tests, other assays are available to define the receptor affinities of these agents. Such tests include:

Antagonist Assays (72)

Opiate receptor (mu) antagonism is a property characteristic of Ag/Ant analgesics and pure antagonists. The tests utilized *in vivo* have therefore concentrated mainly on antagonism of mu agonist activities.

Dependence Model

The morphine-dependent mouse (17) and cyclozocine-dependent monkey (16) have been used to detect antagonists that will induce withdrawal signs in these dependent animals. Pure antagonists, Ag/Ant and partial mu agonists can be detected with these models.

RTF

Antagonism of morphine analgesia as measured by the RTF can also be used to detect pure antagonists and Ag/Ant agents (72).

Mouse Straub Tail

A rapid and sensitive index of mu antagonist activity can be obtained by monitoring morphine-induced Straub tail in the mouse after pretreatment with test compounds (72).

Discriminative Stimulus Testing

The discriminative stimulus properties of opiates have been studied in primates (36,88,101), and indicate that these animals can distinguish between mu and kappa agonist analgesics. The Ag/Ant agents are not uniform in their behavioral actions with butorphanol, cyclazocine, and nalorphine, generalizing to kappa agonists in this behavioral paradigm. Pentazocine and nalbuphine do not generalize to either morphine or cyclazocine.

Analysis of possible CNS sites responsible for the discriminative stimulus generalization properties of mu agonists indicates involvement of the periaqueductal gray matter (52). This brain site is also very sensitive to mu-dependent analgesia (125), but not kappa-dependent analgesia (119). Therefore, both kappa-induced analgesia and discriminative stimulus actions may involve different neuronal pathways from those involved in these actions of mu agonists.

Dependence Potential

The dependence potential of an analgesic agent also reflects the receptor affinity of the drug. The tests available include:

Precipitated Withdrawal

Both acute (111) and chronic (85) mu narcotic administration will result in withdrawal signs after administration of naloxone. These signs include tremor, teeth-chattering, wet dog shakes, tachycardia, hyperventilation, weight loss, and diarrhea. In this assay, partial mu agonists (111) and kappa agonists (103, Table 5)

TABLE 5. *Naloxone-induced jumping in the mouse after acute opiate injections[a]*

	Drug	mg/kg	Naloxone-induced jumping	
			% Responding	Mean/responder
Saline		–	22	18
Mu:	Morphine	4	56	34
		16	89	44
	Etorphine	0.02	78	27
	Methadone	16	44	39
	Levorphanol	4	89	33
	Phenazocine	2	67	38
Kappa:	EKC	8	0	–
		16	0	–
Sigma:	SKF 10,047	32	0	–
Ag/Ant:	Levallorphan	64	38	32
	Nalorphine	64	11	–
	Pentazocine	64	44	34
	Butorphanol	1	78	19
		5	67	27

[a]Naloxone administered 60 min after narcotic injection and mice observed for 5 min in a plexiglass cylinder (3″ diameter).

are inactive in eliciting withdrawal signs after acute naloxone. Mu agonists (85,107,111) and enkephalin analogs (110) are active.

Chronic administration of the narcotic agonist for this assay as well as for primary dependence and substitutive tests can be achieved by several means: (i) parenteral administration every 12 hr, (ii) intraperitoneal infusion (40,102), (iii) pellet implantation (107), (iv) or intraventricular infusion for peptides which do not cross the blood brain barrier (110).

Primary Dependence

Withdrawal signs on abrupt discontinuance of chronic opiate treatment is characteristic of mu agonists (107). However, withdrawal from kappa and Ag/Ant analgesics is a milder syndrome with fewer autonomic signs (123). No withdrawal syndrome is evident with partial mu agonists (16), presumably as a result of the slow dissociation of these agents from the mu receptor. Similar data have been observed with clinical studies of buprenorphine (46) and profadol (47).

During chronic treatment with narcotic agonists, the development of tolerance can also be monitored with these procedures (107).

Cross-Tolerance

Morphine-dependent animals which develop tolerance to this narcotic also become tolerant to other mu agonists (61), but not to kappa agonists or Ag/Ant (103).

Morphine Substitution

Attenuation of withdrawal signs after cessation of chronic morphine treatment can be used to detect mu agonists (100).

Straub Tail

Mu agonists elicit contraction of the sacrococcygeal dorsalis muscle resulting in Straub tail in the mouse. However, Ag/Ant and kappa agonists are inactive in this behavioral test (92,103). Other agents (e.g., cocaine, caffeine, and nicotine) can also elicit Straub tail, therefore, naloxone reversal should be tested.

Self-Injection

Narcotic-reinforced responding in rodents and primates has been advocated as a reliable and rapid screening procedure for opiates (121). In this protocol, mu agonists, partial mu agonists, and enkephalin analogs are all self-injected, reflecting their dependence potential (121,122). In contrast, kappa agonists (EKC, ketazocine, MR-2034) are not self-injected, whereas Ag/Ant are intermediate between kappa and mu agonists (121,122). This assay would indicate that of the various potent narcotics only kappa agonists are devoid of dependence potential.

NOVEL ANALGESICS

The following is a short list of potentially novel approaches to analgesia and the analgesic tests used to characterize them.

Nefopam

Nefopam is a weak analgesic which demonstrates a ceiling to its analgesic activity, but is well tolerated in man (34). In animal testing procedures, nefopam is active in the MPQW assay but not the RTF test. In the Randall and Selitto procedure (79), nefopam is inactive in the noninflamed foot. The analgesic activities in the MPQW and the hyperalgesia assays are not reversed by naloxone. In addition, nefopam does not displace ^{3}H-naloxone binding to rat brain membranes, indicating a non-narcotic mechanism (54). In sum, these testing procedures correlate with clinical studies demonstrating the moderate analgesic activity of nefopam.

Methotrimeprazine

The tricyclic derivative, methotrimeprazine, is an active analgesic in postoperative and postpartum pain (28,55). However, in animal tests (mouse hot-plate) analgesia is not reversed by naloxone and the drug does not displace ^{3}H-naloxone (95). No cross-tolerance with morphine is present. These data strongly suggest a nonopiate analgesic mechanism for this drug also (62).

Baclofen

In the RTF assay, baclofen possesses analgesic activity which is supraspinal, independent of muscle relaxation, and not reversed by naloxone (76).

Clonidine

The α_2 agonist clonidine is analgesic both in the rat and mouse as tested with the hot-plate assay (56), with electrical stimulation of the tail (66,89), and with the tail-immersion (48°C) assay (57,58). This action appears to be spinal (57,80,94,128). Modulation of enkephalinergic pathways may be involved, because activity in the hot-plate assay is reversed by naloxone (56).

Cholinergics

Physostigmine and oxotremorine have been found to potentiate both morphine and clonidine analgesia, whereas atropine reduced the analgesia of these compounds (57). It therefore appears that muscarinic mechanisms may also modulate enkephalinergic neurons (69). In this regard, stereospecific analgesia has been demonstrated with the MPQW assay for the isomers of the muscarinic agonist acetyl-β-methylcholine (22).

Eseroline, an analog of eserine, which is devoid of anticholinesterase activity is also analgesic (4,49), and is naloxone reversible.

GABAergics

The putative GABA mimetics muscimol, baclofen, and 4,5,6,7-tetrahydroisoxazolo [5,4-C] pyridin-3-ol; (*Drugs of the Future* (1980): 5:257) possess analgesic activity in the MPQW, the mouse hot-plate, the Randall-Selitto, and the monkey shock titration assays (37). However, activity in the RTF assay was not marked, indicating that these agents are not potent analgesics. GABA transaminase inhibitors also elicit naloxone resistant analgesia which correlates with CNS GABA accumulation (106).

Enkephalinase Inhibitors

Enkephalinase is a key enzyme involved in the degradation of enkephalins (82). Therefore, potential inhibitors of this enzyme have been proposed as potential analgesic agents. Such an enkephalinase inhibitor, thiorphan, is inactive in the tail withdrawal assay (48°C) but does potentiate i.vt. enkephalin-dependent analgesia (82).

ACKNOWLEDGMENTS

I wish to express my gratitude to my co-workers Dr. R. Hudgin, Dr. M. Stotland, Mr. J. Richard, Ms. A. Rackham, and Mrs. S. Charleston who have all contributed to the establishment of the rationale for Table 3.

REFERENCES

1. Amodei, N., and Paxinos, G. (1980): Unilateral knife cuts produce ipsilateral suppression of responsiveness to pain in the formalin test. *Brain Res.*, 193:85–94.
2. Andersen, R. K., Lund, J. P., and Puil, E. (1978): Enkephalin and substance P effects related to trigeminal pain. *Can. J. Physiol. Pharmacol.*, 56:216–222.
3. Audigier, Y., Mazarguil, H., Gont, R., and Cros, J. (1980): Structure-activity relationships of enkephalin analogues at opiate and enkephalin receptors: Correlation with analgesia. *Eur. J. Pharmacol.*, 63:35–46.
4. Bartolini, A., Renzi, G., Galli, A., Aiello, P. M., and Bartolini, R. (1981): Eseroline: A new antinociceptive agent derived from physostigmine with opiate receptor agonist properties. Experimental in vivo and in vitro studies on cats and rodents. *Neurosci. Lett.*, 25:179–183.
5. Belcher, G. (1979): The effects of intra-arterial bradykinin, histamine, acetylcholine and prostaglandin E[1] on nociceptive and non-nociceptive dorsal horn neurones of the cat. *Eur. J. Pharmacol.*, 56:385–395.
6. Blumberg, H. B., Wolf, P. S., and Dayton, H. B. (1965): Use of writing test for evaluating analgesic activity of narcotic antagonists. *Proc. Soc. Exp. Biol. Med.*, 118:763–766.
7. Bonnet, K. A., and Peterson, K. E. (1975): A modification of the jump-flinch technique for measuring pain sensitivity in rats. *Pharmacol. Biochem. Behav.*, 3:47–55.
8. Burns, R. B. P., Alioto, N. J., and Hurley, K. E. A. (1968): A modification of the bradykinin-induced writing test for analgesia. *Arch. Int. Pharmacodyn. Ther.*, 175:41–53.
9. Carlson, R. P., Dagle, G. E., and Van Arman, C. G. (1973): Inflammatory response in dogs given intra-articular injection of Mycobacterium butyricum mineral oil adjuvant. *Am. J. Vet. Res.*, 34:515–519.
10. Carmon, A., and Frostig, R. (1981): Noxious stimulation of animals by brief intense laser induced heat: Advantages to pharmacological testing of analgesics. *Life Sci.*, 29:11–16.
11. Carroll, M. N., and Lim, R. K. S. (1960): Observations on the neuropharmacology of morphine and morphine-like analgesia. *Arch. Int. Pharmacodyn. Ther.*, 125:383–403.
12. Chernov, H. I., Wilson, D. E., Fowler, F., and Plummer, A. J. (1967): Nonspecificity of the mouse writing test. *Arch. Int. Pharmacodyn. Ther.*, 167:171–178.
13. Collier, H. O., Dinneen, J., Johnson, L. C., Johnson, C. A., and Schneider, C. (1968): The abdominal constriction response and its suppression by analgesic drugs in the mouse. *Br. J. Pharmacol.*, 32:295–310.
14. Colpaert, F. C. (1979): Can chronic pain be suppressed despite purported tolerance to narcotic analgesia? *Life Sci.*, 24:1201–1210.
15. Colpaert, F. C., De Witte, P., Maroli, A. N., Awonters, F., Niemegeers, C. J. E., and Janssen, P. A. J. (1980): Self-administration of the analgesic suprofen in arthritic rats: Evidence of mycobacterium butyricum-induced arthritis as an experimental model of chronic pain. *Life Sci.*, 27:921–928.
16. Cowen, A. (1974): Evaluation of nonhuman primates: Evaluation of the physical dependence capacities of oripavine-thebaine partial agonists in Patas monkeys. *Adv. Biochem. Psychopharm.*, 8:427–438.
17. Cowan, A. (1976): Use of the mouse jumping test for estimating antagonistic potencies of morphine antagonists. *J. Pharm. Pharmacol.*, 27:177–182.
18. Cowan, A., Lewis, J. W., and MacFarlane, I. R. (1977): Agonist and antagonist properties of buprenorphine, a new antinociceptive agent. *Br. J. Pharmacol.*, 60:537–545.
19. D'Amour, F. E., and Smith, D. L. (1941): A method for determining loss of pain sensation. *J. Pharmacol. Exp. Ther.*, 72:74–79.
20. Dennis, S. G., and Melzack, R. (1979): Self-mutilation after dorsal rhizotomy in rats: Effects of prior pain and pattern of root lesions. *Exp. Neurol.*, 65:412–421.
21. Dennis, S. G., Melzack, R., Gutman, S., and Boncher, F. (1980): Pain modulation by adrenergic agents and morphine as measured by three pain tests. *Life Sci.*, 16:1247–1259.
22. Dewey, W. L., Cocolas, G., Daves, E., and Harris, L. S. (1980): Stereospecificity of intraventricularly administered acetylmethylcholine antinociception. *Life Sci.*, 17:9–10.
23. Dubuisson, D., and Dennis, G. (1977): The formalin test: A quantitative study of the analgesic effects of morphine, meperidine, and brain stem stimulation in rats and cats. *Pain*, 4:161–174.
24. Dykstra, L. A. (1979): Effects of morphine, pentazocine and cyclazocine alone and in combination

with naloxone on electric shock tiltration in the squirrel monkey. *J. Pharmacol. Exp. Ther.*, 211:722–732.

25. Emele, J. F., and Shanaman, J. (1963): Bradykinin writing: A method for measuring analgesia. *Proc. Soc. Exp. Biol. Med.*, 114:680–682.

26. Evans, W. O. (1961): A new technique for the investigation of some analgesic drugs on a reflexive behavior in the rat. *Psychopharmacology, (Berlin)*, 2:318–321.

27. Evans, W. O. (1962): A comparison of the analgesic potency of some analgesics as measured by the "flinch-jump" procedure. *Psychopharmacology (Berlin)*, 3:51–54.

28. Fraser, H. F., and Rosenberg, D. E. (1963): Observations on the human pharmacology and addictiveness of methotrimeprazine. *Clin. Pharmacol. Ther.*, 4:596–601.

29. Gacel, G., Fournie-Zaluski, M-C., and Rogues, B. P. (1980): Tyr-D-Ser-Gly-Phe-Leu-Thr, a highly preferential ligand for δ-opiate receptors. *FEBS Lett.*, 118:245–247.

30. Giesler, G. J., and Liebeskind, J. C. (1976): Inhibition of visceral pain by electrical stimulation of the periaqueductal gray matter. *Pain*, 2:43–48.

31. Gilfoil, T. M., Klavins, I., and Grumbach, L. (1963): Effects of acetylsalicylic acid on the edema and hyperesthesia of the experimentally inflamed rat's paw. *J. Pharmacol. Exp. Ther.*, 142:1–5.

32. Gray, W. D., Osterberg, A. C., and Scuto, T. J. (1970): Measurement of the analgesic efficacy and potency of pentazocine by the D'Amour and Smith Method. *J. Pharmacol. Exp. Ther.*, 172:154–162.

33. Grotto, M., and Sulman, F. G. (1967): Modified receptacle method for animal analgesimetry. *Arch. Int. Pharmacodyn. Ther.*, 165:152–159.

34. Heel, R. C., Brogden, R. N., Pakes, G. E., Speight, T. M., and Avery, G. S. (1980): Nefopam: A review of its pharmacological properties and therapeutic efficacy. *Drugs*, 19:249–267.

35. Hendershot, L. C., and Forsaith, J. (1959): Antagonism of the frequency of phenylquinone-induced writhing in the mouse by weak analgesics and non-analgesics. *J. Pharmacol. Exp. Ther.*, 125:237–240.

36. Herling, S., and Woods, J. H. (1981): Discriminative stimulus effects of narcotics: Evidence for multiple receptor-mediated actions. *Life Sci.*, 28:1571–1584.

37. Hill, R. C., Maurer, R., Buescher, H-H., and Roemer, D. (1981): Analgesic properties of the GABA-mimetic THIP. *Eur. J. Pharmacol.*, 69:221–224.

38. Hirose, J., and Jyogama, H. (1971): Measurement of arthritic pain and effects of analgesics in the adjuvant-treated rat. *Jpn. J. Pharmacol.*, 21:717–720.

39. Houde, R. W. (1979): Analgesic effectiveness of the narcotic agonist-antagonists. *Br. J. Clin. Pharmacol.*, 7:297S–308S.

40. Howes, J. F. (1981): A simple, reliable method for predicting the physical dependence liability of narcotic antagonist analgesics in the rat. *Pharmacol. Biochem. Behav.*, 14:689–692.

41. Hughes, J. (1975): Isolation of an endogenous compound from the brain with pharmacological properties similar to morphine. *Brain Res.*, 88:295–308.

42. Imrie, R. C. (1976): Animal models of arthritis. *Lab Anim. Sci.*, 26:345–351.

43. Jaffe, J. H., and Martin, W. R. (1980): Opioid analgesics and antagonists. In: *The Pharmacological Basis of Therapeutics*, edited by A. G. Gilman, L. S. Goodman, and A. Gilman, pp. 494–534. MacMillan, New York.

44. James, G. W. L., and Church, M. K. (1978): Hyperalgesia after treatment of mice with prostaglandins and arachidonic acid and its antagonism by anti-inflammatory-analgesic compounds. *Arzneimittel-forsch.*, 28:804–807.

45. Janssen, P. A. J., Niemegeers, C. J. E., and Dony, J. G. H. (1963): The inhibitory effect of fentanyl and other morphine-like analgesics on the warm water induced tail withdrawal reflex in rats. *Arzneimittel-forsch.*, 13:502–507.

46. Jasinski, D. R., Pevnick, J. S., and Griffith, J. D. (1978): Human pharmacology and abuse potential of the analgesic buprenorphine. *Arch. Gen. Psychiatry*, 35:501–516.

47. Jasinski, D. R. (1979): Effects in man of partial morphine agonists. In: *Agonist and Antagonist Actions of Narcotic Analgesic Drugs*, edited by H. W. Kosterlitz, H. O. J. Collier, and J. E. Villarreal, pp. 94–103. University Park Press, Baltimore.

48. Jessell, T. M., and Iversen, L. L. (1977): Opiate analgesics inhibit substance P release from rat trigeminal nucleus. *Nature*, 268:549–551.

49. Jhamandas, K., Elliott, J., and Sutak, M. (1981): Opiatelike actions of eseroline, an eserine derivative. *Can. J. Physiol Pharmacol.*, 59:307–310.

50. Koster, R., Anderson, M., and de Beer, E. J. (1959): Acetic acid for analgesic screening. *Fed. Proc.*, 18:412.
51. Kosterlitz, H. W., and Waterfield, A. A. (1975): In vitro models in the study of structure-activity relationships of narcotic analgesics. *Annu. Rev. Pharmacol. Toxicol.*, 15:29–47.
52. Krynock, G. M., and Rosecrans, J. A. (1979): Morphine as a discriminative stimulus: Role of periaqueductal gray neurons. *Res. Commun. Chem. Pathol. Pharmacol.*, 23:49–60.
53. Kuzana, S., and Kawni, K. (1975): Evaluation of analgesic agents in rats with adjuvant arthritis. *Chem. Pharm. Bull. (Tokyo)*, 23:1184–1191.
54. Kvam, D. C. (1979): Nefopam hydrochloride: A survey of preclinical pharmacology. *Clin. Ther. (Suppl. B)*, 2:1–12.
55. Lasagna, L., and DeKornfeld, T. J. (1961): Methotrimeprazine. A new phenothiazine derivative with analgesic properties. *J. A. M. A.*, 178:119–122.
56. Lin, M. T., Chi, M. L., Chandra, A., and Tsay, B. L. (1980): Serotonergic mechanisms of beta-endorphin and clonidine-induced analgesia in rats. *Pharmacology*, 20:323–328.
57. Lipman, J. J., and Spencer, P. S. J. (1979): Further evidence for a central site of action for the antinociceptive effect of clonidine-like drugs. *Neuropharmacology*, 18:731–733.
58. Lipman, J. J., and Spencer, P. S. J. (1980): A comparison of muscarinic cholinergic involvement in the antinociceptive effects of morphine and clonidine in the mouse. *Eur. J. Pharmacol.*, 64:249–258.
59. Lombard, M. C., Nashold, B. S. Jr., and Albe-Fessard, D. (1979): Deafferentation hypersensitivity in the rat after dorsal rhizotomy: A possible animal model of chronic pain. *Pain*, 6:163–174.
60. Loux, J. J., Smith, S., and Salem, H. (1978): Comparative analgesic testing of various compounds in mice using writhing techniques. *Arzneimittelforsch.*, 28:1644–1647.
61. Martin, W. R., Eades, C. G., Thompson, J. A., Huppler, R. E., and Gilbert, P. E. (1976): The effects of morphine- and nalorphine-like drugs in the non-dependent chronic spinal dog. *J. Pharmacol. Exp. Ther.*, 197:517–532.
62. Maxwell, D. R., Palmer, H. T., and Ryall, R. W. (1961): A comparison of the analgesic and some other central properties of methotrimeprazine and morphine. *Arch. Int. Pharmacodyn. Ther.*, 132:60–73.
63. McKenzie, J. S., and Beechey, N. R. (1962): A method of investigating analgesic substances in mice, using electrical stimulation of the tail. *Arch. Int. Pharmacodyn. Ther.*, 35:376–392.
64. Metcalf, G., Rees, J. M. H., and Ward, S. J. (1979): In vivo antagonism of analgesia and respiratory depression induced by proposed μ and K opiate agonists. *Br. J. Pharmacol.*, 66:473–474.
65. Nilsen, P. L. (1961): Studies on algesimetry by electrical stimulation of the mouse tail. *Acta Pharmacol. Toxicol.*, 18:10–22.
66. Paalzow, L. (1974): Analgesia produced by clonidine in mice and rats. *J. Pharm. Pharmacol.*, 26:361–363.
67. Pardo, E. G., and Rodriguez, R. (1966): Reversal by acetylsalicylic acid of pain induced functional impairment. *Life Sci.*, 5:775–781.
68. Pearl, J., Stander, H., and McKean, D. B. (1969): Effects of analgesics and other drugs on mice in phenylquinone and rotorod tests. *J. Pharmacol. Exp. Ther.*, 167:9–13.
69. Pedigo, N. W., Dewey, W. L., and Harris, L. S. (1975): Determination and characterization of the antinociceptive activity of intraventricularly administered acetylcholine in mice. *J. Pharmacol. Exp. Ther.*, 193:845–852.
70. Pert, A., and Yaksh, T. L. (1974): Sites of morphine induced analgesia in the primate brain: Relation to pain pathways. *Brain Res.*, 80:135–140.
71. Pert, C. B., and Snyder, S. H. (1973): Properties of opiate-receptor binding in rat brain. *Proc. Natl. Acad. Sci. (U.S.A.)*, 70:2243–2247.
72. Pierson, A. K., (1974): Assays for narcotic antagonist activity in rodents. *Adv. Biochem. Psychopharmacol.*, 8:245–261.
73. Pierson, A. K., and Rosenberg, F. J. (1976): WIN 35,197-2, another benzomorphan with a unique analgesic profile. In: *Report to the Committee on Problems of Drug Dependence*, pp. 949–965. National Academy of Science, Washington, D.C.
74. Pircio, A. W., Fedele, C. T., and Bierwagen, M. E. (1975): A new method for the evaluation of analgesic activity using adjuvant-induced arthritis in the rat. *Eur. J. Pharmacol.*, 31:207–215.
75. Pircio, A. W., Gylys, J. A., Cavanagh, R. L., Buyniski, J. P., and Bierwagen, M. E. (1976): The pharmacology of butorphanol, a 3,14-dihydroxy-morphinan narcotic antagonist analgesic. *Arch. Int. Pharmacodyn. Ther.*, 220:231–257.

76. Proudfit, H. K., and Levy, R. A. (1978): Delimitation of neuronal substrates necessary for the analgesic action of baclofen and morphine. *Eur. J. Pharmacol.*, 47:159–166.
77. Pruss, T. P., Gardocki, J. F., Taylor, R. J., and Muschek, L. D. (1980): Evaluation of the analgesic properties of zomepirac. *J. Clin. Pharmacol.*, 20:216–222.
78. Rance, M. J., and Dickens, J. M. (1978): The influence of drug-receptor kinetics on the pharmacological and pharmacokinetic profiles of buprenorphine. In: *Characteristics and Function of Opioids*, edited by J. M. VanRee and L. Terenius, pp. 65–66. Elsevier, North-Holland Biomedical Press, New York.
79. Randall, L. O., and Selitto, J. J. (1957): A method for measurement of analgesic activity on inflamed tissue. *Arch. Int. Pharmacodyn. Ther.*, 111:409–419.
80. Reddy, S. V. R., Maderdrat, J. L., and Yaksh, T. L. (1980): Spinal cord pharmacology of adrenergic agonist-mediated antinociception. *J. Pharmacol. Exp. Ther.*, 213:525–533.
81. Ronai, A. Z., Berzetei, I. P., Szenkely, J. I., Miglecz, E., Kurgyis, J., and Bajusz, S. (1981): Enkephalin-like character and analgesia. *Eur. J. Pharmacol.*, 69:263–271.
82. Roques, B. P., Fournié-Zaluski, M. C., Soroca, E., Lecomte, J. M., Malfroy, B., Llorens, C., and Schwartz, J-C. (1980): The enkephalinase inhibitor thiorphan shows antinociceptive activity in mice. *Nature*, 288:286–288.
83. Rosenfeld, J. P., and Holzman, B. S. (1977): Differential effect of morphine on stimulation of primary versus higher order trigeminal terminals. *Brain Res.*, 124:367–372.
84. Rosenfeld, J. P., Broton, J. G., and Clavier, R. M. (1978): A reliable, facial nociception device for unrestrained, awake animals: Effects of morphine and trigeminal complex lesions. *Physiol. Behav.*, 21:287–290.
85. Saelens, J. K., Granat, F. R., and Sawyer, W. K. (1971): The mouse jumping test - A simple screening method to estimate the physical dependence capacity of analgesics. *Arch. Int. Pharmacodyn. Ther.*, 190:213–218.
86. Satoh, M., Kawajiri, S-I, Shishido, K., Yamamoto, M., and Takagi, H. (1979): Bradykinin-induced flexor reflex of rat hind-limb for evaluating various analgesic drugs. *J. Pharm. Pharmacol.*, 31:184–186.
87. Satoh, M., Kawajiri, S., Yamamoto, M., Foong, F-W., and Masuda, C. (1979): Analgesic action of cyclazocine: Blocking nociceptive responses induced by intra-arterial bradykinin-injection and tooth pulp stimulation. *Arch. Int. Pharmacodyn. Ther.*, 241:300–306.
88. Schaefer, G. J., and Holtzman, S. G. (1981): Morphine-like stimulus effects in the monkey: Opioids with antagonist properties. *Pharmacol. Biochem. Behav.*, 14:241–245.
89. Schmitt, H., LeDonarec, J-C., and Petillot, N. (1974): Antinociceptive effects of soma α-sympathomimetic agents. *Neuropharmacology*, 13:289–294.
90. Sewell, R. D. E., and Spencer, P. S. J. (1976): Antinociceptive activity of narcotic agonist and partial agonist analgesics and other agents in the tail immersion test in mice and rats. *Neuropharmacology*, 15:683–687.
91. Shaw, J. S., Turnbull, M. J., Dutta, A. S., Gormley, J. J., Hayward, C. F., and Stacey, G. J. (1978): A structure-activity study with enkephalin analogues: Further evidence for multiple opiate receptor types. In: *Characteristics and Function of Opioids*, edited by J. M. Van Ree and L. Terenius, pp. 185–195. Elsevier North-Holland Biomedical Press, New York.
92. Shimano, I., and Wendel, H. (1964): A rapid screening test for potential addiction liability of new analgesic agents. *Toxicol. Appl. Pharmacol.*, 6:334–339.
93. Siegmund, E. A., Cadmus, R. A., and Lu, G. (1957): Screening of analgesics, including aspirin-type compound, based upon the antagonism of chemically induced "writhing" in mice. *J. Pharmacol. Exp. Ther.*, 119:184–193.
94. Spaulding, T. C., Venafro, J. J., Mu, M. G., and Fielding, S. (1979): The dissociation of the antinociceptive effect of clonidine from supraspinal structures. *Neuropharmacology*, 18:103–105.
95. St. John, A. B., and Born, C. K. (1979): Characterization of analgesic and activity effects of methotrimeprazine and morphine. *Res. Commun. Chem. Pathol. Pharmacol.*, 26:25–34.
96. Stacker, G., Bauer, P., Steinringer, H., Schreiber, E., and Schmierer, G. (1979): Effects of the synthetic enkephalin analogue FK 33-824 on pain thresholds and pain tolerance in man. *Pain*, 7:159–172.
97. Sweet, W. H. (1981): Animal models of chronic pain: Their possible validation from human experience with posterior rhizotomy and congenital analgesia. *Pain*, 10:275–295.
98. Taber, R. I. (1974): Predictive value of analgesic assays in mice and rats. *Adv. Biochem. Psychopharmacol.*, 8:191–210.

99. Takagi, H., Inukai, T., and Nakama, M. (1966): A modification of Haffner's method for testing analgesics. *Jap. J. Pharmacol.*, 16:287–294.

100. Takemori, A. E., Stesin, A. J., and Tulunay, F. C. (1974): A single-dose suppression test in morphine-dependent mice. *Proc. Soc. Exp. Biol. Med.*, 145:1232–1235.

101. Teal, J. J., and Holtzman, S. G. (1980): Discriminative stimulus effects of prototype opiate receptor agonists in monkeys. *Eur. J. Pharmacol.*, 68:1–10.

102. Teiger, D. G. (1976): Assessment of physical dependence in the rat by continuous intraperitoneal infusion. In: *Report to the Committee on Problems of Drug Dependence*, 38:342–349. National Academy of Science, Washington, D.C.

103. Tepper, P., and Woods, J. H. (1978): Changes in locomotor activity and naloxone-induced jumping in mice produced by WIN 35, 197-2 (ethyl-ketazocine) and morphine. *Psychopharmacology*, 58:125–129.

104. Van Arman, C. G., Carlson, R. P., Risley, E. A., Thomas, R. H., and Nuss, G. W. (1970): Inhibitory effects of indomethacin, aspirin and certain drugs on inflammation induced in rat and dog by carrageenan, sodium urate and ellagic acid. *J. Pharmacol. Exp. Ther.*, 175:459–468.

105. Wagers, P. W., and Smith, C. M. (1960): Responses in dental nerves of dogs to tooth stimulation and the effects of systemically administered procaine, lidocaine and morphine. *J. Pharmacol. Exp. Ther.*, 130:89–105.

106. Wakett, W. W. (1980): Irreversible inhibitors of GABA transaminase induce antinociceptive effects and potentiate morphine. *Neuropharmacology*, 19:715–722.

107. Way, E. L., Loh, H. H., and Shen, F-N. (1969): Simultaneous quantitative assessment of morphine tolerance and physical dependence. *J. Pharmacol. Exp. Ther.*, 167:1–8.

108. Weil-Fugazza, J., Godefray, F., and Besson, J-M. (1979): Changes in brain and spinal tryptophan and 5-hydroxyindoleucetic acid levels following acute morphine administration in normal and arthritic rats. *Brain Res.*, 175:291–301.

109. Wiesenfeld, Z., and Lindblom, U. (1980): Behavioral and electrophysiological effects of various types of peripheral nerve lesions in the rat: A comparison of possible models for chronic pain. *Pain*, 8:285–298.

110. Wei, E. T. (1981): Enkephalin analogs and physical dependence. *J. Pharmacol. Exp. Ther.*, 216:12–18.

111. Wiley, J. N., and Downs, D. A. (1979): Naloxone-precipitated jumping in mice pretreated with acute injections of opioids. *Life Sci.*, 25:797–802.

112. Winter, C. A., and Flataker, L. (1965): Reaction thresholds to pressure in edematous hindpaws of rats and responses to analgesic drugs. *J. Pharmacol. Exp. Ther.*, 150:165–171.

113. Winter, C. A., Fling, P. J., Tocco, D. J., and Tanabe, K. (1979): Analgesic activity of diflunisal (MK-647; 5-(2,4-difluorophenyl) salicylic acid) in rats with hyperalgesia induced by Freund's adjuvant. *J. Pharmacol. Exp. Ther.*, 311:678–685.

114. Wood, P. L., and Stotland, L. M. (1980): Actions of enkephalin, μ and partial agonist analgesics on acetylcholine turnover in rat brain. *Neuropharmacology*, 19:975–982.

115. Wood, P. L. (1981): Multiple opiate receptors: Support of unique mu, delta and kappa sites. *Neuropharmacology*, 21:487–497.

116. Wood, P. L., Charleson, S. E., Lane, D., and Hudgin, R. L. (1981): Multiple opiate receptors: Differential binding of mu, kappa and delta agonists. *Neuropharmacology*, 20:1215–1220.

117. Wood, P. L., Stotland, M., Richard, J. W., and Rackham, A. (1980): Actions of mu, kappa, sigma, delta and agonist/antagonist opiates on striatal dopaminergic function. *J. Pharmacol. Exp. Ther.*, 215:697–703.

118. Wood, P. L., and Rackham, A. (1981): Actions of kappa, sigma and partial mu narcotic receptor agonists on rat brain acetylcholine turnover. *Neurosci. Lett.*, 23:75–80.

119. Wood, P. L., Rackham, A., and Richard, J. (1981): Spinal analgesia: Comparison of the mu agonist morphine and the kappa agonist ethylketazocine. *Life Sci.*, 28:2119–2125.

120. Wood, P. L., and Charleson, S. (1981): High affinity [³H]-ethylketazocine binding: Evidence for specific kappa receptors. *Neuropharmacology*, 21:215–219.

121. Woods, J. H. (1977): Narcotic reinforced responding: A rapid screening procedure. In: *Report to the Committee on Problems of Drug Dependence*, 39:420–437. National Academy of Science, Washington, D.C.

122. Woods, J. H., Hein, D. W., Herling, S., Young, A. M., and Valentino, R. J. (1979): Discriminative and reinforcing effects of some systemically active enkephalin analogues. In: *Endogenous and*

Exogenous Opiate Agonists and Antagonists, edited by E. L. Way, pp. 443–446. Pergamon Press, New York.

123. Woods, J. H., Smith, C. B., Medzihradsky, F., and Swain, H. H. (1979): Preclinical testing of new analgesic drugs. In: *Mechanisms of Pain and Analgesic Compounds,* edited by R. E. Beers Jr. and E. G. Bassett, pp. 429–445. Raven Press, New York.

124. Woolfe, G., and MacDonald, A. D. (1944): The evaluation of the analgesic action of pethidine hydrochloride (Demerol). *J. Pharmacol. Exp. Ther.*, 80:300–307.

125. Yaksh, T. L., Yeung, J. C., and Rudy, T. A. (1976): Systematic examination in the rat of brain sites sensitive to the direct application of morphine: Observations of differential effects within the periaqueductal gray. *Brain Res.*, 114:83–103.

126. Yaksh, T. L., and Rudy, T. A. (1978): Narcotic analgesics: CNS sites and mechanisms of action as revealed by intracerebral injection techniques. *Pain*, 4:299–359.

127. Yanaura, S., Yamatake, Y., and Ouchi, T. (1976): A new analgesic testing method using ultrasonic stimulation I. Effects of narcotics and nonnarcotic analgesics. *Jap. J. Pharmacol.*, 26:301–308.

128. Zemlan, F. P., Corrigan, S. A., and Pfaff, D. W. (1980): Noradrenergic and serotonergic mediation of spinal analgesia mechanisms. *Eur. J. Pharmacol.*, 61:111–124.

Analgesics: Neurochemical, Behavioral, and
Clinical Perspectives, edited by M. Kuhar and
G. Pasternak. Raven Press, New York © 1984.

The Role of Endogenous Nonendorphin Substances in Nociception

D. R. Haubrich, E. R. Baizman, B. A. Morgan, and J. K. Saelens

Sterling-Winthrop Research Institute, Rensselaer, New York 12144

In 1644, the idea of a "centralized" pain pathway was conceived by Descartes as a channel directly connecting the end organ to the brain. The evolution of this concept (190) culminated in the gate-control theory of Melzack and Wall in 1965 (191), who proposed that a mechanism in the dorsal horn of the spinal cord acts as a "gate" which can increase or decrease the flow of nerve impulses from peripheral fibers into the CNS. This theory, involving both primary transmitters of nociceptive information, and secondary mechanisms to either moderate or amplify this information, was propounded a decade before the discovery of the endogenous opioid system, and has achieved considerable heuristic value in current studies of the neurophysiology and neurochemistry of pain. The important role of opioid peptides as inhibitors of nociceptive transmission is discussed in detail in other chapters of this book. The purpose of this chapter is to evaluate the role of other chemical entities as either transmitters or modulators of nociceptive information within the CNS. Attention is focused on two peptides, substance P (SP) and neurotensin (NT), and four nonpeptides, norepinephrine, serotonin, acetylcholine, and gammaaminobutyric acid, for which available data supporting a role in nociception is most convincing.

NEUROPEPTIDES AS TRANSMITTERS OR MODULATORS OF NOCICEPTION

Role of Substance P in Nociceptive Processes

Since its discovery in 1931 (309), much evidence has accumulated linking substance P to the control of nociceptive processing within the spinal cord. In 1953, Pernow (233) first reported that substance P was distributed preferentially within spinal cord dorsal roots. Based largely on this anatomical localization, Lembeck (165) proposed that SP functioned as a transmitter of the primary sensory afferent neuron. After the peptide was characterized (42) and synthesized in 1971 (296), immunocytochemical studies led Hokfelt and colleagues (123,124,211) to conclude that SP was involved in regulating the excitability of spinal neurons in nociceptive pathways. Substance P-like immunoreactivity (SPLI) occurs in 10 to 20% of the cell bodies of dorsal root ganglia, and within small diameter primary afferent processes which travel in the tract of Lissauer and terminate in a dense plexus of immunostaining nerve axons, and terminals in the marginal zone (lamina I) and substantia gelatinosa (lamina II) of the rat, cat, and human spinal cord (39,50, 53,54,119,122,123,124,160,179,180,291). In the dorsal (but not ventral) horn, SPLI was markedly reduced by dorsal root ligation (121,126), dorsal rhizotomy (12,123), or sciatic nerve section (13,144). Thus, some of the SP within the cord originates from primary afferents, principally unmyelinated C- and thinly myelinated A-delta fibers (12,121,123,124,126), which convey noxious information from the periphery. Substance P is also present in intrinsic interneurons within laminae I to III of the rat (12,134) and human spinal cord (160), and occurs in neurons of deeper laminae (IV to VI) (160,179) as well as in fibers seen in the ventral horn (121,160).

Further evidence for association of SP with nociceptive sensory fibers comes from studies of its distribution in the trigeminal nucleus. The substantia gelatinosa of the nucleus caudalis of the trigeminal complex receives nociceptive input (69) and contains SP-positive cell bodies and fibers (50,51,53,123,126,179,180). Most of this immunostaining disappeared after trigeminal nerve sectioning (50,51), Gasserian ganglion lesions (65), or removal of the tooth pulp (218), which supplies only nociceptive afferents to the trigeminal nerve (92). Since release of SPLI has been directly demonstrated in the pulp (26,217), SP is likely to be a sensory transmitter in this system.

Substance P is also found in many higher brain regions proposed to be intimately involved with pain transmission or modulation, including the medullary nucleus raphe magnus and nucleus reticularis gigantocellularis, the mesencephalic periaqueductal gray (124,126), and in the pontine region within the locus ceruleus (238). Thus, numerous studies have outlined an extensive network of SP immunoreactive cell bodies and nerve fibers within the spinal cord, and in discrete pathways and nuclei at higher levels of the neuraxis. This neuroanatomical evidence suggests that SP is strategically localized to transmit or modulate incoming nociceptive information, and is consistent with the hypothesis that it may serve an endogenous role in the perception, transmission, or modulation of pain.

The precise nature of the role of SP in nociceptive information processing is not entirely clear, however, its distribution is consistent with a potential interaction between other systems thought to be intimately involved in nociceptive mechanisms. For example, the close parallel between neuronal systems containing enkephalin and those containing SP, particularly in CNS regions receiving primary sensory input, suggests a functional interrelationship between the two peptides (49,50,53, 120,121,146,264). Although each peptide seems to exist within a separate population of neurons, significant overlap is evident in the distribution of their nerve terminals (49,53,122,126).

In contrast to the distribution of SP, enkephalin-like immunoreactivity is not found within primary afferents. However, the distribution pattern of enkephalin-positive cell bodies in the dorsal horn, located principally in interneurons within laminae I and II (120,133), resembles that of SP neurons and terminals (126). The distribution of enkephalin-like immunoreactivity also correlates well with that of spinal cord opiate receptors, of which about half seem to be localized presynaptically on primary afferent fibers (9,81,161).

The codistribution of SP and enkephalin, together with other evidence cited below, is a finding that has led to the concept that these two peptides may exert opposing physiological roles in the control of nociceptive transmission in the spinal cord. Based on the discovery that opioid agonists could suppress potassium ion-evoked SP release from slices of rat spinal trigeminal nucleus, Jessel and Iversen (142) hypothesized a model SP-enkephalin circuit within laminae I and II of the spinal cord. With this model, they proposed that part of the physiological effect of enkephalin released from substantia gelatinosa interneurons could involve a presynaptic, opioid receptor-mediated inhibition of primary afferent transmission. Incoming nociceptive stimuli would then be blocked before the activation of spinothalamic projection cells in deeper layers.

Although immunocytochemical and ultrastructural studies of the dorsal horn have clarified the presence of SP directly within nerve terminals (12,39,40,237), they have not yet defined the precise anatomical relationship between enkephalin and SP-containing neuronal elements at this level. In this context, primary afferent terminals have been observed in both pre- and postsynaptic axodendritic, axoaxonic, and axosomatic contacts within the marginal zone, substantia gelatinosa, and deeper dorsal horn laminae (12,133,160,237). Similar observations, primarily of axodendritic SP profiles, have been made in the locus ceruleus (238). However, an intensive search of laminae I through III for presynaptic enkephalinergic contacts on primary afferent terminals, which might offer evidence of a structural correlate for the presynaptic (axoaxonic) inhibition of primary sensory transmission, proposed by Jessel and Iversen (142), has not yet been successful (133). Furthermore, because enkephalin-positive terminals have been observed in axosomatic and axodendritic contacts with thalamic projection cells in lamina V (258), some opiate receptors are localized postsynaptically on cell soma and dendrites in this region. Single neurons in laminae I and V receive a dual innervation by both SP and Met-enkephalin in the human spinal cord (160). Taken together, these more recent findings suggest that both neuropeptides may modulate nociceptive sensory information at different postsynaptic sites on the same cell, and provide evidence that enkephalin and SP-containing terminals exist in several different configurations within the dorsal horn. Further complications encountered in probing the synaptic relationships between enkephalin and SP in the dorsal horn involve the large number of interneurons in this region, as well as the presence of enkephalin (127) and SP (38,125) in terminals which originate from descending brainstem projections.

Substance P is also associated with enkephalin in numerous higher brain regions involved with nociceptive sensory processing including the nucleus caudalis of the trigeminal complex (65,126), the nucleus reticularis gigantocellularis in the caudal medulla (126), the nucleus raphe magnus (124), the midbrain periaqueductal gray

(126), and the locus ceruleus (238). The distribution of SP also parallels regions of origin and/or terminal fields of other classical neurotransmitters. Substance P cells synapsing on catecholaminergic neurons within the locus ceruleus (238) are a prime example, suggesting that SP may be involved in modulating noradrenergic output from the locus ceruleus cells. Coexistence of peptides and classical neurotransmitter substances within the same neuron is a fairly common occurrence in the CNS and periphery (122). SP has also been found together with serotonin in neurons supplying a descending projection from the nucleus raphe magnus to the dorsal and ventral horn (38,125). The physiological significance of these observations is unknown, and details of the mechanism of interaction between the peptides and the biogenic amine are lacking.

Thus, the anatomical distribution of SP suggests that it is closely associated with areas of the nervous system that process noxious information. The distribution of SP together with enkephalin, primarily in regions of origin and termination of central pain pathways, strongly implies a functional interaction between the two peptides. Although the detailed neuronal circuitry within the spinal cord dorsal horn relative to their potential interaction is not clearly defined, a variety of neuroanatomical relationships have been observed, which might permit direct or indirect SP-enkephalin modulation of thalamic relay neurons. The anatomical data further suggest that SP may influence the activity of neurons or pathways in higher brain areas, which contain classical neurotransmitter substances, such as norepinephrine and serotonin.

If SP functions as a transmitter of nociceptive information, then its release from appropriate nerve terminals *in vivo* should be induced selectively by noxious stimuli. A number of studies have demonstrated a calcium ion-dependent release of SPLI material from CNS tissue *in vitro*. For example, Otsuka and Konishi (221) found the release of SP in perfusates of isolated rat spinal cords after dorsal (but not ventral) root stimulation. Subsequent studies have shown potassium ion-evoked release of SPLI *in vitro* from various types of neuronal preparations, which was dependent on the presence of calcium ions (2,90,110,111,139,142,143,167,202,268). Results from several studies suggest that the release of SP may be associated with nociceptive processes. For example, enkephalins or other opioids inhibited release of SPLI *in vitro* from structures associated with noxious information processing (2,142,202). Yaksh and co-workers (320) utilized a spinal subarachnoid perfusion technique in the cat to demonstrate *in vivo* the potassium ion-evoked release of SPLI. In this study, sciatic nerve stimulation at high stimulus intensities sufficient to activate A-delta and C-nociceptive afferents elevated levels of SPLI in the perfusate. Lower stimulus intensities, which presumably did not activate nociceptive afferents, were ineffective. Perfusion of the spinal cord with morphine resulted in a naloxone-sensitive inhibition of the stimulation-induced release of SPLI. Of further interest was the finding that spinal perfusion with a pain-inducing substance, capsaicin, also elevated SPLI in the perfusate. These findings provide support for the hypothesis that release of SP from the spinal cord is induced *in vivo* by intense noxious stimuli, and suggest that this release is under inhibitory control of opioids.

Capsaicin (8-methyl-N-vanillyl-6-nonenamide) has been used to study the phys-iological role of SP, as it induces calcium ion-dependent release of SPLI from the spinal cord or spinal cord explants *in vitro* (2,90,295) and *in vivo* (318,320). When administered topically, capsaicin evokes intense local pain (199), while its paren-teral administration to animals induces an insensitivity to noxious thermal and chemical stimuli (89,129,140,204,318), although it has little effect on mechanical nociceptive stimuli (e.g., noxious pinch, 108,318). Studies *in vitro* (2,90,202,295) and *in vivo* (87,108,143,318,320) suggested that the prolonged capsaicin-induced antinociception results from depletion of SP from primary afferent neurons, dorsal roots, and from the dorsal horn of the spinal cord, as well as from the spinal trigeminal nucleus (111). The content of SP in other regions of the CNS was not affected by capsaicin (110). The severity and permanence of the effects of capsaicin depended, in part, on the age of the animals. In neonates, capsaicin-induced depletion of SP from the spinal cord was accompanied by degeneration of primary afferent terminals in the dorsal horn (52,88,129,140,141,143,204), along with a decrease in opiate binding sites (204). In adults, degeneration of primary afferents did not occur (149), but a reversible decrease of SPLI in the spinal cord was observed (87,88,143), without alteration of opiate binding (143). Direct intrathecal administration of capsaicin to adult rats produced substantial (40 to 50%) depletion of spinal cord SP accompanied by prolonged thermal analgesia (318). However, some animals given intrathecal capsaicin injections showed substantial depletion of SP in the cord without changes in thermal nociceptive thresholds (203). These studies suggest that SP can be released by capsaicin, and that depletion of SP may result in antinociception. However, these findings must be interpreted cautiously in view of the findings that treatment with capsaicin may cause nonspecific neu-rotoxic effects within the cord (203), and that depletion of other neuropeptides (e.g., somatostatin) (89) from primary afferents by capsaicin may be involved in its actions. Furthermore, several reports also claim a lack of effect of capsaicin on thermal nociceptive thresholds, despite substantial SP depletion in the cord (27,37,108); thus, the effects of capsaicin probably depend on many variables, including age of the animals, dose, route of administration, nociceptive test(s) or species, and strain of animals used.

Another line of evidence that supports the hypothesis that SP is a nociceptive transmitter is that direct microiontophoretic application of SP or its analogs onto cell bodies deep in the dorsal horn (laminae IV, V, or VI) can selectively excite dorsal horn neurons responsive to noxious thermal cutaneous stimuli (61,113–115, 197,222,223,239,250,266,314,315,334). Cells activated by non-noxious input were unaffected, and occasionally, depression of synaptically-evoked or spontaneous firing was noted. By contrast, opioids or opioid peptides applied into the same region generally inhibited firing of these nociceptively driven neurons in a naloxone-reversible fashion (60,71,73). Neither iontophoretically applied nor intravenously administered morphine depressed SP-induced excitation of nociceptive dorsal horn neurons, indicating that morphine is not an SP antagonist (240).

Not all of the electrophysiological results are consistent with a nociceptive role for SP in the spinal cord. For example, if SP is released by nociceptive stimuli into the substantia gelatinosa region of the cord, which is the principal terminal area for fine diameter primary afferents (173,174), then iontophoretic ejection of the peptide into these superficial layers should excite second-order nociceptive neurons in deeper layers of the dorsal horn. Morphine and opioid peptides administered into the substantia gelatinosa selectively depressed the noxious stimulation-induced firing which was recorded from neurons in laminae IV and V (60,70,71,73). However, iontophoretic ejection of SP into the substantia gelatinosa was found to have no effect (73) or produced either enhancement or depression of synaptically evoked (noxious heat-induced) firing of opioid-sensitive deep dorsal horn neurons (61). The authors suggested that SP may be involved presynaptically to modify transmitter release, or postsynaptically to alter membrane excitability and thus facilitate synaptic activation.

In higher brain centers, excitation was the most frequently observed response after iontophoretic application of SP or its analogs onto neurons. Cells in the cat trigeminal nucleus caudalis, which were activated by tooth pulp stimulation, were selectively depressed by opioids and strongly excited by SP (8). Thus, the responses to SP and to opioids within this brainstem region were similar to those seen in spinal cord studies. Nociceptive (noxious pinch) activation of cells in the nucleus reticularis gigantocellularis of the rat, however, was not altered by iontophoretic application of morphine, Met-enkephalin, or SP (100). Therefore, either these neuropeptides are not directly involved in nociceptive processing within this nucleus, or, as in the spinal cord (315), SP may not activate cells sensitive to noxious mechanical stimuli. In the locus ceruleus, SP excited neurons that contained norepinephrine independently of cholinergic or opioid systems (98). About half the cells tested within the nucleus raphe magnus, excited by electrical stimulation of the periaqueductal gray, also showed excitatory responses to SP (244); however, some cells inhibited by electrical stimulation were excited by SP. The prolonged excitation of substantia nigra neurons evoked by SP and an agonist analog, eledoisin, was similar to that observed in other areas of the CNS (59); and as in isolated tissue studies, tachyphylaxis to repeated iontophoretic application of these peptides was a prominent finding.

The evidence outlined above indicates that SP can selectively increase the electrical activity of dorsal horn neurons responsive to nociceptive stimuli; whereas those neurons responsive to non-noxious input are unaffected. Occasionally, depression of synaptically-evoked or spontaneous firing occurs. Because of inconsistent effects of SP within the substantia gelatinosa, it is not clear if SP is a direct mediator of synaptic transmission at the primary afferent synapse. Furthermore, the results of electrophysiological studies concerning the ionic mechanism(s) by which SP depolarizes cells are controversial (150,210,213,236). Nicoll et al. (210) have argued that the slow time course observed for SP actions on single neurons does not necessarily refute its proposed transmitter role, as the time course of transmitter action released from nociceptive afferents is poorly understood; furthermore, the low transport number of SP may result in its reduced or delayed release from micropipettes (15,99,115,240). Diffusion of SP to distant receptors (e.g., dendritic) may also contribute to the slow response.

If SP has a function in the transmission of nociceptive information, then appropriate administration of SP or SP receptor agonists should elicit a behavioral response indicative of perception of pain. Several studies suggest that injection of SP evokes a specific behavioral syndrome resembling irritation. Acute intracerebral, but not parenteral (241), administration of SP to mice induces a dose-related reciprocal hindlimb scratching (RHLS) response (273). The scratching response is mimicked only by peptides structurally related to SP, is potentiated by naloxone, is inhibited by pure opioid agonists, and is unaffected by mixed agonist-antagonists or inactive enantiomers. Furthermore, repeated administration of SP does not result in tachyphylaxis (67). Other studies employing intracisternal injections of SP in mice (248) have shown that the SP-induced RHLS is due primarily to a spinally-mediated mechanism. In unanesthetized mice, injection of nanogram amounts of SP intrathecally between L5 and L6 spinal segments induced an immediate, caudally-directed biting and RHLS, which was dose-related, and was qualitatively mimicked by low abdominal subcutaneous injection of 0.1 N acetic acid (135,136). This behavioral syndrome was inhibited by subcutaneous pretreatment with morphine, but not by intrathecal morphine administration. The inhibition was reversed by systemic administration of naloxone. A similar, though less intense syndrome has been described in the rat after an intrathecal SP injection (312).

The available data (67) indicate that the SP receptor mediating this "nociceptive response" is similar to the SP receptor found in certain peripheral tissues, such as the guinea pig ileum (29,30,103). Using the RHLS syndrome described by Share and Rackham (273), Dobry and co-workers (67) found that intracranial administration of SP6-11 produced effects similar to those of SP, whereas the pentapeptide, SP7-11, was inactive. Further structure activity data, available from single neuron studies (223,239), also showed that SP sequences down to SP6-11 were effective in exciting SP sensitive spinal motoneurons or dorsal horn cells. These data suggest that similar specific SP receptors are involved in eliciting both the behavioral and electrophysiological actions of SP, and that SP receptors in gut tissue bear a resemblance to those in the CNS.

A corollary of the concept that SP is associated with the transmission of nociceptive information is that the blockade of its effect should result in a reduced sensitivity to pain. Two methods of altering the transmission across SP synapses; presynaptic inhibition by opiates or opioid peptides, and depletion by capsaicin, have been discussed earlier in this chapter. The pharmacological blockade of SP receptors is another way of modifying the action of SP. Recently, Folkers et al. (83) have described two compounds, D-Pro2, D-Phe7, D-Trp9-SP (PFW), and D-Pro2, D-Trp7, 9-SP (PWW), which antagonize the effects of SP in a variety of peripheral tissues (83,163). In the guinea pig ileum, PFW was not an agonist (83), whereas PWW was a partial agonist on the *Taenia coli* and the urinary bladder (163). The excitatory effect of SP on rat locus ceruleus neurons was blocked by

PWW administered at similar ejection currents (76), but the excitations caused by glutamate or ACh were unaffected. Application of PWW alone did not alter locus firing, suggesting that noradrenergic cell activity in this nucleus was not dependent on an excitatory SP input. The response of locus ceruleus neurons to a noxious stimulus (pinching of the contralateral paw) was not blocked by the SP antagonist; thus, the excitation of locus ceruleus neurons by noxious stimuli is apparently not mediated by SP. Rosell et al. (257) have found that PFW blocks the vasodilation induced in the microvasculature of cat dental pulp by electrical stimulation of the inferior alveolar nerve. Because the dental pulp is richly supplied with SP immunoreactive nerve fibers, which release SP immunoreactive material on nociceptive stimulation, blockade by PFW provides further evidence linking SP with nociceptive processing. Antidromic vasodilation in the rat hindpaw, which was induced by electrical stimulation of the saphenous nerve and is associated with the release of SP, was also blocked by PFW (166). Irritant effects of exogenously applied SP in the rabbit eye were inhibited by PWW (128).

The effects of these SP antagonists on nociceptive thresholds have also been evaluated. Intrathecal administration of PFW decreased the response of mice to cutaneous capsaicin application and also blocked the acute scratching response evoked by coadministered SP (242). Unexpectedly, the same dose of PFW administered intrathecally (6.5 nmoles) did not alter nociceptive thresholds in the tail flick or hot-plate tests which are used to measure analgesic "efficacy" equivalent to opiates. Higher doses (20 nmoles) were found to elicit significant hindlimb motor dysfunction. In contrast to these results, Lembeck et al. (166) have reported that SP administered intraspinally shortened tail withdrawal latencies in mice (hot-water stimulus), whereas similar treatment with SP antagonists prolonged response latencies. Using the acetylcholine-induced writhing model in the mouse, Baizman et al. (11) found that intrathecal administration of PFW or PWW produced dose-related antagonism of the writhing response. Although motor dysfunction was again noted at the highest antagonist dose tested (6.5 nmoles), inhibition of writhing was observed at doses that did not evoke hindlimb paralysis.

Several groups have investigated the effects of baclofen [beta-(aminomethyl)-4-chlorobenzenepropanoic acid] on SP-related actions. Although baclofen has been found to antagonize the effects of SP on rat spinal motoneurons (261) and to nonselectively block the response of neurons in the locus ceruleus to SP, glutamate, and ACh (97), it does not appear to interact with SP receptors outside the CNS. Baclofen does not antagonize the myogenic responses of the guinea pig intestine to SP (325), or the effect of SP on single neurons of the guinea pig myenteric plexus (150), nor does it alter the effect of SP on the twitch response of the field-stimulated guinea pig vas deferens (331). Baclofen does block the RHLS behavior that occurs after intracranial injection of SP in the mouse (67); however, this effect is also blocked by a variety of other substances, including amphetamine, chlorpromazine, cyproheptadine, and diazepam. These results suggest either that baclofen is a selective antagonist at central SP receptors, or, more likely, that the compound can function as a physiological antagonist of SP in the CNS.

The effects of SP have been evaluated in classical antinociceptive models. In these studies, which are summarized in Tables 1 and 2, SP has been reported to produce antinociception, hyperalgesia, no effect, or biphasic effects on nociceptive thresholds in mice or rats! Thermal (hot-plate or tail flick) and chemical (acetic acid-induced writhing) stimuli were the principal nociceptive challenges, and SP was administered intraventricularly, intracerebrally, intraspinally, or systemically in doses ranging from a few nanograms to hundreds of micrograms. Effects of SP persisted for as long as 1 to 2 hr after its administration. The alarming inconsistencies and contradictions apparent in this data provide an excellent example of the problems associated with the investigation and interpretation of the pharmacology of peptides. The variable responses to SP may be the result of instability after its administration, its inability to penetrate to the site of action, or both. Substance P is degraded quickly in the blood (31) and plasma (20), and like other peptides, probably has a limited ability to penetrate the CNS after parenteral administration (228).

The studies most easily interpreted with regard to the central actions of SP are those in which the peptide was administered directly into the CNS. Frederickson et al. (84) found that SP produced naloxone-reversible analgesia in mice when very small (1 to 5 ng) doses were injected intraventricularly. These effects were variable and never approached the efficacy achieved with morphine (85). Higher doses of SP had no significant effect, but enhanced the hyperalgesia produced by systemic naloxone injection.

The antinociceptive effects reported for SP *in vivo* are obviously difficult to reconcile with the hypothesis that it may be a nociceptive mediator. However, several explanations can be envisaged for these findings. Administration of relatively large amounts of SP into the CNS might induce a prolonged and persistent desensitization of SP receptors, thus leading to a reduced responsiveness of CNS neurons to nociceptive stimuli. *In vitro* desensitization of peripheral systems to SP is a well-recognized consequence of contact with high concentrations of the peptide. Alternatively, SP administered intracerebrally or intrathecally may be acting on descending bulbospinal pathways, proposed to play a major role in modulating nociceptive processes (80,319). It is conceivable that the presence of serotonin within these descending axons, which also contain SP (38,122,125,147) could modify the responses to activation of nociceptive afferents.

Since naloxone has been found to antagonize SP-induced antinociception in many studies, alternative possibilities, which must be considered, are that the peptide acts *in vivo* to release endogenous opioids. Although no such evidence is currently available from *in vitro* studies, results of one study suggest that such release may occur *in vivo* (205). A direct interaction of SP with opioid receptors is unlikely; it is ineffective in depressing electrically-evoked contractions of the guinea pig ileum (45), or mouse vas deferens (84,270), and is a weak inhibitor of the binding of radiolabeled dihydromorphine (294) or naloxone (289). Furthermore, morphine does not alter the post-synaptic effects of iontophoretically applied SP (240) or the contractile effects of SP in the unstimulated guinea pig ileum (30,45,256).

TABLE 1. *Effects of substance P on nociceptive reflex responses in the mouse*

Dose	Route	Nociceptive test(s)	Effect	Time course or pretreatment interval (min)	Comments	References
2 ng 5 ng 1 µg	i.c. i.p. i.p.	Hot-plate	Antinociception	Onset: 30 Peak: 60–90 Dur: 90–120	Antagonized by naloxone (60 ng/mouse i.p.) Cross-tolerance to i.p. morphine Depression of locomotor activity	285
1 µg	i.p.	Hot-plate	Antinociception	Onset: 30 Peak: 60 Dur: 30	Depression of spontaneous locomotor activity 200 µg morphine i.p. = 1 µg SP.	
5 µg	i.p.				No eff. on morphine withdrawal jumping. Incr. DA turnover, dec. 5HT turnover	284
1.25-5 ng	i.c.v.	Hot-plate	Antinociception	Onset: 15 Duration: 60	Naloxone-reversible. Peak efficacy minor and variable comp. to morphine.	84, 85
50-1,000 ng	i.c.v.	Hot-plate	No effect or hyperalgesia (jumping)		Hyperalgesia seen only in combination with naloxone (0.2 mg/kg s.c.) Reverts to analgesia w/ baclofen (5 mg/kg s.c.)	

Dose	Route	Test	Effect	Timing	Comments	Ref.
10 µg	i.v.	Hot-plate	Antinociception	Test: 60	Antag. by naloxone (0.4 mg/kg i.p.)	214, 215
0.01-0.5 mg	i.v.	Hot-plate	Hyperalgesia	Test: 20	Hot-plate effects depended on control latencies	
.02-.2 µg	i.v.	Acetic acid writhing	Antinociception			
1.0 µg	i.v.	Acetic acid writhing	Hyperalgesia			
0.02-20 µg	i.p.	Hot-plate	No effect	Test: 30, 60, 90	Hyperalgesia at 60 after 200 µg of SP	93
200 µg	i.p.	Hot-plate	Hyperalgesia			
1-5 µg	i.p.	Hot-plate	No effect	Test: 15, 30, 60, 90	—	95
2 ng-2 µg	i.c.v.	Hot-plate	No antinociception	Test: 30, 60, 90	Tremors, depression of locomotor activity	107
0.8 µg	i.cist.	Tail immersion	Hyperalgesic	Onset: 15 Dur: 100	Accompanied by hyperthermia	208
1 ng-10 µg	i.c.v.	Acetic acid writhing	Antinociception-5 ng	Test: 10	Antagonized by naloxone (1 mg/kg i.p.)	156
0.2 mg	i.p.	Acetic acid writhing	No effect > 100 ng i.c.v.			
250 µg	i.p.	Hot-plate	Antinociception	Test: 60 (SP)	Antinociception abolished by PCPA. $pGlu^6SP_{6-11}$ equimolar doses to SP, active	193
500 µg	i.p.			Test: 30 ($pGlu^6SP_{6-11}$)		
0.3 µg	i.c.v.	Tail flick	No effect	Test: 5	—	67
17.5 ng	i.c.v.	Tail flick and hot-plate	No effect	—	—	241
297 ng	i.s.					

TABLE 2. *Effects of substance P on nociceptive reflex responses in the rat*

Dose	Route	Nociceptive test(s)	Effect	Time course or pretreatment interval (min)	Comments	References
0.3–10 µg	i.c. (PAG)	Tail flick	Antinociception	Onset: 1 Peak: 3 Duration: 30	ED_{50} = 0.7 µg/rat Antagonized by naloxone (20–40 mg/kg i.p.) Molar potency = 25 × morphine No effect with 25 µg	182
40 µg	i.c. (PAG)	Tail flick	2 sec increase in latency	Onset: 3 Peak: 10 Duration: 20		183
100–400 µg	i.c.v. i.p.	Hot plate and tail flick	No effect No effect (hot-plate) i.p./i.c.		Morphine (5 µg) produced cutoff (>15 sec) latencies 8–40 µg i.p. inactive in TF or HP	198
1 µg	i.c. (PAG)		Antinociception (tail flick)—i.p./i.c.	Onset: 10 Peak: 30 Duration: 30		
1 ng–10 µg	i.t.	Paw pressure Tail immersion Hot-plate Tail flick	Transient hyperalgesia (hot-plate) No effect (pressure, tail immersion) No effect	Onset: 3 Duration: <10 Test: 30	No effect in other nociceptive tests at 3, 10, or 30 min postinjection	107
0.2–60 µg 0.5 µg	i.p. i.c.v.	Tail flick Tail compression	No effect Antinociception and hyperalgesia during recovery	Onset: 45 Peak 15; duration: 30	Antinociception abolished by raphe lesions pGlu⁶SP₆₋₁₁ inactive (0.275)	93 193
20–200 µg	i.a. (carotid)	Pseudoaffective Response (forelimb flexion; head dextrorotation)	Variable (3/9 responders)	—	Pseudoaffective behavior antagonized by chlorpheniramine	156
0.1–100 µg	i.t. (lumbar)	Tail flick	Antinociception	Onset: 10 Peak: 20 Duration: 30	ED_{50} = 1.5 µg/rat Also seen in spinalized rats Antagonized by naloxone (5 µg i.t. and 5.0 mg/kg i.v.)	68
10 µg	i.v.t.	Vocalization, vocalization after discharge	Elevated electrical thresholds	Onset: 5 Duration: 10	Effects potentiated by i.v.t. bacitracin Effects abolished by anti-Met-enkephalin antibody injections	205

In conclusion, considerable neuroanatomical, electrophysiological, and pharmacological evidence supports the hypothesis that SP plays an important role in the transmission, modulation, or perception of certain types of nociceptive stimuli. The peptide may directly transmit noxious information from the periphery via classical release and trans-synaptic diffusion across the first central synapse within the spinal cord. Substance P may also modulate the excitability of cells deep in the dorsal horn, which project to higher centers, thereby regulating perception of noxious stimuli. Opioid peptides, activating opioid receptors appear to exert an opposing inhibitory influence on SP release within the cord, although the precise neuronal circuitry involved remains unknown. The presence of SP at higher levels of the neuraxis within structures and pathways presumed to participate in nociceptive sensory processing suggests an even broader influence over CNS function.

The recognition that SP plays a role in the control of nociceptive information processing suggests the possibility that manipulation of SP in the dorsal horn may have clinical implications. For example, lowered SP levels (coupled with reduced populations of primary afferents) in the substantia gelatinosa were associated with reduced sensitivity to pain in patients with familial dysautonomia (229). Furthermore, the discovery of peptide analogs of SP, which block SP receptors in the CNS and peripheral tissues, may provide useful tools for the development of potent SP antagonists as nonopioid analgesics. Such compounds will also facilitate the exploration of other areas of SP biology, such as its hypotensive and vasodilator actions.

Role of Neurotensin in Nociceptive Processes

The tridecapeptide, neurotensin (NT: pyroGlu-Leu-Tyr-Glu-Asn-Lys-Pro-Arg-Arg-Pro-Tyr-Ile-Leu-OH) exhibits a broad spectrum of biochemical, behavioral, and pharmacological properties that support its role as a neurotransmitter or neuromodulator (23,34,35,78,164,206,207,280,304,305). Like SP, neurotensin displays a heterogenous distribution in the CNS (36,154,298,300–302,328,329) is present within nerve terminals (300,302,303), and is concentrated selectively in a number of brain regions concerned with nociceptive sensory processing. Although the actions of this peptide have not been examined as comprehensively as those of SP, the available neuroanatomical, electrophysiological, and pharmacological studies generally support the concept that one physiological function of NT may involve modulation of pain transmission.

Within the spinal cord, neurotensin-like immunoreactivity (NTLI) has been localized within cell perikarya, terminals, and fibers in cord regions receiving primary afferent input. A dense band of immunoreactive terminals and fibers is concentrated throughout lamina II of the dorsal horn with lower densities in laminae I and III (301,302). In a more recent comprehensive immunohistochemical study of the rat dorsal horn, Hunt and co-workers (134) found discrete subgroups of NT-containing cell bodies lying along a narrow border between laminae II and III with dendritic branches extending into laminae I, II, and III. Nerve terminals rich in NT were also observed in a dense inner band, deep in lamina IV, and a less dense band within laminae I and II.

In parallel with these light microscopic observations, ultrastructural analysis of the rat lumbosacral cord has confirmed high densities of NT-containing terminals, varicosities, and cell bodies within laminae II and III (272). In this study, neurotensin was found in large granular vesicles within axons and terminals of apparently intrinsic spinal cord neurons.

These studies suggest that NT found within the substantia gelatinosa overlaps with the distribution of both SP and enkephalin systems as well as that of opiate receptors (9,10,126,281,299). In contrast to the distribution of SP, however, NT cell bodies have not been found within dorsal root ganglia (39), or in dorsal root fibers (305). Thus, the presence of neurotensin within primary sensory neurons originating from the periphery is unlikely. Furthermore, the NT receptor density in the dorsal horn did not change after dorsal root sectioning (212), suggesting that NT receptors, unlike some opiate receptors (81,161), are not located on primary afferent terminals. Neurotensin perikarya intrinsic to the spinal cord have also been described in the dorsal horn (281).

The distribution of neurotensin in selected higher brain areas is also consistent with a role in nociceptive processing. For example, in the caudal medulla, NT has been visualized in the medial region of the substantia gelatinosa of the spinal trigeminal nucleus (300), whereas enkephalin and SP were found concentrated in its lateral aspect (65,120,126,298,300). In these studies, the lateral medullary reticular formation, the gray matter of the floor of the fourth ventricle and the locus ceruleus were noted to be particularly rich in NT. Cell bodies and nerve terminals which contain NT were found in ventral tegmentum, the periaqueductal gray matter, and the dorsal raphe nuclei (300), all of which have been proposed to be involved in nociception (80,322).

Thus, the neuroanatomical distribution of NT, and its correspondence with the central distribution of enkephalin and SP, suggest that NT may function directly or indirectly within pain pathways. The peptide is localized within dorsal horn laminae receiving primary sensory input, but unlike SP, NT is not present within primary afferent fibers. Immunocytochemical and ultrastructural studies agree that a population of intrinsic interneurons within the dorsal horn probably contains NT, as well as SP and enkephalins. Therefore, NT may be involved at the spinal cord level as a modulator of CNS sensory function. Furthermore, numerous higher brain regions associated with the processing of noxious input also contain high concentrations of NT.

Studies of the actions of NT on single neurons have been performed in attempts to further characterize its potential role as an endogenous substance involved with nociceptive processing. Neurotensin, like SP, should therefore alter the activity of central neurons which selectively respond to noxious stimulation. Miletic and Randic (196) addressed this issue and found that iontophoresis of NT induced a slow, moderate excitation of about two-thirds of the cells studied within laminae I to III of the cat spinal cord, but did not excite neurons in deeper layers. However, in marked contrast to the actions of SP and opioids, NT showed a lack of specificity; neurons excited by either peripheral noxious or innocuous stimuli each responded to NT with slight to moderate excitation. Neurotensin evokes antinociception when given to animals. If the peptide were to modulate nociceptive input by inhibition at the level of the spinal cord, neurotensin-containing cells may be exciting other inhibitory interneurons in this region of the dorsal horn. In another work, NT was found to excite frog spinal cord motoneurons (209). This effect was blocked by tetrodotoxin, suggesting again that NT may be acting indirectly, perhaps by suppression of inhibitory interneurons.

Unlike SP, which consistently increased cell firing in the CNS, iontophoresis of NT onto single units in higher brain regions produced contradictory effects. Zieglgansberger et al. (333) found that NT excited certain brainstem neurons. Guyenet and Aghajanian (97) reported that NT was inactive on five cells tested in the locus ceruleus which responded to SP (excitation) and Met-5-enkephalin (depression). In contrast, Young et al. (330) found inhibition of firing in about half the locus ceruleus cells examined, whereas adjacent regions were much less responsive to the peptide. Although methodological and sampling differences may account for these discrepancies, the latter study suggests that NT may play an inhibitory role in this brain region. Pressure ejection of NT, but not its iontophoretic application, evoked depressant effects on cerebellar Purkinje neurons (186), suggesting that delivery of NT by some iontophoretic systems may be questionable.

Thus, a limited amount of electrophysiological evidence is available to relate the actions of NT with nociceptive neurons. Since the peptide excited dorsal horn cells responding to either noxious or non-noxious stimuli, no conclusions can be drawn as to the relevance of these excitatory actions in the selective transmission or modulation of nociception. No evidence is available to suggest that the electrophysiological actions of NT in higher brain regions may be related to noxious information processing.

The effects of NT have been examined on nociceptive reflex responses in animals. Intracisternal administration of nanogram amounts of NT produced dose-related elevations in response latencies of mice tested on the hot-plate, and inhibited acetic acid-induced writhing, whereas intravenous injections of the peptide were ineffective (47). These antinociceptive effects, evident 30 min after injection, and persisting for up to 1 to 2 hr, were unaffected by systemic naloxone pretreatment. In a subsequent study, NT was found to be about 100 times more potent in antagonizing mouse writhing than in elevating hot-plate latencies, but was about equipotent with Dala2 Met-5-enkephalinamide in the hot-plate test (47). Although hypothermia (also noted previously by Bissette et al., 24) and reductions in locomotor activity accompanied the antinociceptive effects, these actions did not appear to be responsible for the reduced sensitivity to noxious stimuli. A variety of classical receptor antagonists did not block the NT response. In the rat, intracisternal injections of NT were effective in the hot-plate test, but not the tail flick test (48).

The results of Nemeroff et al. and Osbahr et al. have essentially been confirmed more recently using the tail immersion, hot-plate, and writhing models (208,220). These studies agree that the actions of NT in several standard antinociceptive models, although dose-related, were apparently independent of the opioid system.

Although hypothermia accompanied the antinociceptive effects, other hypothermic agents were inactive in these models, suggesting dissociation of the two actions. Since NT was inactive after systemic administration, it seems unable to reach central receptors mediating antinociception from the peripheral circulation, a conclusion supported by the absence of any effect of the systemically injected peptide on body temperature (208).

Direct injections of NT into the periaqueductal gray produce antinociceptive effects in both hot-plate and tail flick tests (286). Neurotensin was about three times more potent than morphine on a molar basis, and naloxone was ineffective in reversing the analgesia. When administered into the mesencephalic reticular formation, NT also elevated hot-plate, but not tail flick latencies.

In contrast to the similarities between the central effects of NT and those of SP, several aspects of the pharmacology of these two peptides are clearly different. For example, in the study of Nemeroff et al. (208), SP elicited hyperthermia and hyperalgesia in doses equimolar to antinociceptive doses of NT. Furthermore, the RHLS elicited in mice by intracerebral or intrathecal injections of SP did not occur when NT was administered (136,241,273).

Although the pharmacologic effects of NT can be clearly distinguished from those of SP in the *in vivo* studies discussed above, *in vitro* evidence is available which suggests that a pharmacologic interaction may occur between the two peptides. Neurotensin-induced contractions in the guinea pig ileum may result in part from release of SP (200); opioids were found to block NT-induced contractions in the atropinized ileum (201,332). In view of the lack of effect of NT in the SP scratching models, and the opposite effects of these peptides on temperature regulation and nociception as discussed above, a similar interaction between NT and SP systems within the CNS seems unlikely.

Thus, the central actions of NT, specifically its role in nociception, have been less well characterized than those of SP. However, some evidence does exist to support a role for the tridecapeptide in mediating antinociception. The mechanism of this effect remains unclear, although direct involvement of opiate receptors in this effect is unlikely. Neurotensin, like SP, exerts its effects by binding to receptors which are presumed responsible for its physiological actions. Radiolabeled NT added to brain homogenates (162), brain slices (329), or synaptosomal fractions (162), binds to specific receptors with high affinity (151–153,297,303). These studies generally agree that the C-terminal five or six amino acids of NT are involved in its binding affinity and biological activity, and confirm that NT binding sites are heterogeneously distributed in the CNS, primarily in those areas possessing high immunoreactive concentrations of the peptide.

The available evidence supporting a role for NT in nociceptive processes needs to be extended. For example, a few studies have shown that NT can be released from CNS regions *in vitro*. Potassium-induced depolarization of superfused rat hypothalamic slices (138) or hypothalamic fragments (181) evokes a calcium ion-dependent release of NT. Studies on the release of NT from spinal cord *in vitro* or *in vivo*, or spinal trigeminal nucleus after appropriate stimulation have not yet been reported.

Several workers have described the presence of soluble and membrane-bound peptidases in brain homogenates which degrade NT (74,297) and which are partially inhibited by bacitracin (181). No information is available on their specificity of cleavage, nor their differential distribution in brain areas enriched in NT and NT receptors. An active uptake system for NT has not been demonstrated (305).

In conclusion, neurotensin, like substance P and enkephalin, is heterogeneously distributed within the CNS such that it could function in the modulation of pain. However, iontophoretic studies of the actions of neurotensin on single units in the spinal cord are inconclusive, because neurotensin excited, rather than inhibited neurons in the dorsal horn which were sensitive to both nociceptive and non-nociceptive peripheral stimuli. These latter experiments could be complicated by problems of NT delivery from micropipettes. Furthermore, the role of NT remains uncertain in higher brain centers which contain specific NT receptors as well as high levels of immunoreactive peptides. Evidence for the direct release of NT *in vivo* in response to appropriate nociceptive input has not been obtained.

The data of Clineschmidt and co-workers (47,48), Nemeroff et al. (208), and more recently Sullivan and Pert (286), showing that central administration of NT produced dose-related antinociception in several standard models, are the most compelling evidence that NT plays a role in nociceptive processes. Antinociceptive effects were not reversed by naloxone, clearly excluding opioid receptor involvement. Although the mechanism by which NT evokes antinociception is unclear, it probably acts via receptors in the brain and spinal cord which have been shown to bind radiolabeled peptides.

The development of a specific agonist of neurotensin receptors in the CNS would greatly aid in clarifying its role in nociception. Although little progress in this area has been reported to date, results from recent *in vitro* studies of NT analogs on preparations of vascular tissue seem encouraging (253). An evaluation of the effects of these modified NT analogs on nervous tissue has not been reported.

NONPEPTIDES AS TRANSMITTERS OR MODULATORS OF NOCICEPTION

Role of Monoamines in Nociceptive Processes

Endogenous monoamines, particularly norepinephrine and 5-hydroxytryptamine (5-HT), have been implicated in the regulation of the nociceptive threshold and in the mechanism of action of opiate analgesia (187,192,311,322). The monoaminergic pathways that have been most convincingly implicated in the regulation of the nociceptive threshold are those that descend from the medial brainstem to the spinal cord (bulbospinal pathways). Direct evidence for the existence of such pathways was obtained in the mid 1960s, when Dahlstrom and Fuxe (57,58) demonstrated, by means of a histochemical fluorescence technique, the existence of 5-HT-containing neurons located within the medial medullary reticular formation which project to the spinal cord. The nucleus raphe magnus is one of the 5-HT-containing nuclei that has been studied most extensively. Neurons that contain norepinephrine also descend from the brainstem to the spinal cord. The nuclei of origin for the noradrenergic bulbospinal neurons are located primarily in the pontine medullary reticular formation (57). Fibers of both the serotonergic and noradrenergic systems descend in the lateral funiculi and terminate in the dorsal horn. Ascending noradrenergic fiber tracts, e.g., those originating in the locus ceruleus, have also been implicated in the control of the nociceptive threshold, although this regulation may be mediated indirectly via a tryptaminergic projection. A detailed anatomical description of these pathways is presented elsewhere within this volume (*see* chapter by Basbaum).

The involvement of descending monoamine pathways in the control of the nociceptive threshold has been known or suspected since the late 1950s. The evidence to be summarized below suggests that descending tryptaminergic and noradrenergic pathways, when activated, can produce a significant elevation in the nociceptive threshold. In 1959, Eccles and Lundberg (75) demonstrated that decerebration of cats leads to tonic inhibition of the flexor reflex afferents. This finding has been confirmed and extended by other investigators (33), who have demonstrated that this inhibition is abolished by spinal transection, reduced by administration of monoamine receptor antagonists, and mimicked by the administration of either 5-hydroxytryptophan (5-HTP) or L-DOPA (5,6), which stimulate the rate of synthesis of 5-HT and norepinephrine, respectively. These observations provide indirect evidence that monoaminergic neuronal pathways originating in the brain exert an inhibitory influence over incoming sensory information at the level of the spinal cord.

The importance of these monoaminergic pathways in the control of the nociceptive threshold is revealed by various types of physiological and pharmacological evidence. For example, electrical stimulation (1,72,75,171,188) or injection of morphine (159,290,316) into specific regions of the brain led to marked inhibition of spinal pain transmission. Inhibition of 5-HT synthesis by administration of parachlorophenylalanine (a tryptophan hydroxylase inhibitor) reduced stimulation-produced analgesia (SPA; 3, 4), and SPA could be restored by administration of 5-HTP (4). In addition, depletion of brain 5-HT by administration of 5,6- or 5,7-dihydroxytryptamine or parachlorophenylalanine antagonized the antinociceptive action of either clonidine or the opioid peptide, beta-endorphin (175). Furthermore, the efficacy of acupuncture analgesia has been shown to vary inversely with the presumed functional activity of spinal tryptaminergic neurons (41,102).

Direct stimulation of the nucleus raphe magnus caused marked analgesia which was reversed by antagonists of 5-HT receptors (219,246). In addition, selective destruction of 5-HT-containing neurons of the nucleus raphe magnus, the nucleus raphe pallidus, or the dorsolateral funiculus of the spinal cord (the latter region contains the descending axons of the nucleus raphe magnus projecting to the dorsal horn of the spinal cord) blocked morphine-induced (245) or SPA elicited by stimulation of the periaqueductal gray (14). These findings suggest that spinal inhibition induced by stimulation of the periaqueductal gray, which lacks significant connections to the spinal cord, is mediated via descending 5-HT neurons (80).

Depletion of 5-HT with parachlorophenylalanine (293) or 5,6-dihydroxytryptamine (308) partially blocked morphine analgesia, and administration of cinanserin (a 5-HT receptor antagonist) antagonized analgesia caused by morphine injected directly into periaqueductal sites (317). Depletion of both norepinephrine and 5-HT with tetrabenazine (3,4) almost completely abolished analgesia elicited by stimulation of this region. Lesions in the spinal cord of rats produced by injection of 5,7-dihydroxytryptamine caused a 70% decrease in the concentration of 5-HT and attenuated morphine analgesia (64).

The studies cited above support the hypothesis that descending monoaminergic pathways are involved in the regulation of spinal reflexes. In an effort to define specifically the neurotransmitters involved within bulbospinal pathways and the anatomical regions mediating the elevations in nociceptive thresholds, investigators have administered monoamine receptor agonists or antagonists directly into the spinal cord of awake animals. For example, administration of methysergide or phentolamine to block receptors for 5-HT and norepinephrine, respectively, attenuated the antinociceptive effect of morphine given directly into the periaqueductal gray (316). On the other hand, Kuriashi et al. (158), in a similar experiment, found that only the adrenergic antagonist was effective against morphine administered into the nucleus reticularis gigantocellularis, and, based on this finding, ruled out the importance of descending tryptaminergic pathways emanating from that particular site of injection of morphine. Furthermore, the increase in tail flick latency caused by electrical stimulation of this same brainstem nucleus was also antagonized more effectively by intrathecal phentolamine than by methysergide (319). These findings point to a high degree of neuroanatomical specificity regarding activation of descending tryptaminergic or noradrenergic pathways.

In further support of an antinociceptive role for monoamines exerted at the level of the spinal cord, studies have shown that the iontophoretic administration of 5-HT or norepinephrine into the substantia gelatinosa (16,109) or the dorsal spinal grey matter (19) depresses the discharge of nociceptive dorsal horn neurons in the cat. The inhibitory effects of monoamines are antagonized by monoamine receptor antagonists, but not by naloxone (94,109), thus indicating that the bulbospinal monoamine pathways do not exert their effects on the nociceptive threshold exclusively through an opiate mechanism.

In unanesthetized animals, the intrathecal administration of tryptaminergic or alpha-adrenergic agonists elicited an increase in the nociceptive threshold in a variety of species (158,251,252,310,324). The antinociceptive effect of intrathecal 5-HT was antagonized by blockade of 5-HT receptors with cyproheptidine or methysergide, but not by phentolamine or naloxone, and was potentiated by blockade of 5-HT reuptake (324). The antinociceptive effect of alpha-adrenergic agonists was antagonized by phentolamine, but not by methysergide or naloxone. These findings provide evidence for the role of both adrenergic and tryptaminergic mechanisms within the spinal cord involved in the control of pain threshold in intact, awake animals.

A role for spinal monoaminergic neurons in the control of nociception is also suggested by results showing a correlation between the antinociceptive effects of certain physiological and pharmacological manipulations, and an increase in the rate of turnover or release of monoamines within the spinal cord. Thus, an increase in the turnover rate of norepinephrine (276) or 5-HT (25,275) occurred in the spinal cord of rats after central administration of morphine or electrical stimulation of bulbospinal tryptaminergic or noradrenergic systems. Furthermore, an enhanced rate of release of 5-HT into superfusates of rat spinal cord occurred when morphine was injected into the periaqueductal gray (323). Electrical stimulation of the nucleus reticularis gigantocellularis resulted in antinociception accompanied by an enhanced rate of release of serotonin, but not norepinephrine, into superfusates of awake rats. These findings are consistent with the neuroanatomical selectivity of bulbo-spinal tryptaminergic and catecholaminergic pathways, and suggest that opiates activate the same or similar descending systems which are activated by electrical stimulation.

Although it seems well established that activation of noradrenergic terminals descending into the spinal cord leads to an increase in the nociceptive threshold, studies of the nociceptive role of noradrenergic terminals, which synapse at higher centers within the brain, seem contradictory. For example, several lines of evidence indicate that activation of neurons in the locus ceruleus produces an antinociceptive effect. Thus, electrical stimulation of this nucleus reportedly leads to an increase in the nociceptive threshold (185,262). Consistent with these findings, lesions of the locus ceruleus were found to decrease the nociceptive threshold when measured after 8 to 10 days (96,155). Antinociception elicited by electrical stimulation of the nucleus locus ceruleus was attenuated by treatment with methysergide, cypro-heptidine, or parachlorophenylalanine, which suggests the possibility that stimulation of the locus ceruleus activates descending tryptaminergic systems to increase the pain threshold.

On the other hand, there are studies which suggest that inhibition of locus firing would increase the pain threshold. For example, lesions of the locus ceruleus have also been shown to increase the threshold for the nociceptive response when measured 20 days after lesioning (265). Furthermore, administration of phentoam-ine into the nucleus raphe magnus has been shown to elicit an increase in the nociceptive threshold (101,260). This result can be explained by presuming that phentolamine antagonizes an inhibitory noradrenergic input to the tryptaminergic neurons. In support of this hypothesis, Sagen and Proudfit (260) found that the increase in nociceptive threshold induced by microinjection of phentolamine into the nucleus raphe magnus was blocked by intrathecal injection of methysergide, but not by naloxone. These findings suggest that there are two types of inhibitory noradrenergic fibers; those that impinge on and inhibit the nucleus raphe magnus, and those that descend into the spinal cord to directly regulate the threshold for spinal reflexes. Studies from which an antinociceptive role for stimulation of higher noradrenergic systems may be inferred, e.g., those of Gamulka et al. (96), Kostowski et al. (155), Margalit and Segal (185), and Sandberg and Segal (262), presumably involve noradrenergic pathways that descend directly into the spinal cord and regulate the threshold for incoming information. In contrast, those studies that imply an antinociceptive effect caused by inhibition of adrenergic fibers (101,265) suggest the intermediate involvement of raphe tryptaminergic systems which are under inhibitory noradrenergic control. Thus, removal of the noradrenergic inhibition leads to activation of descending tryptaminergic terminals in the spinal cord with a consequent increase in the threshold for the nociceptive response.

Whether the discovery that descending monoaminergic pathways control the pain threshold will have therapeutic consequences remains to be determined. Based on current knowledge, adrenergic and tryptaminergic agonists would be expected to possess antinociceptive activity; however, the only such compound used for this purpose is xylazine (269), an alpha adrenergic agonist used in veterinary medicine to elicit antinociception and sedation. Clonidine, an antihypertensive drug related both structurally and pharmacologically to xylazine, has been studied more extensively than xylazine for its antinociceptive and sedative properties in animals (224,225,227). Clonidine is considerably more potent than xylazine (189) or morphine in certain antinociceptive testing procedures (79,282), and administration of clonidine has been reported to ameliorate some of the symptoms of narcotic withdrawal in both rodents (79) and humans (43). However, the spinal antinociceptive actions of clonidine are relatively weak compared with those of other adrenergic agonists (251) or morphine (321), and it is known that clonidine elicits a more potent antinociceptive effect when given into the cerebrospinal fluid than when administered by intrathecal injection (32,176). These findings suggest a predominantly supraspinal site of action of clonidine; however, a study by Spaulding et al. (283), showing that spinal transection of mice failed to alter the ED_{50} for clonidine, seems to contradict this conclusion.

Clonidine is known to preferentially stimulate alpha-2 adrenergic receptors, which leads to inhibition of norepinephrine release from neurons (7), and a reduction of noradrenergic neuronal activity in the locus ceruleus (287). These findings suggest that clonidine and xylazine may act at higher centers to reduce noradrenergic activity, and that this action leads to supraspinally mediated antinociception.

The possible role of opiate systems in the antinociceptive activity of clonidine is not yet certain. Alpha-2 adrenergic receptors are located in proximity to opiate receptors in the brain (306). Furthermore, *in vitro* studies have shown that clonidine releases beta-endorphin from brain slices (157) or pituitary cultures (235), and that this effect was blocked by yohimbine. In addition, simultaneous administration of doses of clonidine and morphine, which, by themselves, are ineffective, have been shown to elicit marked antinociceptive activity in rodents (282). A similar potentiation of morphine antinociception was observed to occur in monkeys when the narcotic was given intrathecally together with ST-91, an analog of clonidine (321). Although the studies cited above suggest a strong interaction between alpha-2 adrenergic and endorphin subsystems, clonidine apparently does not evoke an increase in the pain threshold by an opiate mechanism; it neither binds to opiate receptors *in vitro*, nor is its antinociceptive effect antagonized by administration of naloxone (79,282). It is not yet certain if cross-tolerance develops between morphine and clonidine (225,282). Thus, current evidence would suggest that alpha-2 adrenergic mechanisms may be involved in regulation of antinociception. It may be possible to exploit this involvement to develop newer types of analgesic agents to be used alone or in combination with low doses of morphine, such that the undesirable side effects of both drugs may be eliminated.

Role of Acetylcholine in Nociceptive Processes

Numerous studies have implicated central cholinergic systems in nociception and in the mechanism of action of narcotic analgesics. For example, various cholinomimetic agents displayed antinociceptive activity in a variety of tests and species. These agents include oxotremorine (91,105,132,168,194,226,243), arecoline (116, 130,194,249), pilocarpine (63,130), physostigmine (63,106,112,137,178,243,249, 277), and acetylcholine (given intraventricularly) (231). The antinociceptive action of many of these muscarinic agonists was antagonized by treatment with centrally acting antimuscarinic agents such as scopolamine or atropine (63,130,137,194).

Studies of the possible role of opioid mechanisms in the antinociceptive action of acetylcholine (44,104,106,132,137,243) have yielded contradictory results. In one of the more thorough studies, Pedigo and Dewey (230) found that, although the antinociceptive response to either morphine or acetylcholine injected into the cerebral ventricles was antagonized by naloxone, different pA2 values were obtained for naloxone versus the two antinociceptive treatments (suggesting noncompetitive inhibition). The Schild plot showed a slope greater than unity for acetylcholine versus a slope of unity for morphine. Furthermore, in a similar study, the stereoselectivity for narcotic antagonists (pentazocine and cyclazocine) to antagonize the antinociception induced by morphine was reversed compared to that for blockade of acetylcholine-induced antinociception (66,231). These observations strongly suggest that intraventricular acetylcholine does not elicit its antinociceptive effect through an endogenous opiate mechanism.

The possible role of monoamines as mediators of the antinociceptive action of acetylcholine has also been studied (131). Depletion of both catechol- and indoleamines by reserpine and tetrabenazine has been shown to markedly antagonize the antinociceptive activity of intraventricular acetylcholine (230). More selective depletors of catecholamines were either without effect (alpha-methyltyrosine), or slightly attenuated (parachlorophenylalamine) the antinociceptive activity of acetylcholine. Intraventricular administration of 6-hydroxydopamine antagonized the antinociceptive action of oxotremorine (278).

These studies suggest that acetylcholine is an endogenous antinociceptive compound which may act through monoaminergic systems. Additional studies are required to elucidate the neuronal pathways involved in mediating this response, and to determine if the effect of acetylcholine involves activation of the descending monoaminergic pathways discussed above. The possibility that these spinal pathways may mediate the response to acetylcholine is suggested by the finding that the increase in tail flick latency observed in mice treated with cholinomimetic agents was markedly attenuated by spinal transection (66).

The potential therapeutic consequences of this action of ACh and muscarinic agents also remain to be determined. Because of peripheral muscarinic side effects associated with the use of cholinergic agonists, it seems unlikely that such compounds will be clinically useful to induce analgesia. However, it is known that cholinomimetic drugs potentiate the action of narcotic analgesics in laboratory animals (21,132,137,243,267,292) and in man (46,82,232,279), which raises the possibility of combined treatment with low doses of cholinomimetics and narcotics to avoid some of the undesirable side effects of each.

Paradoxically, some reports suggest that blockade of cholinergic systems results in an antinociceptive effect. For example, Van Eick and Bock (307) reported antinociceptive effects of anticholinergic compounds in rodents using the hot-plate test. In the primate, scopolamine was found to be antinociceptive (130), and Migdal and Frumin (195) claimed that centrally acting anticholinergic drugs were analgesic in man. In a study in which both cholinomimetic and anticholinergic drugs were compared in rhesus monkeys, Pert (234) found that both scopolamine and physostigmine were effective in elevating shock thresholds, and in potentiating the antinociceptive effect of morphine, but the effect of physostigmine given alone could not be separated from its nonspecific depressant action. In the same study, methscopolamine (peripheral antimuscarinic), mecamylamine (antinicotinic), hexamethonium (antinicotinic), and the cholinomimetics pilocarpine, nicotine, and arecoline were inactive in the shock titration task.

The suggestion that antinociception may be associated with a decrease in cholinergic tone is consistent with the fact that morphine is a potent inhibitor of the release of acetylcholine from the guinea pig ileum. In addition, administration of morphine inhibits the release of acetylcholine from cat cerebral cortex *in vivo*, and this effect is reversed by naloxone (17,145). Furthermore, treatment of rats with morphine and other narcotics caused a decrease in the turnover rate of acetylcholine in the rat cortex and hippocampus, but not in the corpus striatum (336). These later observations suggest that part of the antinociceptive actions of the narcotic analgesics may be associates with a selective inhibition of central cholinergic neuronal pathways. The paradoxical finding that both cholinomimetic and anticholinergic drugs have antinociceptive effects in certain animal models may be explained by the fact that the release of acetylcholine is controlled by receptors located on presynaptic terminals ("autoreceptors"). Stimulation of these "autoreceptors" by cholinergic agonists leads to inhibition of the release of acetylcholine (288). Thus, depending on the experimental conditions, administration of either cholinomimetics or anticholinergic drugs could attenuate the functional activity at cholinergic synapses, thereby causing an increase in the pain threshold.

Role of Gamma-Aminobutyric Acid in Nociceptive Processes

Numerous studies have been performed in an effort to assess the possible role of gamma-aminobutyric acid (GABA) in the control of nociceptive processes. This amino acid is present throughout the mammalian central nervous system and is estimated to comprise as much as 40% of all neurons (254).

Nociceptive information reaches thalamic and then cortical (conscious) centers of the brain via synaptic relays in the periaqueductal gray, located in the dorsal midbrain. The caudal periaqueductal gray is known to be sensitive to the antinociceptive effect of morphine (322) and to contain appreciable amounts of enkephalins (126). In addition, this nucleus also contains substantial concentrations of GABA and the neuronal elements associated with its uptake and metabolism (18,77,263). Sherman and Gebhart (274) have reported an elevation in GABA in the periaqueductal gray in animals exposed to nociceptive stimuli, and inferred a role of GABA in nociceptive information processing in the periaqueductal gray. Sandner et al. (263) identified the origin of a GABAergic input in the periaqueductal gray to arise from cell bodies in the ipsilateral medial hypothalamus. A direct connection between the GABAergic neurons arising from the medial hypothalamus and the enkephalinergic neurons is unlikely, because the GABAergic neurons are located rostrally, whereas the enkephalinergic neurons are found caudally in the periaqueductal gray. Sandner et al. (263) further noted that the medial hypothalamus and periaqueductal gray are components of the periventricular system, or "punishment system" characterized by classical experimental psychologists (216). This association suggests that the GABAergic system in the brain may involve the secondary aversive internal and external perceptions associated with pain, such as apprehension and anxiety, as well as the specific recognition of the origin and type of nociceptive stimuli.

The amino acid may also be involved as a modulator of spinal relay systems in pathways that carry nociceptive information from the periphery to the CNS. The concentration of GABA is highest in the dorsal horn of the spinal cord (148) where it is a major inhibitory transmitter. This suggests a GABAergic input to the functionality of primary afferent terminals. Presynaptic inhibition by GABA of primary afferent terminals may attenuate the propagation of nociceptive information from sensory nerve endings at their point of entry into the spinal cord. Therefore, based on its anatomical location within the spinal cord, and the fact that it is a presynaptic inhibitory transmitter elsewhere in the spinal cord, GABA could be considered a valid candidate for the transmitter which controls the processing of nociceptive information postulated in the "gate theory" of Melzack and Wall (191), discussed previously in this chapter and elsewhere in this volume.

The anatomical and biochemical evidence summarized above suggests a role for GABA in both supraspinal and spinal sites of nociceptive information processing. However, pharmacological information obtained using agents which mimic, antagonize, or manipulate levels and presumably the functional activity of GABAergic neurons, has produced inconsistent results.

Gamma-aminobutyric acid-alpha ketoglutarate transaminase (GABA-T) is the enzyme which metabolizes and thereby inactivates GABA. Yoneda et al. (327) showed that amino-oxyacetic acid (ADAA), a GABA-T inhibitor by virtue of its ability to complex with its coenzyme, pyridoxal phosphate, extended the antinociceptive action of morphine at a dose which increased GABA levels by 180%. In the same study, semicarbazide and bicuculline, agents which block the formation and receptors of GABA, respectively, attenuated the antinociceptive effect of morphine. In contrast, Ho et al. (118) found that ADAA antagonized the antinociceptive activity of morphine and enhanced the development of tolerance and physical dependence in mice. Both studies utilized mice, and the dose of ADAA was the same. The difference between the two studies appeared to be in the nociceptive stimulus. Yoneda et al. (327) used a tail compression, whereas Ho et al. (118) used a tail flick (heat) test. Four years later, Liebman and Pastor (172) showed a similar differentiation of antinociceptive activity for the GABA agonist, muscimol, in analogous tests in the rat.

In an attempt to resolve the issue, Buckett (28) administered two irreversible inhibitors of GABA-T; alpha-vinyl GABA and alpha-acetylenic GABA alone and in combination with morphine in mice using a hot-plate as a nociceptive stimulus. The alpha-vinyl GABA is reported to be the more selective of the two inhibitors (177). Both GABA-T inhibitors were antinociceptive by themselves at low nociceptive stimulus intensity (hot-plate at 52°C) and the alpha-vinyl GABA markedly potentiated the effects of morphine on the 56°C hot-plate (high nociceptive stimulus intensity where alpha-vinyl GABA by itself was inactive). Antinociception induced by administration of GABA-T inhibitors was not naloxone reversible and the time of peak activity coincided with the maximal increase in GABA levels in the mouse brain (4 to 6 hr). These data suggest it is not heat as a stimulus, but rather the use of the tail flick reflex itself (a spinal reflex) which gave rise to the conflicting results. Perhaps an additional action at another site (other than a nociceptive pathway) is involved in the tail flick reflex response to morphine.

The reported interaction of morphine and GABA prompted Sethy and Bombardt (271) to study the effects of morphine and naloxone (both 3 to 30 mg/kg, s.c.) on the regional concentrations of GABA in the rat brain. No significant differences were found between control and drug treated animals with regard to cortical, striatal, or midbrain GABA levels. Yoneda et al. (326) did find a modest increase in GABA in the ventrolateral thalamus after morphine administration, and used this thalamic area to show convergence for nociceptive information carried by lateral spinothalamic and ventral trigeminothalamic tracts.

Zonta et al. (335) and Mantegazza et al. (184) presented some intriguing interactions between morphine and drugs that mimic or augment the action of GABA. Using the tail flick test, these investigators found that nipecotic acid (300 μg, i.c.v.) and guvacine (300 μg, i.c.v.) two inhibitors of neuronal GABA uptake, both attenuated the effect of morphine. Intraventricular administration of muscimol (0.25 μg, i.c.v.), and isoguvacine (5 μg, i.v.c.), two GABA agonists, also antagonized the effect of morphine in the tail flick test. This was in marked contrast to the report of Biggio et al. (22), who showed that parenterally administered muscimol potentiated the antinociceptive effect of morphine in both mice and rats subjected to either hot-plate or tail flick tests. Muscimol itself failed to produce antinociception in either model. Hill and co-workers (117) examined the effects of muscimol and its structurally rigid analog 4,5,6,7-tetrahydroisoxazolo-(5,4-c) pyridin-3-ol (THIP) in a wide variety of tests. In agreement with the findings of other investigators, THIP and muscimol were inactive in the tail flick test, but active in the phenylquinone writhing test and hot-plate test in mice, arthritis (paw flexion) and paw pressure test in rats, and shock titration in the rhesus monkey.

Liebman and Pastor (172) demonstrated an antinociceptive effect (vocalization and motor response to pinch) of GABA after microinjection into the lateral ventricle of rats (1,500 μg). Similar results were found for muscimol (0.5 μg). Like Zonta et al. (335) and Hill et al. (117), Liebman and Pastor (172) did not demonstrate an increase in tail flick latency with muscimol. The investigations of Liebman and Pastor were particularly informative, because (a) they demonstrated an antinociceptive effect of GABA and (b) they showed that muscimol was antinociceptive in one animal model (vocalization and motor response to pinch), but not in another (tail flick) in the same species and by the same route of administration.

There has been considerable interest in the antinociceptive effects of the GABA analog, beta-(parachlorophenyl)-gamma-aminobutyric acid or baclofen. The mechanism of action of baclofen is unknown at this time, but it is unlikely that it is a GABA agonist. It does not act directly on GABA receptors (86), and its effects are not antagonized by known GABA receptor antagonists (55,62). Baclofen has been shown to have an antinociceptive effect in a wide variety of animal models by a number of investigators (56,117,169,170,172,247,259,313). The antinociceptive effect of baclofen can be demonstrated when the drug is given orally or parenterally, is not reversed by naloxone (169,259), and can be discriminated from morphine in drug discrimination studies (259). Like other GABA agonists, baclofen was inactive in the tail flick procedure when administered by the intraventricular route (172,259), although this finding is in dispute (170). Interestingly, baclofen and other GABAmimetics such as muscimol and diazepam significantly attenuate naloxone precipitated jumping in morphine-dependent mice (255,259), suggesting that interactions between the GABA system and morphine are not restricted to neuronal pathways that process nociceptive information.

Taken together, the biological evidence suggests that facilitation of gabergic transmission attenuates the transmission of nociceptive information. However, because of the ubiquitous role of GABAergic neurons in inhibition in the CNS of mammals, manipulation of GABAergic transmission in order to attenuate pain is almost invariably accompanied by other changes in brain function, which usually include sedation, motor deficits, and other forms of CNS depression. If more selective GABA agonists or GABAmimetics could be prepared, perhaps selective for a yet to be discovered subset of GABA receptors subserving nociceptive pathways, medically useful analgesics could emerge.

REFERENCES

1. Adams, J. E. (1976): Naloxone reversal of analgesia produced by brain stimulation in the human. *Pain*, 2:161–166.
2. Akagi, H., Otsuka, M., and Yanagisawa, M. (1980): Identification by high-performance liquid chromatography of immunoreactive substance P released from isolated rat spinal cord. *Neurosci. Lett.*, 20:259–263.
3. Akil, H., and Mayer, D. J. (1972): Antagonism of stimulation-produced analgesia by p-CPA, a serotonin synthesis inhibitor. *Brain Res.*, 44:692–697.
4. Akil, H., and Liebeskind, J. C. (1975): Monoaminergic mechanisms of stimulation-produced analgesia. *Brain Res.*, 94:279–296.
5. Anden, N.-E., Jukes, M. G. M., and Lundberg, A. (1964): Spinal reflexes and monoamine liberation. *Nature (Lond.)*, 202:1222–1223.
6. Anden, N.-E., Jukes, M. G. M., Lundberg, A., and Vyklicky, L. (1966): The effect of DOPA on the spinal cord. I. Influence in transmission from primary afferent. *Acta Physiol. Scand.*, 67:373–386.
7. Anden, N. E., Grabowska, M., and Strombom, A. (1976): Different alpha-adrenoreceptors in the central nervous system mediating biochemical and functional effects of clonidine and receptor blocking agents. *Naunyn Schmiedebergs Arch. Pharmacol.*, 292:43–52.
8. Anderson, R. K., Lund, J. P., and Puil, E. (1978): Enkephalin and substance P effects related to trigeminal pain. *Can. J. Physiol. Pharmacol.*, 56:216–222.
9. Atweh, S. F., and Kuhar, M. J. (1977): Autoradiographic localization of opiate receptors in rat brain. I. Spinal cord and lower medulla. *Brain Res.*, 124:53–67.
10. Atweh, S. F., and Kuhar, M. J. (1977): Autoradiographic localization of opiate receptors in rat brain. II. The brain stem. *Brain Res.*, 129:1–12.
11. Baizman, E. R., LoPresti, D. M., Meo, N. J., Pierson, A. K., and Morgan, B. A. (1982): In vitro and in vivo studies of substance P (SP) and two putative SP antagonists. *Soc. Neurosci. (Abstr.)*, 8:986.
12. Barber, R.P., Vaughn, J. E., Slemmon, J. R., Salvaterra, P. M., Roberts, E., and Leeman, S. E. (1979): The origin, distribution and synaptic relationships of substance P axons in rat spinal cord. *J. Comp. Neurol.*, 184:331–352.
13. Barbut, D., Polak, J. M., and Wall, P. D. (1981): Substance P in spinal cord dorsal horn decreases following peripheral nerve injury. *Brain Res.*, 205:289–298.
14. Basbaum, A. I., Marley, N. J. E., O'Keefe, J., and Clanton, C. H. (1977): Reversal of morphine and stimulus-produced analgesia by subtotal spinal cord lesions. *Pain*, 3:43–56.
15. Belcher, G., and Ryall, R. W. (1977): Substance P and Renshaw cells: A new concept of inhibitory synaptic interactions. *J. Physiol. (Lond.)*, 272:105–119.
16. Belcher, G., Ryall, R. W., and Schaffner, R. (1978): The differential effects of 5-hydroxytryptamine, noradrenaline and raphe stimulation on nociceptive and non-nociceptive dorsal horn interneurones in cat. *Brain Res.*, 151:307–321.
17. Beleslin, D., and Polak, R. L. (1965): Depression by morphine and chloralose of acetylcholine release from the cat's brain. *J. Physiol. (Lond.)*, 177:411–419.
18. Belin, M. F., Aguera, M., Tappaz, M., McRae-Deguenice, A., Bobillier, P., and Pujol, J. F. (1979): GABA-accumulating neurons in the nucleus raphe dorsalis and periaqueductal gray in the rat: a biochemical radioautographic study. *Brain Res.*, 170:279–297.
19. Bell, J. A., and Matsumiya, T. (1981): Inhibitory effects of dorsal horn and excitant effects of ventral horn intraspinal microinjections of norepinephrine and serotonin in the cat. *Life Sci.*, 29:1507–1514.
20. Berger, H., Fechner, K., Albrecht, E., and Niedrich, H. (1979): Substance P: In vitro inactivation by rat brain fractions and human plasma. *Biochem. Pharmacol.*, 28:3173–3180.
21. Bhargava, H. N., and Way, E. L. (1972): Acetylcholinesterase inhibition and morphine effects in morphine tolerant and dependent mice. *J. Pharmacol. Exp. Ther.*, 183:31–40.
22. Biggio, G., Della Bella, D., Frigeni, V., and Guidotti, A. (1977): Potentiation of morphine analgesia by muscimol. *Neuropharmacology*, 16:149–150.
23. Bissette, G., Manberg, P., Nemeroff, C. B., and Prange, A. J., Jr. (1978): Neurotensin, a biologically active peptide. *Life Sci.*, 23:2173–2182.
24. Bissette, G., Nemeroff, C. B., Loosen, P. T., Prange, A. J., Jr., and Lipton, M. A. (1976):

Hypothermia and intolerance to cold induced by intracisternal administration of the hypothalamic peptide, neurotensin. *Nature (Lond.)*, 262:607–609.

25. Bourgoin, S., Oliveras, J. L., Bruxell, J., Hamon, M., and Besson, J. M. (1980): Electrical stimulation of the nucleus raphe magnus in the rat. Effect of 5-HT metabolism in the spinal cord. *Brain Res.*, 194:377–389.

26. Brodin, E., Gazelius, B., Olgart, L., and Nilsson, G. (1981): Tissue concentration and release of substance P-like immunoreactivity in the dental pulp. *Acta Physiol. Scand.*, 111:141–149.

27. Buck, S. H., Miller, M. S., and Burks, T. F. (1982): Depletion of primary afferent substance P by capsaicin and dihydrocapsaicin without altered thermal sensitivity in rats. *Brain Res.*, 233:216–220.

28. Buckett, W. R. (1980): Induction of analgesia and morphine potentiation by irreversible inhibitors of GABA-transaminase. *Br. J. Pharmacol.*, 68:129–130.

29. Bury, R. W., and Mashford, M. L. (1976): Biological activity of C-terminal partial sequences of substance P. *J. Med. Chem.*, 19:854–856.

30. Bury, R. W., and Mashford, M. L. (1977): A pharmacological investigation of synthetic substance P on the isolated guinea pig ileum. *Clin. Exp. Pharmacol. Physiol.*, 4:453–461.

31. Bury, R. W., and Mashford, M. L. (1977): The stability of synthetic substance P in blood. *Eur. J. Pharmacol.*, 45:257–260.

32. Cahusac, P., Hayes, A. G., Skingle, M., and Tyers, M. B. (1981): Studies on the antinociceptive effects of clonidine and 4-hydroxyclonidine in the rat. *Br. J. Pharmacol.*, 74:963.

33. Carpenter, D., Engberg, I., and Lundberg, A. (1965): Differential supraspinal control of inhibitory and excitatory actions from the FRA to ascending spinal pathways. *Acta Physiol. Scand.*, 63:103–110.

34. Carraway, R., and Leeman, S. E. (1973): The isolation of a new hypotensive peptide, neurotensin, from bovine hypothalami. *J. Biol. Chem.*, 248:6854–6861.

35. Carraway, R., and Leeman, S. E. (1975): Structural requirements for the biological activity of neurotensin, a new vasoactive peptide. In: *Peptides: Chemistry, Structure and Biology. Proceedings of the 4th American Peptide Symposium*, edited by R. Walter and J. Meienhofer, pp. 679–685. Ann Arbor Science Publisher, Ann Arbor, Michigan.

36. Carraway, R., and Leeman, S. E. (1976): Characterization of radioimmunoassayable neurotensin in the rat; its differential distribution in the central nervous system, small intestine and stomach. *J. Biol. Chem.*, 251:7045–7052.

37. Cervero, F., and McRitchie, H. A. (1981): Neonatal capsaicin and thermal nociception: A paradox. *Brain Res.*, 215:414–418.

38. Chan-Palay, V., Jonsson, G., and Palay, S. L. (1978): Serotonin and substance P coexist in neurons of the rats' central nervous system. *Proc. Natl. Acad. Sci., U.S.A.*, 75:1582–1586.

39. Chan-Palay, V., and Palay, S. L. (1977): Immunocytochemical identification of substance P cells and their processes in rat sensory ganglia and their terminals in the spinal cord: Light microscopic studies. *Proc. Natl. Acad. Sci., U.S.A.*, 74:3597–3601.

40. Chan-Palay, V., and Palay, S. L. (1977): Ultrastructural identification of substance P cells and their processes in rat sensory ganglia and their terminals in the spinal cord by immunocytochemistry. *Proc. Natl. Acad. Sci., U.S.A.*, 74:4050–4054.

41. Chang Chen-yu, Tu Huan-Chi, Chao, Yen-fang, Pai Yao-hui, Ku Hsi-kon, Cheng, Jui-Kang, Shan Hong-Ying, and Yang Fu-yao. (1979): Effects of electrolytic lesions or intracerebral injections of 5,6-dihydroxytryptamine in raphe nuclei on acupuncture analgesia in rats. *Chinese Med. J.*, 92:129–136.

42. Chang, M. M., Leeman, S. E., and Niall, H. D. (1971): Amino acid sequence of substance P. *Nature (Lond.)*, 232:86–87.

43. Charney, D. S., Sternberg, D. E., Kleber, H. D., Heninger, G. R., and Redmond, D. E. (1981): The clinical use of clonidine in abrupt withdrawal from methadone. *Arch. Gen. Psychiatry*, 38:1273–1277.

44. Chen, G. (1958): The antitremorine effect of some drugs as determined by Haffner's method of testing analgesia in mice. *J. Pharmacol. Exp. Ther.*, 124:73–76.

45. Chipkin, R. E., Stewart, J. M., and Morris, D. H. (1978): Substance P and opioid interaction on stimulated and non-stimulated guinea pig ileum. *Eur. J. Pharmacol.*, 53:21–27.

46. Christensen, E. M., and Gross, E. G. (1948): Analgesic effects in human subjects of morphine, meperidine and methadone. *J.A.M.A.*, 137:594–598.

47. Clineschmidt, B. V., and McGuffin, J. C. (1977): Neurotensin administered intracisternally inhibits responsiveness of mice to noxious stimuli. *Eur. J. Pharmacol.*, 46:395–396.
48. Clineschmidt, B. V., McGuffin, J. C., and Bunting, P. B. (1979): Neurotensin: Antinocisponsive action in rodents. *Eur. J. Pharmacol.*, 54:129–139.
49. Cuello, A. C. (1978): Enkephalin and substance P containing neurons in the trigeminal and extrapyramidal systems. *Adv. Biochem. Psychopharmacol.*, 18:111–123.
50. Cuello, A. C., Emson, P., Del Fiacco, M., Gale, J., Iversen, L. L., Jessel, T. M., Kanazawa, I., Paxinos, G., and Quik, M. (1978): Distribution and release of substance P in the central nervous system. In: *Centrally Acting Peptides*, edited by J. Hughes, pp. 135–155. University Park Press, Baltimore.
51. Cuello, A. C., Del Fiacco, M., and Paxinos, G. (1978): The central and peripheral ends of the substance P-containing sensory neurons in the rat trigeminal system. *Brain Res.*, 152:499–509.
52. Cuello, A.C., Gamse, R., Holzer, P., and Lembeck, F. (1981): Substance P immunoreactive neurons following neonatal administration of capsaicin. *Naunyn Schmiedebergs Arch. Pharmacol.*, 315:185–194.
53. Cuello, A. C., and Kanazawa, I. (1978): The distribution of substance P immunoreactive fibers in the rat central nervous system. *J. Comp. Neurol.*, 178:129–156.
54. Cuello, A. C., Polak, J., and Pearse, A. G. E. (1976): Substance P: A naturally occurring transmitter in human spinal cord. *Lancet*, 2:1054–1056.
55. Curtis, D. R., Game, C. J. A., Johnston, G. A. R., and McCulloch, R. M. (1974): Central effects of beta-(p-chlorophenyl)-gamma-aminobutyric acid. *Brain Res.*, 70:493–499.
56. Cutting, P. A., and Jordan, C. C. (1975): Alternative approaches to analgesia: Baclofen as a model compound. *Br. J. Pharmacol.*, 54:171–179.
57. Dahlstrom, A., and Fuxe, K. (1964): Evidence for the existence of monoamine-containing neurons in the central nervous system. I. Demonstration of monoamines in the cell bodies of brain stem neurons. *Acta Physiol. Scand. (Suppl. 232)*, 62:1–55.
58. Dahlstrom, A., and Fuxe, K. (1965): Evidence for the existence of monoamine neurons in the central nervous system. II. Experimentally induced changes in the intraneuronal amine levels of bulbospinal neuron systems. *Acta Physiol. Scand. (Suppl.)*, 247, 64:5–36.
59. Davies, J., and Dray, A. (1976): Substance P in the substantia nigra. *Brain Res.*, 107:623–627.
60. Davies, J., and Dray, A. (1978): Pharmacological and electrophysiological studies of morphine and enkephalin on rat supraspinal and cat spinal neurones. *Br. J. Pharmacol.*, 63:87–96.
61. Davies, J., and Dray, A. (1980): Depression and facilitation of synaptic responses in cat dorsal horn by substance P administered into substantia gelatinosa. *Life Sci.*, 27:2037–2042.
62. Davies, J., and Watkins, J. E. (1974): The action of beta-phenyl-GABA derivatives on neurones of the cat cerebral cortex. *Brain Res.*, 70:501–505.
63. Dayton, H. E., and Garrett, R. L. (1973): Production of analgesia by cholinergic drugs. *Proc. Soc. Exp. Biol. Med.*, 142:1011–1013.
64. Deakin, J. F., and Dostrovsky, L. P. (1978): Involvement of the periaqueductal gray matter and spinal 5-hydroxytryptaminergic pathways in morphine analgesia: Effects of lesions and 5-hydroxytryptamine depletion. *Br. J. Pharmacol.*, 63:159–165.
65. Del Fiacco, M., and Cuello, A. C. (1980): Substance P and enkephalin-containing neurons in the rat trigeminal system. *Neuroscience*, 5:803–815.
66. Dewey, W. L., Snyder, J. W., Harris, L. S., and Howes, J. F. (1969): The effect of narcotics and narcotic antagonists on the tail flick response in spinal mice. *J. Pharm. Pharmacol.*, 21:548–555.
67. Dobry, P. J. K., Piercey, M. F., and Schroeder, L. A. (1981): Pharmacological characterization of scratching behavior induced by intracranial injection of substance P and somatostatin. *Neuropharmacology*, 20:267–272.
68. Doi, T., and Jurna, I. (1981): Intrathecal substance P depresses the tail flick response—antagonism by naloxone. *Naunyn Schmiedebergs Arch. Pharmacol.*, 317:135–139.
69. Dubner, R., and Hays, R. L. (1979): Pain mechanisms in the trigeminal system. In: *Mechanisms of Pain and Analgesic Compounds*, edited by R. F. Beers and E. G. Bassett, pp. 157–169. Raven Press, New York.
70. Duggan, A. W., Hall, J. G., and Headley, P. M. (1976): Morphine, enkephalin and the substantia gelatinosa. *Nature (Lond.)*, 264:456–458.
71. Duggan, A. W., Hall, J. G., and Headley, P. M. (1977): Suppression of transmission of nociceptive impulses by morphine: Selective effects of morphine administered in the region of the substantia gelatinosa. *Br. J. Pharmacol.*, 61:65–76.

72. Duggan, A. W., and Griersmith, B. T. (1979): Inhibition of the spinal transmission of nociceptive information by supraspinal stimulation in the cat. *Pain*, 6:147–161.
73. Duggan, A. W., Griersmith, B. T., Headley, P. M., and Hall, J. G. (1979): Lack of effect by substance P at sites in the substantia gelatinosa where met-enkephalin reduces the transmission of nociceptive impulses. *Neurosci. Lett.*, 12:313–317.
74. Dupont, A., and Merand, Y. (1978): Enzymic inactivation of neurotensin by hypothalamic and brain extracts of the rat. *Life Sci.*, 22:1623–1630.
75. Eccles, R. M., and Lundberg, A. (1959): Supraspinal control of interneurones mediating spinal reflexes. *J. Physiol. (Lond.)*, 147:565–584.
76. Engberg, G., Svensson, T. H., Rosell, S., and Folkers, K. (1981): A synthetic peptide as an antagonist of substance P. *Nature (Lond.)*, 293:222–223.
77. Falm, S. (1976): Regional distribution studies of GABA and other putative neurotransmitters and their enzymes. In: *GABA in Nervous System Function, KROC Foundation Series, Vol. 5*, edited by E. Roberts, T. N. Chase, and D. B. Towers, pp. 169–186. Raven Press, New York.
78. Fernstrom, M. H., Carraway, R. E., and Leeman, S. E. (1980): Neurotensin. In: *Frontiers in Neuroendocrinology*, edited by L. Martini and W. F. Ganong, pp. 103–127. Raven Press, New York.
79. Fielding, S., Wilker, J., Hynes, M., Szewczak, M., Novick, W. J., and Lal, H. (1978): A comparison of clonidine with morphine for antinociceptive and withdrawal actions. *J. Pharmacol. Exp. Ther.*, 207:899–905.
80. Fields, H. L., and Basbaum, A. I. (1978): Brainstem control of spinal pain-transmission neurons. *Annu. Rev. Physiol.*, 40:217–248.
81. Fields, H. L., Emson, P. C., Leigh, B. K., Gilbert, R. F. T., and Iversen, L. L. (1980): Multiple opiate receptor sites on primary afferent fibers. *Nature (Lond.)*, 284:351–353.
82. Floodmark, S., and Wramner, T. (1945): The analgetic action of morphine, eserine and prostigmine studied by a modified Hardy-Wolff-Goodell method. *Acta Physiol. Scand.*, 9:88–96.
83. Folkers, K., Horig, J., Rosell, S., and Bjorkroth, U. (1981): Chemical design of antagonists of substance P. *Acta Physiol. Scand.*, 111:505–506.
84. Frederickson, R. C. A., Burgis, V., Harrell, C. E., and Edwards, J. D. (1978): Dual actions of substance P on nociception: Possible role of endogenous opioids. *Science*, 199:1359–1362.
85. Frederickson, R. C. A., and Gesellchen, P. D. (1980): Analgesic and other activities of substance P and fragments. In: *Neuropeptides and Neural Transmission*, edited by C. A. Marsan and W. Z. Traczyk, pp. 111–120. Raven Press, New York.
86. Fukuda, H., Kudo, T., and Ono, H. (1977): Effect of beta-(p-chlorophenyl)-GABA (baclofen) on spinal synaptic activity. *Eur. J. Pharmacol.*, 44:17–24.
87. Gamse, R., Holzer, P., and Lembeck, F. (1980): Decrease of substance P in primary afferent neurons and impairment of neurogenic plasma extravasation by capsaicin. *Br. J. Pharmacol.*, 68:207–213.
88. Gamse, R., Lackner, D., Gamse, G., and Leeman, S. E. (1981); Effect of capsaicin pretreatment on capsaicin-evoked release of immunoreactive somatostatin and substance P from primary sensory neurons. *Naunyn Schmiedebergs Arch. Pharmacol.*, 316:38–41.
89. Gamse, R., Leeman, S. E., Holzer, P., and Lembeck, F. (1981): Differential effects of capsaicin on the content of somatostatin, substance P and neurotensin in the nervous system of the rat. *Naunyn Schmiedebergs Arch. Pharmacol.*, 317:140–148.
90. Gamse, R., Molnar, A., and Lembeck, F. (1979): Substance P release from spinal cord slices by capsaicin. *Life Sci.*, 25:629–636.
91. George, R., Haslett, W. L., and Jenden, D. J. (1962): The central action of a metabolite of tremorine. *Life Sci.*, 1:361–363.
92. Gobel, S., and Buck, J. M. (1977): Degenerative changes in primary trigeminal axons and in neurons in nucleus caudalis following tooth pulp extirpations in the cat. *Brain Res.*, 132:347–354.
93. Goldstein, J. M., and Malick, J. B. (1979): Lack of analgesic activity of substance P following intraperitoneal administration. *Life Sci.*, 25:431–436.
94. Griersmith, B. T., and Duggan, A. W. (1980): Prolonged depression of spinal transmission and nociceptive information by 5-HT administered in the substantia gelatinosa: Antagonism by methysergide. *Brain Res.*, 187:231–236.
95. Growcott, J. W., and Shaw, J. S. (1979): Failure of substance P to produce analgesia in the mouse. *Br. J. Pharmacol.*, 66:129.
96. Gumulka, W., Meszaros, J., Tarchalska, B., Gajewska, S., and Szreniawski, Z. (1978): Lesions

of the locus coeruleus: The effect of pethidine and pentazocine analgesia. *Pol. J. Pharmacol. Pharm.*, 30:775–780.

97. Guyenet, P. G., and Aghajanian, G. K. (1977): Excitation of neurons in the locus coeruleus by substance P and related peptides. *Brain Res.*, 136:178–184.

98. Guyenet, P. G., and Aghajanian, G. K. (1979): ACh, substance P and met-enkephalin in the locus coeruleus: Pharmacological evidence for independent sites of action. *Eur. J. Pharmacol.*, 53:319–328.

99. Guyenet, P. G., Mroz, E. A., Aghajanian, G. K., and Leeman, S. E. (1979): Delayed iontophoretic ejection of substance P from glass micropipettes: Correlation with time course of neuronal excitation in vivo. *Neuropharmacology*, 18:553–558.

100. Haigler, H. J., and Spring, D. D. (1980): Substance P, morphine and methionine-enkephalin: Effects on spontaneous and evoked neuronal firing in the nucleus reticularis gigantocellularis of the rat. *Eur. J. Pharmacol.*, 67:65–74.

101. Hammond, D. L., Levy, R. A., and Proudfit, H. K. (1980): Hypoalgesia following microinjection of noradrenergic antagonists in the nucleus raphe magnus. *Pain*, 9:85–101.

102. Han, C-S., Chou, P-H., Lu, C-C., Lu, L-H., Yang, T-H., Jen, M-F. (1979): The role of central 5-hydroxytryptamine in acupuncture analgesia. *Scientia Sinica*, 12:91–104.

103. Hanley, M. R., and Iversen, L. L. (1980): Substance P receptors. In: *Neurotransmitter Receptors, Part I, (Vol. 9: Receptors and Recognition, Series B)*, edited by S. J. Enna and H. I. Yamamura, pp. 73–103. Chapman and Hall, London.

104. Harris, L. S., and Dewey, W. L. (1972): Role of cholinergic systems in the central action of narcotic agonists and antagonists. In: *Agonist and Antagonist Actions of Narcotic Analgesic Drugs*, edited by H. W. Kosterlitz, H. O. J. Collier, and J. E. Villarreal, pp. 198–206. MacMillan Press, London.

105. Harris, L. S., Dewey, W. L., and Howes, J. F. (1968): The tail-flick test, cholinergic mechanisms. *Fed. Proc.*, 27:753.

106. Harris, L. S., Dewey, W. L., Howes, J. F., Kennedy, J. S., and Pars, H. (1969): Narcotic-antagonist analgesics: Interactions with cholinergic systems. *J. Pharmacol. Exp. Ther.*, 169:17–22.

107. Hayes, A. G., and Tyres, M. B. (1979): Effects of intrathecal and intracerebroventricular injections of substance P on nociception in the rat and mouse. *Br. J. Pharmacol.*, 66:488.

108. Hayes, A. G., and Tyers, M. B. (1980): Effects of capsaicin on nociceptive heat, pressure and chemical thresholds and on substance P levels in the rat. *Brain Res.*, 189:561–564.

109. Headley, P. M., Duggan, A. W., and Griersmith, B. T. (1978): Selective reduction by noradrenaline and 5-hydroxytryptamine of nociceptive responses of cat dorsal horn neurones. *Brain Res.*, 145:185–189.

110. Helke, C. J., DiMicco, J. A., Jacobowitz, D. M., and Kopin, I. J. (1981): Effect of capsaicin administration to neonatal rats on the substance P content of discrete CNS regions. *Brain Res.*, 222:428–431.

111. Helke, C. J., Jocobowitz, D. M., and Thoa, N. B. (1980): Substance P release from the nucleus tractus solitarius and trigeminal spinal nucleus in vitro. *Neurosci. Abstr.*, 6:619.

112. Hendershot, L. C., and Forsaith, J. (1959): Antagonism of the frequency of phenylquinone-induced writhing in the mouse by weak analgesics and nonanalgesics. *J. Pharmacol. Exp. Ther.*, 125:237–240.

113. Henry, J. L. (1976): Effects of substance P on functionally identified units in cat spinal cord. *Brain Res.*, 114:439–451.

114. Henry, J. L. (1977): Substance P and pain: A possible relation in afferent transmission. In: *Substance P*, edited by U. S. von Euler and B. Pernow, pp. 231–240. Raven Press, New York.

115. Henry, J. L., Krnjevic, K., and Morris, M. E. (1975): Substance P and spinal neurons. *Can. J. Physiol. Pharmacol.*, 53:423–432.

116. Herz, A. (1962): Wirkungen des arecolins auf das zentral nervensystem. *Arch. Exp. Pathol. Pharmacol.*, 242:414–429.

117. Hill, R. C., Mauer, R., Buescher, H. H., and Roemer, D. (1981): Analgesic properties of the GABA-mimetic THIP. *Eur. J. Pharmacol.*, 69:221–224.

118. Ho, I. K., Loh, H. H., and Way, E. L. (1976): Pharmacological manipulation of gamma-aminobutyric acid (GABA) in morphine analgesia, tolerance and physical dependence. *Life Sci.*, 18:1111–1124.

119. Hokfelt, T., Elde, R., Johansson, O., Luft, R., Nilsson, G., and Arimura, A. (1976): Immuno-

histochemical evidence for separate populations of somatostatin-containing and substance P-containing primary afferent neurons in the rat. *Neuroscience*, 1:131–136.

120. Hokfelt, T., Elde, R., Johansson, O., Terenius, L., and Stein, L. (1977): The distribution of enkephalin immunoreactive cell bodies in the rat central nervous system. *Neurosci. Lett.*, 5:25–31.

121. Hokfelt, T., Johansson, O., Kellerth, J. O., Ljungdahl, A., Nilsson, G., Nygards, A., and Pernow, B. (1977): Immunohistochemical distribution of substance P. In: *Substance P*, edited by U. S. von Euler and B. Pernow, pp. 117–145. Raven Press, New York.

122. Hokfelt, T., Johansson, O., Ljungdahl, A., Lundberg, J. M., and Schultzberg, M. (1980): Peptidergic neurons. *Nature (Lond.)*, 284:515–521.

123. Hokfelt, T., Kellerth, J. O., Nilsson, G., and Pernow, B. (1975): Experimental immunohistochemical studies on the localization and distribution of substance P in cat primary sensory neurons. *Brain Res.*, 100:235–252.

124. Hokfelt, T., Kellerth, J. O., Nilsson, G., and Pernow, B. (1975): Substance P: Localization in the central nervous system and in some primary sensory neurons. *Science*, 190:889–890.

125. Hokfelt, T., Ljungdahl, A., Steinbusch, H., Verhofstad, A., Nilsson, G., Brodin, E., Pernow, B., and Goldstein, M. (1978): Immunohistochemical evidence of substance P-like immunoreactivity in some 5-hydroxytryptamine-containing neurons in the rat central nervous system. *Neuroscience*, 3:517–538.

126. Hokfelt, T., Ljungdahl, A., Tienius, L., Elde, R., and Nilsson, G. (1977): Immunohistochemical analysis of peptide pathways possibly related to pain and analgesia: Enkephalin and substance P. *Proc. Natl. Acad. Sci. U.S.A.*, 74:3081–3085.

127. Hokfelt, T., Terenius, L., Kuypers, H. G., and Dann, O. (1979): Evidence for enkephalin immunoreactive neurons in the medulla oblongata projecting to the spinal cord. *Neurosci. Lett.*, 14:55–60.

128. Holmdahl, G., Hakanson, R., Leander, S., Rosell, S., Folkers, K., and Sundler, F. (1981): A substance P antagonist, D-Pro2, D-Trp7,9 SP inhibits inflammatory responses in the rabbit eye. *Science*, 214:1029–1031.

129. Holzer, P., Jurna, I., Gamse, R., and Lembeck, F. (1979): Nociceptive thresholds after neonatal capsaicin treatment. *Eur. J. Pharmacol.*, 58:511–514.

130. Houser, V. P. (1976): Modulation of the aversive qualities of shock through a central inhibitory cholinergic system in the rat. *Pharmacol. Biochem. Behav.*, 4:561–568.

131. Houser, V. P., and Houser, F. L. (1973): The alteration of aversive thresholds with cholinergic and adrenergic agents. *Pharmacol. Biochem. Behav.*, 1:433–444.

132. Howes, J. F., Harris, L. S., Dewey, W. L., and Voyda, C. A. (1969): Brain acetylcholine levels and inhibition of the tail flick reflex in mice. *J. Pharmacol. Exp. Ther.*, 169:23–28.

133. Hunt, S. P., Kelly, J. S., and Emson, P. C. (1980): The electron microscopic localization of methionine-enkephalin within the superficial layers (I and II) of the spinal cord. *Neuroscience*, 5:1871–1890.

134. Hunt, S. P., Kelly, J. S., Emson, P. C., Kimmel, J. R., Miller, R. J., and Wu, J.-Y. (1981): An immunohistochemical study of neuronal populations containing neuropeptides or gamma-amino butyrate within the superficial layers of the rat dorsal horn. *Neuroscience*, 6:1883–1898.

135. Hylden, J. L. K., Cleary, C. J., and Wilcox, G. L. (1980): Spinal analgesia and hyperalgesia in the mouse. *Soc. Neurosci. (Abstr.)*, 6:434.

136. Hylden, J. L. K., and Wilcox, G. L. (1981): Intrathecal substance P elicits a caudally-directed biting and scratching behavior in mice. *Brain Res.*, 217:212–215.

137. Ireson, J. D. (1970): A comparison of the antinociceptive actions of cholinomimetic and morphine-like drugs. *Br. J. Pharmacol.*, 40:92–101.

138. Iversen, L. L., Iversen, S. D., Bloom, F., Douglas, C., Brown, M., and Vale, W. (1978): Calcium-dependent release of somatostatin and neurotensin from rat brain in vitro. *Nature (Lond.)*, 273:161–163.

139. Iversen, L. L., Jessel, T., and Kanazawa, I. (1976): Release and metabolism of substance P in rat hypothalamus. *Nature (Lond.)*, 264:81–83.

140. Jansco, G., Kiraly, E., and Jansco-Gabor, A. (1977): Pharmacologically induced selective degeneration of chemosensory primary neurons. *Nature (Lond.)*, 270:741–743.

141. Jansco, G., Kiraly, E., and Jansco-Gabor, A. (1980): Chemosensitive pain fibers and inflammation. *Int. J. Tiss. React.*, 11:57–66.

142. Jessel, T. M., and Iversen, L. L. (1977): Opiate analgesics inhibit substance P release from rat trigeminal nucleus. *Nature (Lond.)*, 268:549–551.
143. Jessel, T. M. Iversen, L. L., and Cuello, A. C. (1978): Capsaicin-induced depletion of substance P from primary sensory neurons. *Brain Res.*, 152:183–188.
144. Jessell, T., Tsunoo, A., Kanazawa, I., and Otsuka, M., (1979): Substance P: Depletion in the dorsal horn of rat spinal cord after section of the peripheral processes of primary sensory nerves. *Brain Res.*, 168:247–259.
145. Jhamandas, K., Phillis, J. W., and Pinsky, C. (1971): Effects of narcotic analgesics and antagonists on the in vivo release of acetylcholine from the cerebral cortex of the cat. *Br. J. Pharmacol.*, 43:53–66.
146. Johansson, O., Hokfelt, T., Elde, R. P., Schultzberg, M., and Terenius, L. (1978): Immunohistochemical distribution of enkephalin neurons. *Adv. Biochem. Psychopharmacol.*, 18:51–70.
147. Johansson, O., Hokfelt, T., Pernow, B., Jeffcoate, S. L., White, N., Steinbusch, H. W. M., Verhofstad, A. A. J., Emson, P. C., and Spindel, E. (1981): Immunohistochemical support for three putative transmitters in one neuron: Co-existence of 5-hydroxytryptamine, substance P and thyrotropin releasing hormone-like immunoreactivity in medullary neurons projecting to the spinal cord. *Neuroscience*, 6:1857–1881.
148. Johnston, G. A. R. (1968): The intraspinal distribution of some depressant amino acids. *J. Neurochem.*, 15:1013–1017.
149. Joo, F., Szolcsanyi, J., and Jansco-Gabor, A. (1969): Mitochondrial alterations in the spinal ganglion cells of the rat accompanying substance P release induced by capsaicin. *Life Sci.*, 8:621–626.
150. Katayama, Y., North, R. A., and Williams, J. T. (1979): The action of substance P on neurones of the myenteric plexus of the guinea pig small intestine. *Proc. R. Soc. Biol.*, 206:191–206.
151. Kitabgi, P., Carraway, R., Van Reitschoten, J., Granier, C., Morgat, J., Menez, A., Leeman, S. E., and Freychet, P. (1977): Neurotensin: Specific binding to synaptic membranes from rat brain. *Proc. Natl. Acad. Sci. U.S.A.*, 74:1846–1850.
152. Kitabgi, P., and Freychet, P. (1978): Effects of neurotensin on isolated intestinal smooth muscles. *Eur. J. Pharmacol.*, 50:349–357.
153. Kitabgi, P., Poustis, C., Granier, C., Van Reitschoten, J., Rivier, J., Morgat, J.-L., and Freychet, P. (1980): Neurotensin binding to extraneural and neural receptors: Comparison with biological activity and structure-activity relationships. *Mol. Pharmacol.*, 18:11–19.
154. Kobayashi, R., Brown, M. R., and Vale, W. (1977): Regional distribution of neurotensin and somatostatin in rat brain. *Brain Res.*, 126:584–588.
155. Kostowski, W., Jerlicz, M., Bidzinski, A., and Hauptmann, M. (1978): Reduced analgesic effects of morphine after bilateral lesions of the locus coeruleus in rats. *Pol. J. Pharmacol. Pharm.*, 30:49–53.
156. Kotani, Y., Oka, M., Yonehara, N., Kudo, T., and Inoki, R. (1981): Algesiogenic and analgesic activities of synthetic substance P. *Jpn. J. Pharmacol.*, 31:315–321.
157. Kunos, G., Farsang, C., and Ramirez-Gonzales, M. D. (1980): Beta-endorphin: Possible involvement in the antihypertensive effect of central alpha-receptor activation. *Science*, 211:82–84.
158. Kuriashi, Y., Harada, Y., and Takagi, H. (1979): Noradrenaline regulation of pain-transmission in the spinal cord mediated by alpha-adrenoceptors. *Brain Res.*, 174:333–337.
159. Kuriashi, Y., Harada, Y., Satoh, M., and Takagi, H. (1979): Antagonism by phenoxybenzamine of the analgesic effect of morphine injected into the nucleus reticulogigantocellularis of the rat. *Neuropharmacology*, 18:107–110.
160. LaMotte, C. C., and de Lanerolle, N. C. (1981): Human spinal neurons: Innervation by both substance P and enkephalin. *Neuroscience*, 6:713–723.
161. LaMotte, C., Pert, C. B., and Snyder, S. H. (1976): Opiate receptor binding in primate spinal cord: Distribution and changes after dorsal root section. *Brain Res.*, 112:407–412.
162. Lazarus, L. H., Brown, M. R., and Perrin, M. H. (1977): Distribution, localization, and characteristics of neurotensin binding sites in the rat brain. *Neuropharmacology*, 16:625–629.
163. Leander, S., Hakanson, R., Rosell, S., Folkers, K., Sundler, F., and Tornqvist, K. (1981): A specific substance P antagonist blocks smooth muscle contractions induced by noncholinergic, non-adrenergic nerve stimulation. *Nature (Lond.)*, 294:467–469.
164. Leeman, S. E., Mroz, E. A., and Carraway, R. E. (1977): Substance P and neurotensin. In: *Peptides in Neurobiology*, edited by H. Gainer, pp. 99–144. Plenum Press, New York.
165. Lembeck, F. (1953): Zur frage der zentralen ubertragung afferenter impulse III. Mitteilung, das

vorkommen und die bedentung der substanz P in den dorsal wurzeln des ruckenmarks. *Naunyn Schmiedebergs Arch. Pharmacol.*, 219:197–213.

166. Lembeck, F., Folkers, K., and Donnerer, J. (1981): Analgesic effect of antagonists of substance P. *Biochem. Biophys. Res. Commun.*, 103:1318–1321.

167. Lembeck, F., Mayer, N., and Schindler, G. (1977): Substance P in rat brain synaptosomes. *Naunyn Schmiedebergs Arch. Pharmacol.*, 301:17–22.

168. Leslie, G. B. (1969): The effect of anti-parkinsonian drugs on oxoremorine-induced analgesia in mice. *J. Pharm. Pharmacol.*, 21:248–250.

169. Levy, R. A., and Proudfit, H. K. (1977): The analgesic action of baclofen (beta-4-chlorophenyl-gamma-aminobutyric acid). *J. Pharmacol.*, 202:437–445.

170. Levy, R. A., and Proudfit, H. K. (1979): Analgesia produced by microinjection of baclofen and morphine at brain stem sites. *Eur. J. Pharmacol.*, 57:43–55.

171. Liebeskind, J. C., Guilbaud, G., Besson, J. M., and Oliveras, J.-L. (1973): Analgesia from electrical stimulation of the periaqueductal gray matter in the cat: Behavioral observations and inhibitory effects on spinal cord interneurons. *Brain Res.*, 50:441–446.

172. Liebman, J. M., and Pastor, G. (1980): Antinociceptive effects of baclofen and muscimol upon intraventricular administration. *Eur. J. Pharmacol.*, 61:225–230.

173. Light, A. R., and Perl, E. R. (1979): Re-examination of the dorsal root projection to the dorsal horn including observations on the differential termination of coarse and fine fibers. *J. Comp. Neurol.*, 186:117–132.

174. Light, A. R., and Perl, E. R. (1979): Spinal termination of functionally-defined neurons in the marginal zone and substantia gelatinosa of the spinal dorsal horn. *J. Comp. Neurol.*, 186:133–150.

175. Lin, M. T., Chi, M. L., Chandra, A., and Tsay, B. L. (1980): Serotonergic mechanisms of beta-endorphin- and clonidine-induced analgesia in rats. *Pharmacology*, 20:323–328.

176. Lipman, J. J., and Spencer, P. S. J. (1979): Further evidence for a central site of action for the antinociceptive effect of clonidine-like drugs. *Neuropharmacology*, 18:731–733.

177. Lippert, B., Metcalf, B. W., Jung, M. J., and Casara, P. (1977): 4-Aminobutyric-acid aminotransferase in mammalian brain. *Eur. J. Biochem.*, 74:441–445.

178. Little, H. J., and Rees, J. M. H. (1974): Tolerance development to the antinociceptive actions of morphine, amphetamine, physostigmine and 2-aminoindane in the mouse. *Experientia*, 30:930–932.

179. Ljungdahl, A., Hokfelt, T., and Nilssen, G. (1978): Distribution of substance P-like immunoreactivity in the central nervous system of the rat. I. Cell bodies and nerve terminals. *Neuroscience*, 3:861–943.

180. Ljungdahl, A., Hokfelt, T., Nilsson, G., and Goldstein, M. (1978): Distribution of substance P-like immunoreactivity in the central nervous system of the rat. II. Light microscopic localization in relation to catecholamine-containing neurons. *Neuroscience*, 3:945–976.

181. Maeda, K., and Frohman, L. A. (1981): Neurotensin release by rat hypothalmic fragments in vitro. *Brain Res.*, 210:261–269.

182. Malick, J. B., and Goldstein, J. M. (1978): Analgesic activity of substance P following intracerebral administration in rats. *Life Sci.*, 23:835–844.

183. Malthe-Sorensen, D., Cheney, D. L., and Costa, E. (1978): Modulation of acetylcholine metabolism in the hippocampal cholinergic pathway by intraseptally injected substance P. *J. Pharmacol. Exp. Ther.*, 206:21–28.

184. Mantegazza, P., Tammiso, R., Vicentini, L., Zambotti, F., and Zonta, N. (1979): Nipecotic acid and guvacine antagonism on morphine analgesia in rats. *Pharmacol. Res. Commun.*, 11:657–662.

185. Margalit, P., and Segal, M. (1979): A pharmacologic study of analgesia produced by stimulation of the nucleus locus coeruleus. *Psychopharmacologia*, 62:169–173.

186. Marwaha, J., Hoffer, B., and Freedman, R. (1980): Electrophysiological actions of neurotensin in rat cerebellum. *Regul. Peptides*, 1:115–125.

187. Mayer, D. J., and Price, D. D. (1976): Central nervous system mechanisms of analgesia. *Pain*, 2:379–404.

188. Mayer, D. J., Wolfle, T. L., Aril, H., Carder, B., and Liebeskind, J. C. (1971): Analgesia from electrical stimulation in brainstem of the rat. *Science*, 174:1351–1354.

189. McCleary, P. E., and Leander, J. D. (1981): Clonidine analgesia and suppression of operant responding: Dissociation of mechanism. *Eur. J. Pharmacol.*, 69:63–69.

190. Melzack, R., (1973): The evolution of pain theories. In: *The Puzzle of Pain*, edited by R. Melzack, pp. 125–152. Basic Books, Inc., New York.
191. Melzack, R., and Wall, P. D. (1965): Pain mechanisms: A new theory. *Science*, 150:971–979.
192. Messing, R. B., and Lytle, L. D. (1977): Serotonin-containing neurons: Their possible role in pain and analgesia. *Pain*, 4:1–21.
193. Meszaros, J., Tarchalska, B., Gajewska, S., Janicki, P., Duriasz, H., and Szreniawski, S. (1980): Substance P, hexapeptide pGlu6(SP6-11), analgesia and serotonin depletion. *Pharmacol. Biochem. Behav.*, 14:11–15.
194. Metys, J., Wagner, N., Metysova, J., and Herz, A. (1969): Studies on the central antinociceptive action of cholinomimetic agents. *Int. J. Neuropharmacol.*, 8:413–425.
195. Migdal, W., and Frumin, J. J. (1963): Amnesic and analgesic effects in man of centrally acting anticholinergics. *Fed. Proc.*, 22:188.
196. Miletic, V., and Randic, M. (1979): Neurotensin excites cat spinal neurones located in laminae I-III. *Brain Res.*, 169:600–604.
197. Miletic, V., and Randic, M. (1982): Neonatal rat spinal cord slice preparation: Postsynaptic effects of neuropeptides on dorsal horn neurons. *Dev. Brain Res.*, 2:432–438.
198. Mohrland, J. S., and Gebhart, G. F. (1979): Substance P-induced analgesia in the rat. *Brain Res.*, 171:556–559.
199. Molnar, J. (1965): Die pharmakologischen wirkungen des capsaicins, des scharf schmeckenden wirkstoffes im paprika. *Arzneimittelforsch.*, 15:718–727.
200. Monier, S., and Kitabgi, P. (1980): Substance P induced autodesensitization inhibits atropine resistant neurotensin-stimulated contractions in guinea-pig ileum. *Eur. J. Pharmacol.*, 65:461–462.
201. Monier, S., and Kitabgi, P. (1981): Effects of beta-endorphin, met-enkephalin and somatostatin on the neurotensin-induced neurogenic contraction in the guinea-pig ileum. *Regul. Peptides*, 2:31–42.
202. Mudge, A. W., Leeman, S. E., and Fishbach, G. D. (1979): Enkephalin inhibits release of substance P from sensory neurons in culture and decreases action potential duration. *Proc. Natl. Acad. Sci. U.S.A.*, 76:526–530.
203. Nagy, J. F., Emson, P. C., and Iversen, L. L. (1981): A re-evaluation of the neurochemical and antinociceptive effects of intrathecal capsaicin in the rat. *Brain Res.*, 211:497–502.
204. Nagy, J. I., Vincent, J. R., Staines, W. A., Fibiger, H. C., Reisine, T. D., and Yamamura, H. I. (1980): Neurotoxic actions of capsaicin on spinal substance P neurons. *Brain Res.*, 186:435–444.
205. Naranjo, J. R., Sanchez-Franco, F., Garzon, J., and del Rio, J. (1982): Analgesic activity of substance P in rats: Apparent mediation by met-enkephalin release. *Life Sci.*, 30:441–446.
206. Nemeroff, C. B., Bissette, G., Manberg, P. J., Osbahr, A. J., III, Breese, G. R., and Prange, A. J., Jr. (1980): Neurotensin-induced hypothermia: Evidence for an interaction with dopaminergic systems and the hypothalamic-pituitary thyroid axis. *Brain Res.*, 195:69–84.
207. Nemeroff, C. B., Bissette, G., Prange, A. J., Jr., Loosen, P. T., Barlow, T. S., and Lipton, M. A. (1977): Neurotensin: Central nervous system effects of a hypothalamic peptide. *Brain Res.*, 128:485–496.
208. Nemeroff, C. B., Osbahr, A. J., II, Manberg, P. J., Ervin, G. N., and Prange, A. J., Jr. (1979): Alterations in nociception and body temperature after intracisternally administered neurotensin, beta-endorphin, other endogenous peptides and morphine. *Proc. Natl. Acad. Sci. U.S.A.*, 76:5368–5371.
209. Nicoll, R. A. (1978): The action of thyrotropin-releasing hormone, substance P and related peptides on frog spinal motoneurons. *J. Pharmacol. Exp. Ther.*, 207:817–824.
210. Nicoll, R. A., Schenker, C., and Leeman, S. E. (1980): Substance P as a transmitter candidate. *Annu. Rev. Neurosci.*, 3:227–268.
211. Nilsson, G., Hokfelt, T., and Pernow, B. (1974): Distribution of substance P-like immunoreactivity in the rat central nervous system as revealed by immunohistochemistry. *Med. Biol.*, 52:424–427.
212. Ninkovic, M., Hunt, S. P., and Kelly, J. S. (1981): Effect of dorsal rhizotomy on the autoradiographic distribution of opiate and neurotensin receptors and neurotensin-like immunoreactivity within the rat spinal cord. *Brain Res.*, 230:111–119.
213. Nowak, L. M., and MacDonald, R. L. (1981): Substance P decreases a potassium conductance of spinal cord neurons in cell culture. *Brain Res.*, 214:416–423.
214. Oehme, P., Hecht, K., Piesche, L., Hilse, H., Morgenstern, E., and Poppei, M. (1980): Substance

P as a modulator of physiological and pathological processes. In: *Neuropeptides and Neural Transmission*, edited by C. A. Marsan and W. Z. Traczyk, pp. 73–84. Raven Press, New York.

215. Oehme, P., Hilse, H., Morgenstern, E., and Gores, E. (1980): Substance P: Does it produce analgesia or hyperalgesia? *Science*, 208:305–307.

216. Olds, M. E., and Olds, J. (1963): Approach-avoidance analysis of the rat diencephalon. *J. Comp. Neurol.*, 120:259–295.

217. Olgart, L., Gazelius, B., Brodin, E., and Nilsson, G. (1977): Release of substance P-like immunoreactivity from the dental pulp. *Acta Physiol. Scand.*, 101:510–512.

218. Olgart, L., Hokfelt, T., Nilsson, G., and Pernow, B. (1977): Localization of substance P-like immunoreactivity in nerves in the tooth pulp. *Pain*, 4:153–159.

219. Oliveras, J. L., Redjemi, F., Guilbaud, G., and Besson, J. M. (1975): Analgesia induced by electrical stimulation of the inferior centralis of the raphe in the cat. *Pain*, 1:139–145.

220. Osbahr, A. J., III, Nemeroff, C. B., Luttinger, D., Mason, G. A., and Prange, A. J., Jr. (1981): Neurotensin-induced antinociception in mice: Antagonism by thyrotropin-releasing hormone. *J. Pharmacol. Exp. Ther.*, 217:645–651.

221. Otsuka, M., and Konishi, S. (1976): Release of substance P-like immunoreactivity from isolated spinal cord of new-born rat. *Nature (Lond.)*, 264:83–84.

222. Otsuka, M., and Konishi, S. (1976): Substance P: An excitatory transmitter of primary sensory neurons. *Cold Spring Harbor Symp. Quant. Biol.*, 40:135–143.

223. Otsuka, M., and Konishi, S. (1977): Electrophysiological evidence for substance P as a transmitter of primary sensory neurons. In: *Substance P*, edited by U.S. von Euler and B. Pernow, pp. 207–214. Raven Press, New York.

224. Paalzow, L. (1974): Analgesia produced by clonidine in mice and rats. *J. Pharm. Pharmacol.*, 26:361–363.

225. Paalzow, G. (1978): Development of tolerance to the analgesic effects of clonidine in rats. *Naunyn Schmiedebergs Arch. Pharmacol.*, 304:1–4.

226. Paalzow, G., and Paalzow, L. (1975): Antinociceptive action of oxotremorine and regional turnover of rat brain noradrenaline, dopamine and 5-HT. *Eur. J. Pharmacol.*, 31:261–272.

227. Paalzow, G., and Paalzow, L. (1976): Clonidine antinociceptive activity: Effects of drugs influencing central monoaminergic and cholinergic mechanisms in the rat. *Naunyn Schmiedebergs Arch. Pharmacol.*, 292:119–126.

228. Pardridge, W. M., Frank, H. J. L., Cornford, E. M., Braun, L. D., Crane, P. D., and Oldendorf, W. H. (1981): Neuropeptides and the blood-brain barrier. In: *Neurosecretion and Brain Peptides*, edited by J. B. Martin, S. Reichlin, and K. L. Bick, pp. 321–328. Raven Press, New York.

229. Pearson, J., Brandeis, L., and Cuello, A. C. (1982): Depletion of substance P-containing axons in substantia gelatinosa of patients with diminished pain sensitivity. *Nature*, 295:61–63.

230. Pedigo, N. W., and Dewey, W. L. (1981): Comparison of the antinociceptive activity of intraventricularly administered acetylcholine to narcotic antinociception. *Neurosci. Lett.*, 26:85–90.

231. Pedigo, N. W., Dewey, W. L., and Harris, L. S. (1975): Determination and characterization of the antinociceptive activity of intraventricularly administered acetylcholine in mice. *J. Pharmacol. Exp. Ther.*, 193:845–852.

232. Pellanda, C. L. (1933): La geneserine-morphine adjuvant de l'anesthesia generale. *Lyon Med.*, 151:653.

233. Pernow, B. (1953): Studies on substance P: Purification, occurrence and biological actions. *Acta Physiol. Scand.*, 29,105:1–90.

234. Pert, A. (1975): The cholinergic system and antinociception in the primate: Interaction with morphine. *Psychopharmacology*, 44:131–137.

235. Pettibone, D. J., and Mueller, G. P. (1981): Clonidine releases immunoreactive beta-endorphin from rat pars distalis. *Brain Res.*, 221:409–414.

236. Phillis, J. W. (1980): Substance P in the central nervous system. In: *The Role of Peptides in Neuronal Function*, edited by J. L. Barker and T. G. Smith, Jr., pp. 615–652. Marcel Dekker, New York.

237. Pickel, V. M., Reis, D. J., and Leeman, S. E. (1977): Ultrastructural localization of substance P in neurons of rat spinal cord. *Brain Res.*, 122:534–540.

238. Pickel, V. M., Joh, T. H., Reis, D. J., Leeman, S. E., and Miller, R. J. (1979): Electron microscopic localization of substance P and enkephalin in axon terminals related to dendrites of catecholaminergic neurons. *Brain Res.*, 160:387–400.

239. Piercey, M. F., and Einspahr, F. J. (1980): Use of substance P partial fragments to characterize substance P receptors of cat dorsal horn neurons. *Brain Res.*, 187:481–486.
240. Piercey, M. F., Einspahr, F. J., Dobry, P. J. K., Schroeder, L. A., and Hollister, R. P. (1980): Morphine does not antagonize the substance P mediated excitation of dorsal horn neurons. *Brain Res.*, 186:421–434.
241. Piercey, M. F., Dobry, P. J. K., Schroeder, L. A., and Einspahr, F. J. (1981): Behavioral evidence that substance P may be a spinal cord sensory neurotransmitter. *Brain Res.*, 210:407–412.
242. Piercey, M. F., Schroeder, L. A., Folkers, K., Xu, J.-C., and Horig, J. (1981): Sensory and motor functions of spinal cord substance P. *Science*, 214:1361–1363.
243. Pleuvry, B. J., and Tobias, M. A. (1971): Comparison of the antinociceptive activities of physostigmine, oxotremorine and morphine in the mouse. *Br. J. Pharmacol.*, 43:706–714.
244. Pomery, S. L., and Behbani, M. M. (1980): Response of nucleus raphe magnus neurons to iontophoretically applied substance P in rats. *Brain Res.*, 202:464–468.
245. Proudfit, H. K. (1980): Effects of raphe magnus and raphe pallidus lesions on morphine-induced analgesia and spinal cord monoamines. *Pharmacol. Biochem. Behav.*, 13:705–714.
246. Proudfit, H. K., and Anderson, E. G. (1975): Morphine analgesia: Blockade by raphe magnus lesions. *Brain Res.*, 98:612–618.
247. Proudfit, H. K., and Levy, R. A. (1978): Delimitation of neuronal substrates necessary for the analgesic action of baclofen and morphine. *Eur. J. Pharmacol.*, 47:159–166.
248. Rackham, A., Theriault, M., and Wood, P. L. (1981): Substance P: Evidence for spinal mediation of some behavioral effects. *Neuropharmacology*, 20:753–755.
249. Ramabadran, K., and Jacob, J. J. C. (1978): Facilitory effect of naloxone and involvement of specific ligand-opiate receptor systems in the antinociceptive effects of non-opioid drugs. *Arch. Int. Pharmacodyn. Ther.*, 236:27–42.
250. Randic, M., and Miletic, V. (1977): Effect of substance P in cat dorsal horn neurons activated by noxious stimuli. *Brain Res.*, 128:164–169.
251. Reddy, S. V. R., Maderdrut, J. L., and Yaksh, T. L. (1980): Spinal cord pharmacology of adrenergic agonist-mediated antinociception. *J. Pharmacol. Exp. Ther.*, 213:525–533.
252. Reddy, S. V. R., and Yaksh, T. L. (1980): Spinal noradrenergic terminal system mediates antinociception. *Brain Res.*, 189:391–401.
253. Rioux, F., Quirion, R., Regoli, D., Le Blanc, M.-A., and St. Pierre, S. (1980): Pharmacological characterization of neurotensin receptors in the rat isolated portal vein using analogues and fragments of neurotensin. *Eur. J. Pharmacol.*, 66:273–279.
254. Roberts, E., Chase, T. N., and Towers, D. B., editors. (1976): GABA in nervous system function. In: *Kroc Foundation Series, Vol. 5.* Raven Press, New York.
255. Robson, R. D., Saelens, J. K., and Wilson, D. (1977): Suppression of morphine withdrawal symptoms of baclofen (BF) (Liorisol). *Fed. Proc.*, 36:1025.
256. Rosell, S., Bjorkroth, U., Chang, D., Yamaguchi, I., Wan, Y.-P., Rackur, G., Fisher, G., and Folkers, K. (1977): Effects of substance P and analogs on isolated guinea pig ileum. In: *Substance P*, edited by U. S. von Euler and B. Pernow, pp. 83–88. Raven Press, New York.
257. Rosell, S., Olgart, L., Gazelius, B., Panopoulos, P., Folkers, K., and Horig, J. (1981): Inhibition of antidromic and substance P-induced vasodilation by a substance P antagonist. *Acta Physiol. Scand.*, 111:381–382.
258. Ruda, M. A. (1982): Opiates and pain pathways: Demonstration of enkephalin synapses on dorsal horn projection neurons. *Science*, 215:1523–1525.
259. Saelens, J. K., Bernard, P. S., and Wilson, P. E. (1980): Baclofen as an analgesic. *Brain Res. Bull.*, 5:553–557.
260. Sagen, J., and Proudfit, H. K. (1981): Hypoalgesia induced by blockade of noradrenergic projections to the raphe magnus; Reversal by blockade of noradrenergic projections to the spinal cord. *Brain Res.*, 223:391–396.
261. Saito, K., Konishi, S., and Otsuka, M. (1975): Antagonism between Lioresal and substance P in rat spinal cord. *Brain Res.*, 97:177–180.
262. Sandberg, D. E., and Segal, M. (1978): Pharmacological analysis of analgesia and self-stimulation elicited by electrical stimulation of catecholamine nuclei in the rat brain. *Brain Res.*, 152:529–542.
263. Sandner, G., Dessort, D., Schmitt, P., and Karli, P. (1981): Distribution of GABA in the periaqueductal gray matter. Effects of medial hypothalamic lesions. *Brain Res.*, 224:279–290.

264. Sar, M., Stumpf, W. E., Miller, R. J., Chang, K. J., and Cuatrecasas, P. (1978): Immunohisto-chemical localization of enkephalin in rat brain and spinal cord. *J. Comp. Neurol.*, 182:17–38.
265. Sasa, M., Munekijo, K., Osumi, Y., and Takaori, S. (1977): Attenuation of morphine analgesia in rats with lesions of the locus coeruleus and dorsal raphe nucleus. *Eur. J. Pharmacol.*, 42:53–62.
266. Sastry, B. R. (1979): Substance P effects on spinal nociceptive neurons. *Life Sci.*, 24:2169–2177.
267. Saxena, P. N., and Gupta, G. P. (1957): Effect of atropine and hyoscine on morphine induced analgesia. *Indian J. Med. Res.*, 45:319–325.
268. Schenker, C., Mroz, E. A., and Leeman, S. E. (1976): Release of substance P from isolated nerve endings. *Nature (Lond.)*, 264:790–792.
269. Schmitt, H., Le Douarec, J.-C., and Petillot, N. (1974): Antagonism of the antinociceptive action of xylazone, an alpha-sympathomimetic agent by adrenoceptor and cholinoceptor blocking agents. *Neuropharmacology*, 13:295–303.
270. Segawa, T., Murakami, H., Ogawa, H., and Yajima, H. (1978): Effect of enkephalin and substance P on sympathetic nerve transmission in mouse vas deferens. *Jpn. J. Pharmacol.*, 28:13–19.
271. Sethy, V. H., and Bombardt, P. A. (1978): Is GABA involved in analgesia? *Res. Commun. Chem. Pathol. Pharmacol.*, 19:365–368.
272. Seybold, V., and Maley, B. (1981): Ultrastructural localization of neurotensin-like immunoreac-tivity in the dorsal horn of the rat spinal cord. *Soc. Neurosci. Abstr.*, 7:59.
273. Share, N. N., and Rackham, A. (1981): Intracerebral substance P in mice: Behavioral effects and narcotic agents. *Brain Res.*, 211:370–386.
274. Sherman, A. D., and Gebhart, G. F. (1976): Morphine and pain effects on aspartate, GABA and glutamate in four discrete areas of mouse brain. *Brain Res.*, 110:273–281.
275. Shiomi, H., Murakami, H., and Takagi, H. (1978): Morphine analgesia and the bulbospinal serotonergic system: Increase in concentration of 5-hydroxy-indoleacetic acid in the rat spinal cord with analgesics. *Eur. J. Pharmacol.*, 52:335–344.
276. Shiomi, H., and Takagi, H. (1974): Morphine analgesia and bulbospinal noradrenergic system: Increase in the concentration of normetanephrine in the spinal cord of the rat caused by analgesia. *Br. J. Pharmacol.*, 52:519–526.
277. Sitaram, N., Buchsbaum, M. S., and Gillin, J. C. (1977): Physostigmine analgesia and somato-sensory evoked responses in man. *Eur. J. Pharmacol.*, 42:285–290.
278. Slater, P. (1981): The effect of 6-hydroxydopamine on the antinociceptive action of oxotremorine. *Psychopharmacology*, 74:365–368.
279. Slaughter, D., and Munsell, D. (1940): Some new aspects of morphine action; Effects on pain. *J. Pharmacol. Exp. Ther.*, 68:104–112.
280. Snyder, S. H., and Innis, R. B. (1979): Peptide neurotransmitters. *Annu. Rev. Biochem.*, 48:755–782.
281. Snyder, S. H., Uhl, G. R., and Kuhar, M. J. (1978): Comparative features of enkephalin and neurotensin in the mammalian central nervous system. In: *Centrally Acting Peptides*, edited by J. Hughes, pp. 85–97. MacMillan Press, London.
282. Spaulding, T. C., Fielding, S., Venafro, J. J., and Lal, H. (1979): Antinociceptive activity of clonidine and its potentiation of morphine analgesia. *Eur. J. Pharmacol.*, 58:19–25.
283. Spaulding, T. C., Venafro, J. J., Ma, M. G., and Fielding, S. (1979): The dissociation of the antinociceptive effect of clonidine from supraspinal structures. *Neuropharmacology*, 18:103–105.
284. Starr, M. S., James, T. A., and Gaytten, D. (1978): Behavioral depressant and antinociceptive properties of substance P in the mouse: Possible implication of brain monoamines. *Eur. J. Pharmacol.*, 48:203–212.
285. Stewart, J. M., Getto, C. J., Neldner, K., Reeve, E. B., Krivoy, W. A., and Zimmerman, E. (1976): Substance P and analgesia. *Nature (Lond.)*, 262:784–785.
286. Sullivan, T. L., and Pert, A. (1981): Analgesic activity of non-opiate neuropeptides following injections into the periaqueductal gray matter. *Soc. Neurosci. Abstr.*, 7:504.
287. Svensson, T. H., Bunney, P. S., and Aghajanian, C. K. (1975): Inhibition of both noradrenergic and serotonergic neurons in brain by the alpha adrenergic agonist clonidine. *Brain Res.*, 92:291–306.
288. Szerb, J. C. (1979): Autoregulation of acetylcholine release. In: *"Presynaptic Receptors"*, edited by S. Z. Langer, R. Starke, and M. L. Dubocorich, pp. 293–298. Pergamon Press, New York.
289. Szreniawski, Z., Czlunkowski, A., Janicki, P., Libich, J., and Gumulka, S. W. (1980): Substance

P: Pain transmission and analgesia. In: *Neuropeptides and Neuronal Transmission*, edited by C. A. Marson and W. Z. Traczyk, pp. 121–129. Raven Press, New York.

290. Takagi, H., Doi, T., and Akaike, A. (1976): Microinjection of morphine into the medial part of the bulbar reticular formation in rabbit and rat: Inhibitory effects on lamina V cells of spinal dorsal horn and behavioral analgesia. In: *Opiates and Endogenous Opioid Peptides*, edited by H. W. Kosterlitz, pp. 191–198. Elsevier, North-Holland Biomedical Press, Amsterdam.

291. Takahashi, T., and Otsuka, M. (1975): Regional distribution of substance P in the spinal cord and nerve roots of the cat and the effect of dorsal root section. *Brain Res.*, 87:1–11.

292. Takemori, A. E., Tulunary, F. C., and Yano, I. (1975): Differential effects on morphine analgesia and naloxone antagonism by biogenic amine modifiers. *Life Sci.*, 17:21–28.

293. Tenen, S. S. (1968): Antagonism of the analgesic effect of morphine and other drugs by p-chlorophenylalanine, a serotonin depletor. *Psychopharmacology (Berlin)*, 12:278–285.

294. Terenius, L. (1975): Effect of peptides and amino acids on dihydromorphine binding to the opiate receptor. *J. Pharm. Pharmacol.*, 27:450–453.

295. Theriault, E., Otsuka, M., and Jessel, T. M. (1979): Capsaicin-evoked release of substance P from primary sensory neurons. *Brain Res.*, 170:209–213.

296. Tregear, G. W., Niall, H. D., Potts, J. T., Leeman, S. E., and Chang, M. M. (1971): Synthesis of substance P. *Nature (Lond.)*, 232:87–89.

297. Uhl, G. R., Bennett, J. P., Jr., and Snyder, S. H. (1977): Neurotensin, a central nervous system peptide: Apparent receptor binding in brain membranes. *Brain Res.*, 130:299–313.

298. Uhl, G., Goodman, R., Kuhar, M., Childers, S., and Snyder, S. H. (1979): Immunohistochemical mapping of enkephalin containing cell bodies, fibers and nerve terminals in the brainstem of the rat. *Brain Res.*, 166:75–94.

299. Uhl, G., Goodman, R., Kuhar, M. J., and Snyder, S. H. (1978): Enkephalin and neurotensin: Immunohistochemical localization and identification of an amygdalofugal pathway. In: *Endorphins*, edited by E. Costa and M. Trabucci, pp. 71–87. Raven Press, New York.

300. Uhl, G. R., Goodman, R. R., and Snyder, S. H. (1979): Neurotensin-containing cell bodies, fibers and nerve terminals in the brainstem of the rat: Immunohistochemical mapping. *Brain Res.*, 167:77–91.

301. Uhl, G. R., Kuhar, M. J., and Snyder, S. H. (1977): Neurotensin: Immunohistochemical localization in rat central nervous system. *Proc. Natl. Acad. Sci. U.S.A.*, 74:4059–4063.

302. Uhl, G. R., and Snyder, S. H. (1976): Regional and subcellular distribution of brain neurotensin. *Life Sci.*, 19:1827–1832.

303. Uhl, G. R., and Snyder, S. H. (1977): Neurotensin receptor binding, regional and subcellular distributions favor transmitter role. *Eur. J. Pharmacol.*, 41:88–91.

304. Uhl, G., and Snyder, S. H. (1980): Neurotensin. In: *The Role of Peptides in Neuronal Function*, edited by J. L. Barker and T. G. Smith, Jr., pp. 509–543. Marcel Dekker, New York.

305. Uhl, G., and Snyder, S. H. (1981): Neurotensin. In: *Neurosecretion and Brain Peptides*, edited by J. B. Martin, S. Reichlin, and K. L. Bick, pp. 87–106. Raven Press, New York.

306. Unnerstall, J. R., Palacios, J. M., and Kuhar, M. J. (1981): Opiate/alpha-2 interactions: Colocalization of both receptors by radiohistochemistry. *Soc. Neurosci. Abstr.*, 7:501.

307. Van Eick, A., and Bock, J. (1971): Comparisons of analgesic cholinomimetic, anticholinergic and sympathomimetic drugs by means of the hot plate test. *Arc. Int. Pharmacodyn. Ther.*, 189:384–387.

308. Vogt, M. (1973): The effect of lowering the 5-hydroxytryptamine content of the rat spinal cord on analgesia produced by morphine. *J. Physiol. (Lond.)*, 236:483–498.

309. von Euler, U. S., and Gaddum, J. H. (1931): An unidentified depressor substance in certain tissue extracts. *J. Physiol. (Lond.)*, 72:74–87.

310. Wang, J. K. (1977): Antinociceptive effect of intrathecally administered serotonin. *Anesthesiology*, 47:269–271.

311. Way, E. L., and Shen, F.-H. (1971): Interaction of morphine with the catecholamines and 5-hydroxytryptamine. In: *Narcotic Drugs. Biochemical Pharmacology*, edited by D. H. Clouet, pp. 229–253. Plenum Press, New York.

312. Wilcox, G. L., Hylden, J. L. K., and Seybold, V. S. (1981): Behavior elicited in rats after intrathecal administration of peptides. *Soc. Neurosci. (Abstr.)*, 7:60.

313. Wilson, P. R., and Yaksh, T. L. (1978): Baclofen is antinociceptive in the spinal intrathecal space of animals. *Eur. J. Pharmacol.*, 51:323–330.

314. Wright, D. M., and Roberts, M. H. T. (1978): Supersensitivity to a substance P analogue following dorsal root section. *Life Sci.*, 22:19–24.
315. Wright, D. M., and Roberts, M. H. T. (1980): Responses of spinal neurons to a substance P analogue, noxious pinch and bradykinin. *Eur. J. Pharmacol.*, 64:165–167.
316. Yaksh, T. L. (1978): Direct evidence that spinal serotonin and noradrenaline terminals mediate the spinal antinociceptive effects of morphine in the periaqueductal gray. *Brain Res.*, 160:180–185.
317. Yaksh, T. L., DuChateau, J. C., and Rudy, T. A. (1976): Antagonism by methysergide and cinanserin of the antinociceptive action of morphine administered into the periaqueductal gray. *Brain Res.*, 104:367–372.
318. Yaksh, T. L., Farb, D. H., Leeman, S. E., and Jessel, T. M. (1979): Intrathecal capsaicin depletes substance P in the rat spinal cord and produces prolonged thermal analgesia. *Science*, 206:481–483.
319. Yaksh, T. L., Hammond, D. L., and Tyce, G. M. (1981): Functional aspects of bulbospinal monoaminergic projections in modulating processing of somatosensory information. *Fed. Proc.*, 40:2786–2794.
320. Yaksh, T. L., Jessell, T. M., Gamse, R., Mudge, A. W., and Leeman, S. E. (1980): Intrathecal morphine inhibits substance P release from mammalian spinal cord in vivo. *Nature (Lond.)*, 286:155–157.
321. Yaksh, T. L., and Reddy, S. V. R. (1981): Studies in the primate on the analgetic effects associated with intrathecal actions of opiates, alpha-adrenergic agonists and baclofen. *Anesthesiology*, 54:451–467.
322. Yaksh, T. L., and Rudy, T. A. (1978): Narcotic analgetics: CNS sites and mechanisms of action as revealed by intracerebral injection techniques. *Pain*, 4:299–359.
323. Yaksh, T. L., and Tyce, G. M. (1979): Microinjection of morphine into the periaqueductal gray evokes the release of serotonin from the spinal cord. *Brain Res.*, 171:176–181.
324. Yaksh, T. L., and Wilson, P. R. (1979): Spinal serotonin terminal system mediates antinociception. *J. Pharmacol. Exp. Ther.*, 208:446–453.
325. Yau, W. M. (1978): Effect of substance P on intestinal muscle. *Gastroenterology*, 74:228–231.
326. Yoneda, Y., Kuriyama, K., and Kurihar, K. (1977): Morphine alters distribution of GABA in the thalamus. *Brain Res.*, 124:373–378.
327. Yoneda, Y., Takashima, S., and Kuriyama, K. (1976): Possible involvement of GABA in morphine analgesia. *Biochem. Pharmacol.*, 25:2669–2670.
328. Young, W. S., III, and Kuhar, M. J. (1979): Neurotensin receptors: Autoradiographic localization in rat CNS. *Eur. J. Pharmacol.*, 59:161–163.
329. Young, W. S., and Kuhar, M. J. (1981): Neurotensin receptor localization by light microscopic autoradiography in rat brain. *Brain Res.*, 206:273–285.
330. Young, W. S., III, Uhl, G. R., and Kuhar, M. J. (1978): Iontophoresis of neurotensin in the area of the locus coeruleus. *Brain Res.*, 150:431–435.
331. Zetler, G. (1977): Effects of substance P and other peptides on the field stimulated guinea pig vas deferens. In: *Substance P*, edited by U. S. von Euler and B. Pernow, pp. 97–116. Raven Press, New York.
332. Zetler, G. (1980): Antagonism of the gut-contracting effects of bombesin and neurotensin by opioid peptides, morphine, atropine or tetrodotoxin. *Pharmacology*, 21:348–354.
333. Zieglgansberger, W., Siggins, G., Brown, M., Vale, W., and Bloom, F. (1978): Actions of neurotensin upon single neurone activity in different regions of the rat brain. *Seventh Int. Congr. Pharmacol.*, p. 300.
334. Zieglgansberger, W., and Tulloch, I. F. (1979): Effects of substance P on neurons in the dorsal horn of the spinal cord of the cat. *Brain Res.*, 166:273–282.
335. Zonta, N., Zambott, F., Vincentini, L., Tammiso, R., and Mantegazza, P. (1981): Effects of some GABA-mimetic drugs on the antinociceptive activity of morphine and beta-endorphin in rats. *Naunyn Schmiedebergs Arch. Pharmacol.*, 316:231–234.
336. Zsilla, G., Cheney, D. L., Racagni, G., and Costa, E. (1976): Correlation between analgesia and the decrease in acetylcholine turnover rate in cortex and hippocampus elicited by morphine, meperidine, viminol, R2 and azidomorphine. *J. Pharmacol. Exp. Ther.*, 199:662–668.

Analgesics: Neurochemical, Behavioral, and Clinical Perspectives, edited by M. Kuhar and G. Pasternak. Raven Press, New York © 1984.

The Evaluation of Analgesics in Man

Stanley L. Wallenstein

Sloan-Kettering Institute for Cancer Research, New York, New York 10021

In the relatively brief period since World War II, the methodology for evaluating analgesics in man has undergone a quiet but substantial revolution. Pioneered by the work of Beecher (5), the procedural safeguards basic to the measurement of subjective responses are well accepted today. Haphazard administration of analgesics on the hospital wards and casual observation by hospital personnel, at one time the accepted method for evaluating analgesics for clinical use, are no longer satisfactory. The basic requirements for well-designed studies in this area have been extensively detailed (6,44,46,98). Minimal requirements for acceptable studies include the use of active and/or inactive controls, appropriate randomization of patients or subjects to treatments, and the use of double-blind procedures for the administration of test medications. It is recognized, today, that the effects of analgesics may be obscured by the random variation inherent in the clinical situation, and that this may be compounded in studies that are inadequately designed or poorly controlled. Results may be further confounded when inadequate parameters for the measurement of patients' subjective reports are employed.

These basic principles apply equally to laboratory studies involving experimental pain and clinical studies involving pain from disease or surgery. Although situational variables can be more rigidly controlled in the laboratory than in the clinic, and relatively precise measures of stimulus intensity can be obtained, these studies do have their own particular problems relating to the development of adequate experimental pain models for the clinical pain experience.

In recent years, advances have been made in applying psychophysical methods to the measurement of subjective responses, to the scaling of pain both in the clinic and in the laboratory, and in the application of signal detection theory to the laboratory evaluation of pain and relief. In this chapter, I will attempt to critically evaluate the state of the art of clinical and experimental analgesics, highlighting the more recent advances, and discussing areas that remain controversial, such as the relative merits of crossover and parallel group study designs, and scaling subjective pain estimates.

EXPERIMENTAL PAIN MODELS

Threshold Measurements

Almost every conceivable method for inflicting pain, where the intensity can be controlled and measured quantitatively, has been employed in attempts to screen analgesics in man. The list, a tribute to man's ingenuity, consists of a variety of mechanical, thermal, chemical, and electrical stimuli (7,18,23,38,40,41,57,62,78, 85,103). The pioneering work of Hardy et al. (36), in determining quantitative pain thresholds to radiant heat, served as an impetus for many investigations of the effects of a variety of analgesics on the threshold for pain. Some investigators (107,108) reported large increases in pain thresholds after a variety of analgesics, whereas others (4,59) were unable to demonstrate significant threshold changes. Serious questions concerning the constancy of experimental pain threshold and its appropriateness as a model for the pathological pain experience were raised by Beecher (6). The areas of sensory thresholds and the methodology for measuring them has remained in a state of controversy and development. These measures are relatively insensitive to the effects of analgesics, particularly the so-called "simple analgesics" of the aspirin class, even when modern psychophysical measuring techniques for the measurement of thresholds are employed (17).

Suprathreshold Measurements

Radiant Heat and the "Dol" Scale

The landmark studies of Wolff et al. (37,107), with suprathreshold pain, represented the first attempts to apply a psychophysical theory to the measurement of pain sensation. They found that for radiant heat, subjects were able to discriminate 21 "just noticeable differences" (JNDs) for pricking pain, ranging from threshold to ceiling pain sensations. The JNDs roughly followed Weber's law, which, in essence, states that as the intensity of the stimulus increases, the ability to discriminate differences in intensity decreases proportionately. A scale of pain intensity was devised in which each unit (dol), is composed of two JNDs. These investigators (38) also developed a dol scale for aching pain using pressure from a coiled spring esthesiometer on the forehead. They found that aching pain could be matched with pricking pain from radiant heat, and that pain of equal intensity was elicited by evoking pain which was the same number of JNDs above threshold.

Experimental Pain Methods and Analgesia

Pressure algometer

Despite the relative precision of measuring threshold and suprathreshold pain in the laboratory, the effects of analgesics on laboratory pain has been far from clear-cut or consistent. Smith (87) found that aspirin could delay the onset of a burn from ultraviolet light, but was unable to delay the onset of pressure pain from an algometer applied to the finger. Montanari et al. (70) were able to demonstrate graded effects for graded doses of aspirin, metamizol, and ketobemidone by using a device to exert pressure on the soft tissue between the nail and last knuckle of the left thumb. Aspirin was not significantly superior to placebo in this test, although ketobemidone and metamizol were.

Electrical

In a study in which pain was induced by a 60-cycle alternating current to the middle finger of the dominant hand, Dinnerstein et al. (24) found that aspirin actually increased pain sensitivity. Shock detection threshold, levels of moderate discomfort, and maximum tolerated voltage were lowered after aspirin as compared with a placebo. These paradoxical results are in apparent conflict with observed analgesic effects in clinical pain, and highlight the dangers involved in attempting to generalize about the potential clinical value of an analgesic.

Chemical

Employing intraperitoneal bradykinin to induce pain in man, Lim and co-workers (64) found a significant analgesic effect after ingestion of 650 mg of aspirin, but not after 325 mg. Doses larger than 650 mg produced deeper and more prolonged analgesia. They also found that the combination of aspirin and acetaminophen with caffeine was more effective than the combination without caffeine, suggesting that caffeine may act as a potentiator. In their model, oral amphetamine had analgesic activity, whereas meperidine in 100-mg doses was poor, and in 50-mg doses, ineffective.

Coffman (20) found that pain produced by injection of bradykinin into the brachial artery was obtained in all 15 subjects, but was variable from subject to subject, and from time to time. However, the method was able to determine that both sodium and calcium acetylsalicylate reduced pain in the 1st and 2nd hr after ingestion of the drug.

Cold pressor pain and electrical stimulation

Electrical stimulation and cold pressor pain have been employed to evaluate the analgesic activity of many analgesic drugs. Wolff et al. (105) found that morphine produced a significant effect on both pain tolerance and threshold in the electrical model, and a significant effect on pain tolerance with a lesser effect on the threshold after ice water. Aspirin was no different from placebo in either of the tests.

In studies designed to be evaluated in terms of crossover or noncrossover drug comparisons, Wolff and co-workers (106) evaluated aspirin, codeine, secobarbital and placebo, employing electrical stimulation, and ice water as per the cold pressor test, in 56 volunteers. Codeine, aspirin, and secobarbital were all effective in the electrical model. In the cold pressor studies, codeine and aspirin were more effective than secobarbital. Pain tolerance was a more sensitive measure of drug effect than was pain threshold, and the pain sensitivity range (PSR), determined as the difference between threshold and tolerance, was equivocal. The crossover design was more effective for evaluating analgesia than was the single dose design, despite carry-over effects (106). Cold pressor, electrical stimulation, and a pressure algometer were employed to study graded doses of aspirin, codeine, and d-propoxyphene. Graded dose-response information was obtained for d-propoxyphene and codeine with both cold pressor and electric stimulation, but dose responses for aspirin under 1,000 mg were difficult to obtain. Pain tolerance was found to be the most sensitive pain parameter. Both cold pressor and electric stimulation were more sensitive and reliable than the pressure algometer method. Different methods may measure different aspects of pain behavior. Therefore, it is thought that methodology should be selected carefully for analgesic screening, and at least two different methods should be used (104).

Reithe and Wilske (80) employed the threshold of the human tooth to electrical stimulation to compare propiram fumarate and an analgesic combination of aspirin, phenacetin, codeine, and caffeine. Both drugs were found to be significantly better than placebo, with propiram significantly superior to the aspirin, phenacitin, caffeine (APC) combination, with or without codeine, in this test.

Ultrasound

Employing ultrasonic stimulation to the fingers (46 w/cm^2 in a water bath of 35°C), Yanaura et al. (109) measured threshold as time in seconds to the sensation of a sharp prick, at which time the finger was withdrawn, and the circuit of a digital timer was broken. Codeine, aspirin, aminopyrine, and mefenamic acid, all given orally, were significantly superior to a placebo. When graded doses of aspirin were employed, a graded dose-effect response was obtained. As compared with radiant heat, the authors found that the ultrasonic method produces a pure pain sensation without heat or tissue damage. The procedure is simple and rapid, and the endpoint clear-cut.

Ischemic pain

In recent years, perhaps the largest body of research employing experimental pain as an analgesic screening technique has been concerned with suprathreshold measurements of ischemic pain utilizing the submaximal effort tourniquet technique. This area of investigation received considerable stimulation as a result of the work of Smith and Beecher (86). These investigators believed that the deep cramping sensation of suprathreshold ischemic pain may more closely reflect both the physiological and psychological aspects of pathological pain than do superficial threshold measurements. They found the submaximal effort tourniquet technique sensitive to the effects of a variety of analgesics, including aspirin and narcotics, although significant results for aspirin required considerably larger numbers of subjects than did the studies of morphine. Using the measure of tourniquet time, the ratio of aspirin to placebo decreased with increasing pain. The differences were not significant for slight pain, were significant for moderately or very distressing pain, and not significant for unbearable pain.

Other investigators, however, have reported considerably less success with this experimental pain model. Moore et al. (71) were unable to discriminate between the effects of 900 mg of aspirin and a placebo in prisoner volunteers. The prisoners were found to have higher pain thresholds than the students used by Smith and Beecher (86). Repeated pain induction was found to increase the time to pain threshold, but duration of pain to time of pain tolerance was not affected. The authors conclude that "carefully designed and executed clinical studies utilizing pathological pain can be expected to give the best and most reliable information on the analgesic potency of pharmacological agents."

Ferguson (25) reported significant learning effects in subjects in whom repeated ischemic pain tests have been carried out. Oral aspirin and oral flufenisol were compared in graded doses in a crossover comparison in 10 male volunteers. Analgesic data and drug serum levels were obtained before, and at 2 and 8 hr after drug ingestion. No significant differences between drugs were obtained, and carry-over effects, in terms of enhanced pain tolerance, were observed after 8 hr as compared with 2 hr, despite a reduction in serum levels of the drugs. Carry-over effects were also noted in a second study of aspirin and placebo. These studies suggest that a drug-time interaction can occur in the submaximal effort tourniquet test that may confound expected treatment differences.

Adler et al. (1) reported that subjects were better able to discriminate mild analgesics from placebos by using the submaximal effort tourniquet technique when the subjects behaved calmly in the test situation, than when they exhibited prominent arousal reactions. Subjects given benzoctadiene, a tranquilizer, in order to induce relaxation, were better able to discriminate acetaminophen from placebo than those subjects who received the analgesic and placebo alone. The study design, however, does not permit explanation of the mode of this interaction.

In a study with 32 male volunteers, von Graffenried et al. (95) found significant practice effects when employing the submaximal effort tourniquet technique to study the effects of 100 mg of aspirin and placebo. In this study, systematic investigations of practice effect, initial pain sensitivity, and a variety of behavioral and personality factors were carried out. The analgesic activity of aspirin could not be demonstrated, but practice effects were significant, and there was an interaction between the practice effects and the initial pain sensitivity of the subjects to the test. A significant effect of anxiety was also observed. The greater the anxiety, the shorter the time to attain a given pain level. The greater the decrease in anxiety from one trial to the next, the greater was the practice effect. Those subjects who discriminated between aspirin and placebo were calm, had a low degree of anxiety, did not distract themselves from the pain situation, and showed a positive attitude toward the experiment. Factors that determine the ability of subjects to discriminate are variable and largely unpredictable, and even if maximal standardization of methodology is achieved, conventional experimental pain techniques do not seem to be suited for the investigation of mild analgesics.

Similar conclusions were reached by Meyer et al. (67) in studies of aspirin, dipyrone, pentazocine, and codeine. Details of methodology vary from investigator to investigator, and results in many cases are not comparable. Differences in the scaling of pain, or the amount of work required of the subject in the arm being studied, can significantly affect the conclusions. Using a double-blind approach, the authors found no significant differences between active drugs and placebo (67). They conclude that because of the low reliability of the method, the tourniquet technique offers no satisfactory possibility for human pharmacologic testing of analgesic drugs.

Moore et al. (72) studied the effects of different levels of exercise duration and effort on the subjects' reports of pain in the tourniquet test. They found that the manner in which exercise is performed has an important effect on the subjects' ratings of pain, and that the pain ratings do not increase as a linear function of time. Both of these findings warrant precautions in interpreting the results of the submaximal effort tourniquet test.

Bloomfield and Hurwitz (10) performed the tourniquet test in postpartum patients who had received either 1.2 grams of aspirin or placebo for episiotomy pain. The tourniquet test was carried out on the 2nd postpartum day, and again 8 to 12 months later. In these patients, the aspirin significantly relieved the episiotomy pain, but the tourniquet pain, threshold or suprathreshold, was not demonstrably affected by the aspirin either 2 days or 8 to 12 months postpartum. Uncontrolled nondrug variables, such as attention, intelligence, and motivation may influence pain reports and account for the conflicting results. Tourniquet pain was found to be an unsatisfactory test model for evaluating aspirin analgesia in the same subject in whom aspirin had relieved natural pain.

Problems of Measurement

Cross-Modality Matching

Reading the intensity of a stimulus from a dial, or measuring time to threshold or tolerance can be deceptively simple, and may not reflect to any degree of accuracy the meaning of the experience to the patient. The problem of the interaction of pain perception and reaction to pain was recognized by Beecher (6). He felt that threshold measures more or less reflected pure perception, and suprathreshold measures involved reaction, and more closely reflected the experience of pathological pain. Gracely et al. (32) have employed cross-modality matching to scale verbal descriptors of pain, and have applied these descriptive scaling techniques to clinical as well as experimental pain (39). These techniques have not been without controversy (34,31), but do represent a serious effort to understand and evaluate both experimental and clinical pain measurements (28).

Signal Detection Theory

Clark (19) and Chapman (16) have applied signal detection theory to subjective pain reports. They have attempted to separate the subjective *criterion* for pain from indices of *sensitivity* (usually referred to as d') by plotting the receiver operating characteristics (ROC) of responses over a range of stimuli intensities. The ROC thus plots "hits" against "false alarms" in terms of subjective reports of whether a stimulus is or is not painful, or is more painful than a comparison stimulus. Both Rollman (82) and Jones (49) recognize the special methodological and interpretational problems of signal detection theory as particularly applied to pain. Nevertheless, the method remains an interesting, if controversial, attempt to understand the meaning of subjective reports to experimental pain stimuli.

A nonparametric analog of signal detection analysis was used by Buchsbaum et al. (13) with a new electric stimulation pain assessment technique employing the Tursky electrode. The nonparametric analysis of subjects ratings was sensitive to aspirin, morphine, and opiate antagonists. Individual differences remained stable in two testing sessions 7 months apart. Test insensitivity increased with age. Two indices of the pain response were reported: a "response criterion" and an "error" or insensitivity to differences in stimuli intensity. It was found that both morphine and aspirin affected insensitivity rather than response criterion, and this is consistent with the theoretical viewpoints of Clark (19) and Chapman (16).

Experimental Pain as an Analog for Existing Pain

Hardy and Javert (35) attempted to apply the radiant heat dol scale to the measurement of pain intensity in childbirth by having selected, alert, intelligent patients match their labor pains with the pricking pain induced by radiant heat. They reported that, despite the differences in pain quality, patients were able to match pain intensity. Limitations of the method were that measurements could not be made in the face of distraction or lack of cooperation, and that when high pain intensities were being measured, there was a risk of inflicting injuries from burns.

Kast (55) also found a good correlation with verbal categorical estimates of pain when patients matched the intensity of experimentally-induced pressure pain on the fingertip with the pathological pain which they had been experiencing. However, Sternbach et al. (88) found matching pain techniques may well be inappropriate for patients with chronic pain. In a crossover study of morphine, codeine, aspirin, and placebo, 24 patients with somatogenic pain participated in a study matching tourniquet pain with clinical pain. All results were too variable to achieve statistical significance, and clinical pain level scores showed no relationship to the analgesic dose. Pain tolerance scores were appropriately ordered, but pain ratio scores were identical for all analgesics. Pain estimates appropriately followed the analgesic doses, but were not significant. Matching ischemic and clinical pain thus appears to reflect something other than simple magnitude estimates of clinical pain.

Commentary

Despite the existence of many methods for eliciting and studying pain in the laboratory in human subjects, there are, at this time, no generally accepted laboratory techniques for screening analgesic activity in man. Results with both "mild" and narcotic analgesics have been notoriously inconsistent, both within the same laboratory when using different methods, and from laboratory to laboratory even when the same techniques have been employed. Nevertheless, some laboratory techniques are capable of detecting activity, even of aspirin-like drugs, and, in some instances, sensitive enough to pick up graded dose-effect information. The reasons for the inconsistencies in results are not readily apparent. There is probably no single cause, but rather a variety of factors responsible for aberrant results. There is some evidence that personality traits of the subjects, their interactions with the investigators, and their motivation and involvement in the studies are significant factors in the success or failure of any experimental method. Despite objective measurements of the pain stimuli in the laboratory, the pain response remains subjective and influenced by a wide variety of external and internal events. Some of these events are amenable to control in a particular experimental situation; others are not. All of these events may influence the results. Their influence is probably greater in suprathreshold than in threshold pain, yet, paradoxically, the suprathreshold measures appear to offer greater promise for the screening of analgesics. Much remains to be done in attempting to define the variables affecting the measurement of experimental pain. Consistent, reliable, and reproducible analgesic screening methods in the laboratory remain to be developed.

CLINICAL ANALGESIC STUDIES

Background

The reliability of laboratory pain studies can be limited by personality and attitudinal factors among the subjects. The problem is also compounded when evaluating pathological pain in the clinical setting, when situational factors cannot be controlled as well. The potential environmental and personality influences on pain are manifold (93), and a well-controlled clinical analgesic study with precisely-defined measurement criteria will extract only limited subjective information from the experience of the patient. These variables will only be briefly discussed. One significant variable is the interpersonal relationships of the patient with his family, friends, and the health care team. Uncontrollable events, such as marital problems or the loss of a job, may be of overwhelming significance to the patient's interpretation of pain in terms of his or her understanding of the underlying disease or apparent cause of pain. Even the simple act of involving the patient in the study and obtaining an informed consent can significantly influence both attitude and response.

In view of all the possible sources of influence on the pain response, these basics of study design are almost universally accepted. A meaningful clinical analgesic study will include appropriate controls that will serve not only as reference points for comparison with the test drug, but will also serve as a measure of the sensitivity of the method to detect the drug effects under study. Double-blind conditions must be maintained to limit the influence of suggestion either directly on the patient, or indirectly through the observer. There should be appropriate randomization of patients to treatments so that potential biasing influences will be distributed by chance (65,98). Statistical verification of this type of data is essential for positive evidence that we are dealing with a drug effect rather than a chance distribution of external factors which may be large enough to influence results or be otherwise misleading.

Analgesics are employed and evaluated in a variety of painful states in patients of both sexes ranging from the very young to the elderly. Pain may be acute in nature owing to a variety of causes, such as trauma, headache, dental, menstrual, and postoperative pain, trigeminal neuralgia or surgery, or the result of chronic painful states, such as rheumatic disorders, low back pain, chronic neuralgias, or cancer. No single clinical methodology can be expected to be satisfactory for all situations. Within the broad guidelines stated above, experimental methodology will vary with the patient population under study. Limiting factors in the study design will be determined by whether pain is acute or chronic, whether the patient is hospitalized or an outpatient, and whether the immediate effects of single doses or long-term effectiveness of chronic drug administration are being studied. These issues will also determine the type and quality of observations to be made, and whether crossover comparisons or parallel group studies will be designed. Study design will be further modified by the overall objectives of the research. Studies to determine the presence or absence of analgesic effect, assays to evaluate the relative advantages of different drugs, and studies of the relative effectiveness of drug combinations will require different basic designs to answer the specific question or questions under investigation.

Because the effects of "mild" analgesics may not be far above the noise level inherent in the clinical situation, studies of this type of drug may impose limitations on experimental design that may not be present in evaluating more potent analgesics, such as narcotics. Study sensitivity may be limited by variability in absorption of orally administered drugs, and by the fact that dose-effect curves for drugs of the aspirin type tend to be shallow, as compared with those of narcotic drugs, and by the uncertainties as to at what level the ceiling effects for aspirin analgesia occur. Despite these limitations, both mild and potent analgesics have been evaluated in many hospital settings, and in a variety of painful states, including cancer, postoperative pain, postpartum pain, trauma, dental pain, and arthritis.

Pain Measurement

No completely satisfactory substitute for the subjective reports of the patients has been developed for determining the severity of pain and degree of relief. Matching pathological pain with experimental pain has been attempted but remains unpopular because of the difficulty of comparing different types of pain, and because the influence of a second pain on a preexisting pain is not well defined, and can complicate measurement. Nonverbal behavioral methods in man present

difficulties because behavior may be controlled by conditioning, personality, training, and past experience (47).

Verbal Scales

Most commonly employed pain scales are adaptations of the four point scale of
Keele (47,55a), although a variety of quantal and quantitative measures of pain and
pain relief have been utilized (44). The most common quantitative parameters have
involved patient reports of pain severity in four or five categories, varying from
"none" to "severe" or "very severe," or relief reports ranging from "none" to
"complete." Categories are commonly given numerical values on a linear scale,
although the relative size of these differences may indeed not be equal. Amounts
of analgesia are calculated directly from relief scales, and as pain intensity differences (PIDs) for predrug minus postdrug pain intensity. If repeated estimates are
made, estimation of the area under the time-effect curves are obtained by totaling
the scores for the observation period, providing estimates of total pain relief
(TOTPAR) or sum of pain intensity differences (SPID) (98). Good correlation
between TOTPAR and SPID scores have resulted when both measures were obtained simultaneously (44). Evaluation of the peak drug effect using these parameters tends to be less sensitive than the measures of total analgesia because of
limitations of the scale. This tends to be more evident when patients start with less
than severe pain (29,47).

Data obtained employing these scales tend to be skewed, and various transformations may be employed, such as ridit (11,98), to normalize data before analysis.
However, when a crossover design is employed, treatment differences within patients tend to be normally distributed, and deviations from normality have not been
found to significantly affect analysis (98). Fucella et al. (29), in a study of graded
doses of aspirin and indoprofen, employed both parametric and nonparametric
statistical procedures to evaluate analgesic scores derived from semiquantitative
scales. The nonparametric test for quantitative assays was found to be a valid
statistical procedure without implied assumptions about distribution, and this is
thought to be superior to the ridit transformation, which does not always render
homogeneous data.

Quantal measures require no assumptions of normality for statistical analysis.
These measures usually involve a yes or no response in terms of endpoints such as
better-worse, satisfactory-unsatisfactory, pain is-is not at least half gone. The measures, in general, are less sensitive measures of drug effect than the quantitative
verbal scales.

Visual Analog Scales

Graphic rating scales and visual analogs have long been employed for psychological measurements, but only recently have they been recognized as valid instru-
ments for measuring clinical pain and the effects of analgesic drugs. A visual
analog, usually a 10-cm long line, is generally preferred to a graphic scale with

markings, in that the patients tend to use points corresponding to descriptors on the graphic rating scale, thus failing to take advantage of the extra sensitivity of the line itself (47). Scott and Huskisson (84), evaluating a variety of visual analog and rating scales, found these scales to correlate well with pain severity measured by descriptors, and to be more sensitive than the traditional simple descriptive pain scales. The visual analog scales (VAS) and the graphic rating scales, used horizontally, with words spread out along the length of the line, so as not to define a specific point on the line, were found to be the most satisfactory, and the best available method for measuring pain and pain relief. Joyce et al. (50) compared a visual analog and a four-point scale (FPS) for measuring pain and analgesia in patients with chronic inflammatory or degenerative arthropathy. The VAS was found to be no more difficult for the patient to understand and complete, no less valid, and may have been more sensitive and more reliable than the FPS. The VAS was also preferred by patients.

The reliability of the linear analog was evaluated by Revill et al. (81) by asking the patients to recall, on several occasions, the severity of a pain distant in time. A good correlation between the repeated ratings was obtained, and was significantly more consistent than repeated ratings of a random mark on the scale. Pain ratings were also significantly less variable when the length of the analog was 10 to 20 cm, than when it was 5 cm.

Kremer et al. (58) compared visual analog, numerical, and adjectival scales in patients with chronic cancer pain. All patients completed the adjectival scale, but 11% were unable to complete the VAS, and 2% failed at the numerical scale. More patients preferred the adjectival scale, but scale preference did not influence the pain intensity report.

Ohnaus and Adler (74) compared VAS and verbal rating scales (VRS) directly in an analgesic study in 6 patients with malignant disease. The scales were highly correlated, although in this small study, the VRS produced higher F values in drug comparisons, although none of the data were significant. Nevertheless, they claim the VAS is a more accurate reflection of what the patient feels than the VRS.

Scaling Clinical Pain

What the patient actually feels is, of course, highly speculative, especially because there is no objective measure for the intensity of the stimulus for pathological pain. Attempts have been made to relate the pain experience to subjective estimates of other phenomena utilizing a variety of cross-modality matching procedures. Some results have been projected to clinical pain studies and applied to the measurement of drug effect (39,97). Verbal pain descriptors used to describe a power function of intensity in cross-modality matching studies in the laboratory (92), were applied to the measurement of clinical pain, and simultaneous visual analog pain measurements were made. We (43,97) also found a power function relationship of the descriptors to intensity measures of pathological pain on the VAS. Power functions best described the responses of both patients with postoperative pain, and patients with chronic cancer pain. The curves for the two groups diverged at the upper end of the scales, the patients with cancer pain tending to rate the descriptors "strong," "severe," and "excruciating" as less severe on the analog scale than did the postoperative patients. This difference may be the result of the different pain experiences of the two patient groups (43,97).

Swiratanakul et al. (89) also measured commonly employed pain descriptors by having subjects estimate their severities as indicated by their place on an analog scale. However, the subjects for this investigation were volunteers without pain. They also found unequal differences between descriptors usually rated as equidistant on an ordinal scale. They did not attempt to determine if any other relationship would be applicable.

Multidimensional Pain Measures

There are complex psychological and physical interactions between the feeling of pain and other subjective states. Recognizing that reports of pain involve more than measures of severity, other endpoints for pain or analgesia have been employed by some investigators. Calimlim et al. (15) used "global" measures, representing the patients' overall estimates of drug effects in clinical analgesic studies. These estimates may represent a reasonable evaluation of the clinical usefulness of the drug, but have the disadvantage of combining analgesia, mood, and side effects in an unspecified mix. Therefore, the contributions of each part to the overall evaluation cannot be isolated.

An alternate approach has been to attempt to isolate other relevant psychological variables in the pain experience, and analyze them independently (52,91). Melzack recognized pain intensity as a multidimensional entity (66). He developed a self-rating scale, the McGill pain questionnaire, a detailed adjective check list in which the patient rates his pain in terms of sensory, affective, and evaluative descriptors. The scale has proven effective in defining patients according to a variety of pain states. However, the sensitivity of the scale to analgesic drugs remains to be tested. Logic would dictate that changes in pain intensity would influence the quantity and quality of adjectives checked. This offers the potential of discrimination between sensory and affective components of drug action. This has proven to be the case in laboratory studies of Klepac et al. (56) involving cold pressor and electrical tooth pulp pain.

Sources of Variation

Identifiable as well as unidentifiable variables can influence clinical reports of pain and analgesia. Drug evaluation in this area is highly dependent on either accounting for them in the study design or employing appropriate randomization procedures. Thus, any resulting biasing influence they may have on the treatments under study will occur purely as a result of chance. Kremer et al. (58) found, for example, that depressed-anxious patients had reliably higher pain intensity scores than did nondepressed, nonanxious patients. Kaiko (51) performed a retrospective evaluation of postoperative pain patients who had been on analgesic studies in which 8 and 16 mg intramuscular doses of morphine had served as the standard drug. He found analgesic effect to vary significantly with age. Total relief and duration of analgesia increased with age for both doses of the drug. Differences between the extremes of adult age in this population were about twice that obtained by doubling the morphine dose. In additional studies, Kaiko et al. (53) found significantly greater relief for blacks than whites, for moderate than severe pain, dull than sharp pain, for abdominal rather than pain in the chest or arms. Differences in sex, however, were not significant.

Study sensitivity, as well as the validity and reliability of drug comparisons, will depend on design considerations aimed at limiting the likelihood that either known or unknown variables will bias the data. When variables are not known or easily identified, a randomization process of assigning patients to treatments or order of administration will distribute variables by chance, and the likelihood of differences between treatments being owing to differences in effect, or being owing to chance, can be measured statistically.

Crossover and Parallel Group Studies

The most direct method of equating patient groups is to carry out crossover studies, in which each patient serves as his own control, and receives both test and standard study drugs. Patient drug groups are thus automatically matched for age, sex, pain site, and character, and for a variety of immeasurable, or at least difficult to measure, physical and psychological variables. Crossover studies, however, introduce the added variable of time. In some acute pain conditions, the disappearance of pain with time may severely limit the ability to give the patient a second study medication. Moreover, changes in pain with time influence the absolute score obtainable with each drug administration, and are related to the pain level at the time the medication is administered (76). Lasagna claims that crossover design ignores the possibility of confounding time-associated changes within patients, such as pharmacokinetic changes, psychological changes, and severity of pain, especially in studies involving acute pain. He does concede that crossover can be helpful in acute pain, but investigators should be prepared to discard all but first doses, if their assumptions for using crossover are not justified (60).

In a statistical review of the crossover in terms of cost efficiency, Brown (12) claims that the crossover experiment can yield great savings, if the assumptions of no carry-over effect are valid. But, the design should not be used if this assumption is in doubt. This conclusion is based on projected costs employing a crossover design with sufficient power to detect carry-over effects.

This analysis assumes that carry-over effect, when it exists, is only present within the confines of the study itself. However, patients in the clinical situation are generally receiving analgesics and other medications before being placed on the study. This is the case, not only for chronic pain patients, but for patients with acute pain who will receive one or more of a variety of medications before or after surgery or other procedures. Patient populations suitable for pain studies, and who have not had prior medications, which may react with the study drugs, are limited. Thus, the possibility of pharmacological carry-over in clinical studies exists, regardless of the design employed. The singular advantage of the crossover experiment is that it offers an opportunity to measure carry-over, and gain some idea of the extent of its influence on the study. On the other hand, in parallel group studies, it is not possible to determine whether there is or is not carry-over, and if there is, the extent of its influence on study results. If the meaningfulness of the study is the criterion rather than cost efficiency, it would be appropriate to carry out crossover studies, especially when carry-over may be present. Designs for evaluation of analgesic drugs, which capitalize on the advantages of crossover, and allow for the estimation of carry-over as well as treatment period effects, have been developed by Laska and Meisner (63).

It is possible, also, to so design crossover trials to minimize the possible carry-over effects of the previous study medication. Studies at Memorial Sloan-Kettering Cancer Center are routinely carried out as crossover comparisons in both chronic pain and postoperative pain patients. Only one study medication is given per day, and intervening and night-time medications are standard nonstudy drugs. The patients enter each day of the study as if they were new patients in parallel groups, except that they are matched for all patient variables. In our hands, the variance by days or in terms of day-by-day interaction has been consistently insignificant, statistically, for this type of data (100). Evaluation of relative potency, by employing data from the first dose only, yielded results similar to those obtained with complete crossover comparisons, but the crossover comparisons were more efficient and provided narrower confidence limits (99). In a comparison of crossover and parallel group studies of oral analgesics, Wang and Waite (102) found crossover studies advantageous. Patients served as their own controls, and there was less variability in responses in the same patients at different times than among patients; thus, a smaller number of patients is needed to provide statistically significant data. They also found that as long as crossover of treatment medications did not occur within 4 to 6 hr, the problem of carry-over effect of previous medication is insignificant or negligible.

Pharmacokinetic carry-over can be accounted for in appropriately designed crossover studies, but psychological variables are more difficult to control. Kantor et al. (54) found a placebo as a second dose to be functionally dependent on the effectiveness of the previous medication. Psychological variables will, of course, be operating as unknown entities in parallel studies as well.

Carry-over effects, either pharmacological or psychological are additional variables to consider in determining study design. Whether the study will reveal more information or be more efficient as crossover or a parallel group design can only be determined empirically. Where the patient groups are similar, or where the procedure causing pain is more or less uniform from patient to patient, as in dental pain owing to a third molar extraction, parallel groups may indeed be more efficient.

On the other hand, the crossover design may have many advantages in the studies of cancer patients with either chronic or postoperative pain.

Stratification of Variables

Pain severity

Especially when parallel group studies are employed, stratification of certain variables can improve study sensitivity. Stratification may be accomplished as part of the study design when variables can be identified in advance, or post hoc as part of the analysis. Since pain severity may not be predictable in advance, stratification is usually more easily accomplished by the latter method. Comparing aspirin or aspirin with caffeine to a placebo, Jain et al. (48) found both active drugs superior to the placebo for severe but not for moderate pain. In studies of acetophenetidin, acetaminophen, aspirin, and placebo in postpartum patients, Lasagna et al. (61) detailed a technique for analyzing categorical pain intensity and pain relief data. Patients were stratified for pain severity at each interview period, and data are analyzed employing nonparametric tests. By summing deviations and variations over time, slight but consistent differences between drugs become significantly large. This reinforcement may be inappropriate because of nonindependence of the individual observations, but it is not a problem in interpreting individual chi-square calculations for individual time periods. All three drugs benefited patients with slight pain, but only acetaminophen and aspirin helped patients with moderate pain.

In a study of aspirin, meperidine, codeine plus aspirin, phenacetin, and a combination analgesic in four separate studies in postsurgical gynecological patients, Hill and Turner (42) found that neither aspirin nor meperidine could be distinguished from a placebo when the data were analyzed as a whole. Aspirin was superior to placebo in slight or moderate pain, and meperidine was superior in severe pain. Codeine compound and the combination analgesic were superior to placebo in the overall comparison, but were even more effective if initial pain was considered.

Type of pain

Bloomfield et al. (9) claim that aspirin and codeine, when employed as standard analgesics, may have differential effects for pain of different etiologies. In patients with episiotomies or uterine cramping pain, aspirin was significantly better than placebo for either type of pain. Codeine (60 mg) was only superior to a placebo for episiotomy pain, implying that the two pain models may be quantitatively different, and should not be included in the same study without stratification.

Placebos

The inclusion of the placebo in a controlled clinical trial serves to provide a measure of the sensitivity of the method, and the ability of the patients to discriminate among treatment effects. It serves as a base line for measuring the drug effect, but, in addition, it is part of the drug effect in a complex interaction. Placebos can affect physical as well as psychological endpoints (22), and characterization of the personality of the patient on the basis of a reaction to placebo, can lead to confusing contradictions. Placebo reactors have been reported on different occasions as being neurotic and well-adjusted, extroverted and with low ego strength, acquiescent and antagonistic (68). The placebo reaction does not imply that the patient is malingering. Rather, it is a measure of the patient's confidence in his treatment and physician (44).

Graded Doses and Relative Potency

The ability of patients to discriminate graded effects of graded doses of a standard drug can also serve to establish the sensitivity of the analgesic study method. Graded doses of narcotic drugs have consistently been found to produce graded responses (3,44,45,98).

Although the dose-effect curves for drugs of the aspirin class are generally found to be much flatter than those of the narcotics, graded dose studies of this class of drugs have also been carried out successfully, but they require well designed sensitive assays (77,90,94,98). Not all such attempts, however, have been successful (2,8) and, in general, rather wide confidence limits are a characteristic of drug studies of aspirin.

Studies of Multiple Doses

It is recognized that discrepancies can exist between single dose and multiple dose analgesic studies, and that differences in the pharmacokinetic characteristics of the drugs under study may contribute to these differences (96). Analgesic design and reporting requirements for multidose studies will, of course, differ from those of single dose studies. Only in recent years have reasonably well controlled multidose analgesic assays been carried out (69,75,101).

A method for measuring postoperative patients' demands for subsequent analgesics after receiving study medication offers promise for the evaluation of the effects of long-acting analgesics. Bullingham et al. (14) and Gibbs et al. (30) utilized a demand analgesic apparatus in which patients are connected to a device allowing for self-administration of fixed amounts of i.v. analgesic medication, and automatic recording of the patient's demands. Subjective estimates of pain are also recorded at regular intervals. This method has the potential to provide supplemental information on the effects of an analgesic which is often unavailable in acute studies.

Outpatient Studies

Analgesic studies in outpatients have all the possible sources of variability inherent in inpatient studies, in addition to some special ones of their own. Situational influences will be more varied, and particular problems may be encountered in terms of patient compliance with the study protocol, the unauthorized supplementation of analgesia by nonstudy drugs, and failure to report and record the taking of the study drug adequately. In an outpatient study in oral surgery, Green (33) found that only two-thirds of the 200 patient records were valid and usable, and that gross discrepancies were observed in the number of doses reported as taken, compared to the amount of medications returned at the following visit.

Outpatient studies obviously require special care to maximize patient compliance, to check for possible protocol violations, and to insure adequate reporting of results. Patients should be well motivated to cooperate with the investigator and understand what is required of them. They should also be aware of the overall purpose of the research. Lines of communication should be well established. Some patient groups are better motivated than others to cooperate in a given study. Because of their orientation, medical and pharmacy students can constitute such a group. They have been employed successfully in a well-designed outpatient study of mild analgesics for headaches (73). Outpatient studies with patients having dental pain have also been carried out by Ruedy (83), Cooper and Beaver (21), Forbes et al. (26,27), and Quiding et al. (79), among others.

Commentary

The advances in methodology in the evaluation of analgesic drugs have been remarkable. Improvements in study design, the scaling of pain reports, and employment of visual analog scales have all served to increase the sensitivity of studies in this area. With appropriate rigorous controls and sensitive parameters for measuring subjective responses, successful analgesic studies of even the mild analgesics can be carried out in the clinical milieu in either inpatient or outpatient populations.

Areas of disagreement still exist, particularly concerning the relative merits of crossover and parallel group experimental design. Where clinical pain is so short lived that giving only one medication is all that is feasible, the answer is self-evident. In other cases, where two or more medications per patient can readily be administered, the answer should be obtained empirically.

ACKNOWLEDGMENTS

Discussions with Drs. Raymond W. Houde and Robert F. Kaiko and Ms. Ada Rogers have been invaluable and are greatly appreciated.

This work was supported in part by USPHS NIH grant DA-01707.

REFERENCES

1. Adler, R., Gervasi, A., Holzer, B., and Hemmler, W. (1974): Mild analgesics evaluated with the "submaximal effort tourniquet technique" II. Influence of a tranquilizer on their effect. *Psychopharmacologia (Berlin)*, 38:357–362.
2. Bauer, R. O., Baptisti, A., Jr., and Gruber, C. M., Jr. (1974): Evaluation of propoxyphene napsylate compound in postpartum uterine cramping. *J. Med. (Basel)*, 5:317–328.
3. Beaver, W. T., Wallenstein, S. L., Houde, R. W., and Rogers, A. (1977): Comparisons of the

analgesic effects of oral and intramuscular oxymorphone and of intramuscular oxymorphone and morphine in patients with cancer. *J. Clin. Pharmacol.*, 17:186–198.

4. Beecher, H. K. (1953): Pain controlled and uncontrolled. *Science*, 117:164–167.

5. Beecher, H. K. (1957): The measurement of pain. *Pharmacol. Rev.*, 9:59–209.

6. Beecher, H. K. (1959): *Measurement of Subjective Responses.* Oxford University Press, New York.

7. Benjamin, F. B. (1958): The effect of aspirin on suprathreshold pain in man. *Science*, 128:303–304.

8. Bloomfield, S. S., Barden, T. P., and Hille, R. (1970): Clinical evaluation of flufenisal, a long-acting analgesic. *Clin. Pharmacol. Ther.*, 11:747–754.

9. Bloomfield, S. S., Barden, T. P., and Mitchell, J. (1976): Aspirin and codeine in two postpartum pain models. *Clin. Pharmacol. Ther.*, 20:499–503.

10. Bloomfield, S. S., and Hurwitz, H. N. (1970): Tourniquet and episiotomy pain as test models for aspirin-like analgesics. *J. Clin. Pharmacol.*, 10:361–369.

11. Bross, I. D. J. (1958): How to use ridit analysis. *Biometrics*, 14:18–38.

12. Brown, B. W., Jr. (1980): The crossover experiment for clinical trials. *Biometrics*, 36:69–79.

13. Buchsbaum, M. S., Davis, G. C., Coppola, R., and Dieter, N. (1981): Opiate pharmacology and individual differences. 1. Psychophysical pain measurements. *Pain*, 10:357–366.

14. Bullingham, R. E. S., McQuay, H. J., Dwyer, D., Allen, M. C., and Moore, R. A. (1981): Sublingual buprenorphine used postoperatively: Clinical observations and preliminary pharmacokinetic analysis. *Br. J. Clin. Pharmacol.*, 12:117–122.

15. Calimlim, J. F., Wardell, W. M., Phil, D., Davis, H. T., Lasagna, L., and Gillies, A. J. (1977): Analgesic efficacy of an orally administered combination of pentazocine and aspirin with observations on the use of statistical efficiency of GLOBAL subjective efficacy ratings. *Clin. Pharmacol. Ther.*, 21:34–43.

16. Chapman, C. R. (1975): Psychophysical evaluation of acupunctural analgesia: Some issues and considerations. *Anesthesiology*, 43:501–506.

17. Chapman, L. F., Dingman, H. F., and Ginzberg, S. P. (1965): Failure of systemic analgesic agents to alter the absolute sensory threshold for the simple detection of pain. *Brain*, 88:1011–1022.

18. Christensen, E. M., and Gross, E. D. (1948): Analgesic effects of morphine, meperidine, and methadone. *J.A.M.A.*, 137:594–599.

19. Clark, W. C. (1974): Pain sensitivity and the report of pain: An introduction to sensory decision theory. *Anesthesiology*, 40:272–287.

20. Coffman, J. D. (1966): The effect of aspirin on pain and hand blood flow responses to intra-arterial injection of bradykinin in man. *Clin. Pharmacol. Ther.*, 7:26–37.

21. Cooper, S. A., and Beaver, W. T. (1976): A model to evaluate mild analgesics in oral surgery outpatients. *Clin. Pharmacol. Ther.*, 20:241–250.

22. Cousins, N. (1977): The mysterious placebo. How mind helps medicine work. *Saturday Review*, 9–16.

23. Deneau, G. A., Waud, R. A., and Gowdey, C. W. (1953): A method for determining the effects of drugs on the pain threshold of human subjects. *Can. J. Med. Sci.*, 31:387–393.

24. Dinnerstein, A. J., Blitz, B., and Lowenthal, M. (1965): Effects of aspirin on detection and tolerance of electric shock. *J. Appl. Physiol.*, 20:1052–1053.

25. Ferguson, R. K. (1970): Drug-test interaction in the submaximal-effort tourniquet technique. *Proc. Soc. Exp. Biol. Med.*, 134:1015–1019.

26. Forbes, J. A., Calderazzo, J. P., Bowser, M. W., Foor, V. M., Shackleford, R. W., and Beaver, W. T. (1982): A 12-hour evaluation of the analgesic efficacy of diflunisal, aspirin, and placebo in postoperative dental pain. *J. Clin. Pharmacol.*, 22:89–96.

27. Forbes, J. A., White, R. W., White, E. H., and Hughes, M. K. (1980): An evaluation of the analgesic efficacy of proquazone and aspirin in postoperative dental pain. *J. Clin. Pharmacol.*, 20:465–474.

28. Fox, C. D., Steger, H. G., and Jennison, J. H. (1979): Ratio scaling of pain perception with the submaximum effort tourniquet technique. *Pain*, 7:21–29.

29. Fucella, L. M., Corvi, G., Gorini, F., Mandelli, V., Mascellani, G., Nobili, F., Pedronetto, S., Ragni, M., and Vandelli, I. (1977): Application of nonparametric procedure for bioassay to the evaluation of analgesics in man. *J. Clin. Pharmacol.*, 17:177–184.

30. Gibbs, J. M., Johnson, H. D., and Davis, F. M. (1982): Patient administration of I.V. buprenorphine for postoperative pain relief using the "Cardiff" demand analgesic apparatus. *Br. J. Anaesth.*, 54:279–284.

31. Gracely, R. H., and Dubner, R. (1981): Pain assessment in humans—a reply to Hall. *Pain*, 11:109–120.
32. Gracely, R. H., McGrath, P., and Dubner, R. (1977): Validity and sensitivity of ratio scales of sensory and effective verbal pain descriptors: Manipulation of affect by diazepam. *Pain*, 5:19–29.
33. Green, A. E. (1976): A clinical trial of pentazocine and aspirin following minor oral surgery. *Br. Dent. J.*, 141:247–250.
34. Hall, W. (1981): On "ratio scales of sensory affective verbal descriptors." *Pain*, 11:101–107.
35. Hardy, J. D., and Javert, C. T. (1949): Studies on pain: Measurement of pain intensity in childbirth. *J. Clin. Invest.*, 28:153–162.
36. Hardy, J. D., Wolff, H. G., and Goodell, H. (1940): Studies on pain. A new method for measuring pain threshold. Observations on spatial summation of pain. *J. Clin. Invest.*, 19:649–657.
37. Hardy, J. D., Wolff, H. G., and Goodell, H. (1947): Studies on pain: Discrimination of differences in intensity of pain stimulus as a basis for a scale of pain intensity. *J. Clin. Invest.*, 26:1152–1158.
38. Hardy, J. D., Wolff, H. G., and Goodell, H. (1952): *Pain Sensations and Reactions*. The Williams & Wilkins Co., Baltimore.
39. Heft, M., Gracely, R. H., Dubner, A., and McGrath, P. A. (1980): A validation model for verbal descriptor scaling of human clinical pain. *Pain*, 9:363–373.
40. Hill, H. E., Kornetsky, C. H., Flanary, H., and Wikler, A. (1952): Effects of anxiety and morphine on discrimination intensities of pain stimuli. *J. Clin. Invest.*, 31:473–480.
41. Hill, H. E., Kornetsky, C. H., Flanery, H., and Wikler, A. (1952): Studies on anxiety associated with pain. I. Effects of morphine. *Arch. Neurol. Psychiatr.*, 67:612–619.
42. Hill, R. C., and Turner, P. (1969): Importance of initial pain in postoperative assessment of analgesic drugs. *J. Clin. Pharmacol.*, 9:321–327.
43. Houde, R. W. (1982): Methods for measuring clinical pain in humans. *Acta Anaesthesiol. Scand. (Suppl.)*, 74:25–29.
44. Houde, R. W., Wallenstein, S. L., and Beaver, W. T. (1965): Clinical measurement of pain. In: *Analgetics*, edited by G. de Stevens, pp. 75–122. Academic Press, Inc., New York.
45. Houde, R. W., Wallenstein, S. L., Bellville, J. W., Rogers, A., and Escarraga, L. A. (1964): The relative analgesic and respiratory effects of phenazocine and morphine. *J. Pharmacol. Exp. Ther.*, 144:337–345.
46. Houde, R. W., Wallenstein, S. L., and Rogers, A. (1960): Clinical pharmacology of analgesics. 1. A method for studying analgesic effect. *Clin. Pharmacol. Ther.*, 1:163–174.
47. Huskisson, E. C. (1974): Measurement of pain. *Lancet*, 2:1127–1131.
48. Jain, A. K., McMahon, F. G., Ryan, J. R., Unger, D., and Richard, W. (1978): Aspirin and aspirin-caffeine in postpartum pain relief. *Clin. Pharmacol. Ther.*, 24:69–75.
49. Jones, B. (1979): Signal detection theory and pain research. *Pain*, 7:305–312.
50. Joyce, C. R. B., Zutski, D. W., Hrubes, V., and Mason, R. M. (1975): Comparison of fixed interval and visual analogue scales for rating chronic pain. *Eur. J. Clin. Pharmacol.*, 8:415–420.
51. Kaiko, R. F. (1980): Age and morphine analgesia in cancer patients with postoperative pain. *Clin. Pharmacol. Ther.*, 28:823–826.
52. Kaiko, R. F., Wallenstein, S. L., Rogers, A. G., Grabinski, P. Y., and Houde, R. W. (1981): Analgesic and mood effects of heroin and morphine in cancer patients with postoperative pain. *N. Engl. J. Med.*, 304:1501–1505.
53. Kaiko, R. F., Wallenstein, S. L., Rogers, A. G., and Houde, R. W. (1983): Sources of variation in analgesic responses in cancer patients with chronic pain receiving morphine. *Pain*, 15:191–200.
54. Kantor, T. G., Sunshine, A., Laska, E., Meisner, M., and Hopper, M. (1966): Oral analgesic studies: Pentazocine hydrochloride, codeine, aspirin, and placebo, and their influence on response to placebo. *Clin. Pharmacol. Ther.*, 7:447–454.
55. Kast, E. C. (1968): Clinical measurement of pain. *Med. Clin. North Am.*, 52:23–32.
55a. Keele, K. D. (1948): The pain chart. *Lancet*, 2:6–12.
56. Klepac, R. K., Dowling, J., and Hauge, G. (1981): Sensitivity of the McGill pain questionnaire to intensity and quality of laboratory pain. *Pain*, 10:199–207.
57. Kornetsky, C.H. (1954): Effects of anxiety and morphine on the antiception and perception of painful radiant thermal stimulation. *J. Clin. Physiol. Psychol.*, 47:130–132.
58. Kremer, E., Atkinson, J. H., and Ignelzi, R. J. (1981): Measurement of pain: Patient preference does not confound pain measurement. *Pain*, 10:241–248.

59. Kutscher, A. H., and Kutscher, H. W. (1957): Evaluation of the Hardy-Wolff-Goodell pain threshold apparatus and technique. Review of the literature. *Int. Rec. Med.*, 170:202–212

60. Lasagna, L. (1980): Analgesic methodology: A brief history and commentary. *J. Clin. Pharmacol.*, 20:373–376.

61. Lasagna, L., Davis, M., and Pearson, J. W. (1967): A comparison of acetophenetidin and acetaminophen. *J. Pharmacol. Exp. Ther.*, 155:296–300.

62. Lasagna, L., Tetreault, L., and Fallis, N. (1962): Analgesic drugs and experimental ischemic pain. *Fed. Proc.*, 21:326.

63. Laska, E., and Meisner, M. (1983): Crossover design and inference in clinical analgesic trials. *Clin. Pharmacol. Ther.*, 33:214 *(Abstr.)*.

64. Lim, R. K. S., Miller, D. G., Guzman, F., Rodgers, D. W., Rogers, R. W., Wang, S. K., Chas, P. Y., and Shih, T. Y. (1967): Pain and analgesia evaluated by the intraperitoneal bradykinin-evoked pain method in man. *Clin. Pharmacol. Ther.*, 8:521–542.

65. Lutterbeck, P. M., and Triay, S. H. (1972): Measurement of analgesic activity in man. *Int. J. Clin. Pharmacol.*, 64:315–319.

66. Melzack, R. (1975): The McGill pain questionnaire: Major properties and scoring methods. *Pain*, 1:277–299.

67. Meyer, F. P., Grecksch, G., and Walther, H. (1978): Effectiveness of analgesics evaluated with the tourniquet technique. *Int. J. Clin. Pharmacol.*, 16:229–234.

68. Moerman, D. E. (1981): Edible symbols: The effectiveness of placebos. *Ann. N.Y. Acad. Sci.*, 364:256–268.

69. Mok, M., Lippmann, M., and Steen, S. N. (1981): Multidose/observational, comparative clinical analgesic assay of buprenorphine. *J. Clin. Pharmacol.*, 21:323–329.

70. Montanari, C., Sala, P., Ferrari, P., and Gaetani, M. (1976): Experimental evaluation in man of analgesic effects. *Arzneimittelforsch*, 26:1616–1617.

71. Moore, J. D., Weissman, L., Thomas, G., and Whitman, E. N. (1971): Response of experimental ischemic pain to analgesics in prisoner volunteers. *J. Clin. Pharmacol.*, 11:433–439.

72. Moore, P. A., Duncan, G. H., Scott, D. S., Gregg, J. M., and Ghia, J. N. (1979): The submaximal effort tourniquet test: Its use in evaluating experimental and chronic pain. *Pain*, 6:375–382.

73. Murray, W. J. (1967): Evaluation of acetaminophen-salicylamide combinations in treatment of headache. *J. Clin. Pharmacol.*, 7:150–155.

74. Ohnaus, E. E., and Adler, R. (1975): Methodologic problems in the measurement of pain: A comparison between the verbal rating scale and the visual analogue scale. *Pain*, 1:379–384.

75. Oullette, R. D. (1982): Buprenorphine and morphine efficacy in postoperative pain: A double-blind multiple-dose study. *J. Clin. Pharmacol.*, 22:165–172.

76. Parkhouse, J., and Hallinon, P. (1967): A comparison of aspirin and paracetamol. *Br. J. Anaesth.*, 39:146–154.

77. Parkhouse, J., Rees-Lewis, M., Skolinik, M., and Peters, H. (1968): The clinical dose response to aspirin. *Br. J. Anaesth.*, 40:433–441.

78. Procacci, P., Zoppi, M., and Maresco, M. (1979): Experimental pain in man. *Pain*, 6:123–140.

79. Quiding, H., Oksala, E., Happonen, R., Lehtimaki, K., and Ojala, T. (1981): The visual analog scale in multiple-dose evaluation of analgesics. *J. Clin. Pharmacol.*, 21:424–429.

80. Reithe, P., and Wilske, E. (1974): Analgesic effects on the stimulus threshold of the human tooth. *Arzneimittelforsch*, 24:666–671.

81. Revill, S. I., Robinson, J. O., Rosen, M., and Hagg, M. I. J. (1976): The reliability of a linear analogue for evaluating pain. *Anaesthesia*, 31:1191–1198.

82. Rollman, G. B. (1977): Signal detection and theory measurement of pain: A review and critique. *Pain*, 3:187–211.

83. Ruedy, J. (1973): A comparison of the analgesic efficacy of naproxen and acetylsalicylic acid-codeine in patients with pain after dental surgery. *Scand. J. Rheumatol. (Suppl.)*, 2:60–63.

84. Scott, J., and Huskisson, E. C. (1976): Graphic representation of pain. *Pain*, 2:175–184.

85. Sherman, H., Feasconaro, J. E., and Grundfest, H. (1963): Laboratory evaluation of analgesic effectiveness in human subjects. *Exp. Neurol.*, 7:435–456.

86. Smith, G. M., and Beecher, H. K. (1969): Experimental production of pain in man: Sensitivity of a new method to 600 mg of aspirin. *Clin. Pharmacol. Ther.*, 10:213–216.

87. Smith, R. (1967): Experimental pain in general practice. *Proc. R. Soc. Med.*, 60:415–417.

88. Sternbach, R. A., Deems, L. M., Timmermans, G., and Huey, L. Y. (1977): On the sensitivity of the tourniquet pain test. *Pain*, 3:105–110.

89. Swiratanakul, K., Kelvie, B. S., and Lasagna, L. (1982): The quantification of pain: An analysis of words used to describe pain and analgesia in clinical trials. *Clin. Pharmacol. Ther.*, 32:143–148.
90. Sunshine, A., Laska, E., and Slafta, J. (1978): Oral nefopam and aspirin. *Clin. Pharmacol. Ther.*, 24:555–559.
91. Timmermans, G., and Sternbach, R. A. (1974): Factors of human chronic pain: An analysis of personality and pain reaction variables. *Science*, 184:806–808.
92. Tursky, B. (1976): The development of a pain perception profile: A psychophysical approach. In: *Pain: New Perspectives in Therapy and Research*, edited by M. Weisenberg and B. Tursky, pp. 171–194. Plenum Press, New York.
93. Validya, A. B., Sheth, M. S., Manghani, K. K., Schroff, P., Vora, K. K., and Sheth, U. K. (1974): Double-blind trial of mefanamic acid, aspirin, and placebo in patients with postoperative pain. *Indian J. Med. Sci.*, 28:532–536.
94. Ventafridda, V., Martino, G., Mandelli, V., and Emanueli, A. (1975): Indoprofen, a new analgesic and antiinflammatory drug in cancer pain. *Clin. Pharmacol. Ther.*, 17:284–289.
95. von Graffenreid, B., Adler, R., Abt, K., Nuesch, E., and Spiegel, R. (1978): The influence of anxiety and pain sensitivity on experimental pain in man. *Pain*, 4:253–263.
96. Waife, S. O., Gruber, C. M., Jr., Rodda, B. E., and Nash, J. F. (1975): Problems and solutions to single dose testing of analgesics. Comparisons of propoxyphene, codeine, and fenoprofen. *Int. J. Clin. Pharmacol.*, 107:202–212.
97. Wallenstein, S. L., Heidrich, G., III., Kaiko, R., and Houde, R. W. (1980): Clinical evaluation of mild analgesics: The measurement of clinical pain. *Br. J. Clin. Pharmacol.*, 10:319S–327S.
98. Wallenstein, S. L., and Houde, R. W. (1975): The clinical evaluation of analgesic effectiveness. In: *Methods in Narcotics Research*, edited by S. Ehrenpreis and A. Neidle, pp. 127–145. Marcel Dekker, New York.
99. Wallenstein, S. L., Kaiko, R. F., Rogers, A. G., and Houde, R. W. (1981): Clinical analgesic assay of sublingual buprenorphine and intramuscular morphine. In: *National Institute on Drug Abuse and Research Monograph #41: Problems of Drug Dependence*, edited by L. S. Harris, pp. 288–293. U.S. Government Printing Office, Washington, D.C.
100. Wallenstein, S. L., Rogers, A., Kaiko, R. F., Heidrich, G., III, and Houde, R. W. (1979): Clinical analgesic assay of oral zomepirac and intramuscular morphine. In: *National Institute on Drug Abuse Research Monograph #27: Problems of Drug Dependence*, edited by L. S. Harris, pp. 261–267. U.S. Government Printing Office, Washington, D.C.
101. Wang, R. I., Johnson, R. P., Robinson, N., and Waite, E. (1981): The study of analgesics following single and repeated doses. *J. Clin. Pharmacol.*, 21:121–125.
102. Wang, R. I., and Waite, E. (1981): Crossover and parallel study of oral analgesics. *J. Clin. Pharmacol.*, 21:162–168.
103. Williams, M. W. (1959): Ischemic arm pain and narcotic analgesics. *Toxicol. Appl. Pharmacol.*, 1:590–597.
104. Wolff, B. B., Kantor, T. G., and Cohen, P. (1976): Laboratory pain induction methods for human analgesic assays. In: *Advances in Pain Research and Therapy*, edited by J. J. Bonica and D. A.-Fessard, pp. 363–367. Raven Press, New York.
105. Wolff, B. B., Kantor, T. G., Jarvik, M. E., and Laska, E. (1966): Responses of experimental pain to analgesic drugs. 1. Morphine, aspirin, and placebo. *Clin. Pharmacol. Ther.*, 7:224–238.
106. Wolff, B. B., Kantor, T. G., Jarvik, M. E., and Laska, E. (1969): Response of experimental pain to analgesic drugs. 3. Codeine, aspirin, secobarbital, and placebo. *Clin. Pharmacol. Ther.*, 10:217–228.
107. Wolff, H. G., Hardy, J. D., and Goodell, H. (1940): Studies on pain. Measurement of the effect of morphine, codeine, and other opiates on the pain threshold and an analysis of their relation to the pain experience. *J. Clin. Invest.*, 19:659.
108. Wolff, H. G., Hardy, J. D., and Goodell, H. (1941): Studies on pain. Measurement of the effect of pain threshold of acetylsalicylic acid, acetanilid, acetophenetidin, aminopyrine, ethyl alcohol, trichlorethylene, a barbiturate, quinine, ergotamine tartrate, and caffeine: An analysis of their relation to the pain experience. *J. Clin. Invest.*, 20:63–80.
109. Yanaura, S., Yamatake, Y., and Misawa, H. (1977): Clinical assessment of analgesics using ultrasonic stimulation. A new method. *Jpn. J. Pharmacol.*, 27:501–508.

*Analgesics: Neurochemical, Behavioral, and
Clinical Perspectives*, edited by M. Kuhar and
G. Pasternak. Raven Press, New York © 1984.

Narcotic Analgesics in the Management of Pain

*†Charles E. Inturrisi and *,**,†Kathleen M. Foley

*Departments of Pharmacology and **Neurology, Cornell University Medical College
†Pain Research Program, Memorial Sloan-Kettering Cancer Center,
New York, New York 10021

Drug therapy represents the mainstay of medical therapy in the management of patients with acute and chronic pain. The analgesic drugs commonly used can be divided into three major groups: group I, aspirin and the nonsteroidal anti-inflammatory drugs which act peripherally and produce analgesia through their ability to alter the prostaglandin system; group II, the narcotic type analgesics which bind to discrete opiate receptors and activate an endogenous pain suppression system; group III, the "adjuvant" analgesic drugs such as amitriptyline and methotrimeprazine, which act centrally to produce analgesia in certain pain states through endogenous analgesic systems. These systems are not well understood as yet, but probably involve many different neurotransmitters. The effective use of these analgesic drugs should be part of every physicians armamentarium in managing patients with pain (22,23,27). The choice of the specific drug approach is based on: a full assessment of the type of pain, acute versus chronic; the definition of the specific pain syndrome; and an understanding of the clinical pharmacology of the drug prescribed.

TYPES OF CLINICAL PAIN STATES

In the management of any patient with pain, it is of paramount importance to recognize that pain is only a symptom not a diagnosis. Pain perception then is not simply a function of the amount of physical injury sustained by the patient. Rather, it is a complex state determined by multiple factors including age, sex, cultural, and environmental influences, and multiple psychological factors. The methods of pain management and the goals of adequate therapy vary for each individual patient. Patients suffering from pain can be divided into two major groups, those with acute pain and those with chronic pain (19). The point at which acute pain becomes chronic is not well-defined, but is generally considered to be 6 months. Patients with acute pain are characterized by a well-defined temporal pattern of pain onset, usually associated with subjective and objective physical signs. The objective signs are commonly associated with hyperactivity of the autonomic nervous system, including tachycardia, hypertension, diaphoresis, mydriasis, and pallor, and substantiate to the physician the complaint of severe pain. In contrast, in chronic pain, the symptoms persist after a less well-defined temporal onset, and the signs of autonomic nervous system hyperactivity are absent. Thus, evaluation of the severity of chronic pain is often difficult because the physician has limited objective signs. This lack of a useful diagnostic tool to confirm the severity of pain makes pain such a difficult symptom to evaluate and treat. Distinguishing between acute and chronic pain is particularly important, however, in the management of patients, because their response to treatment often differs. Acute pain is relatively easy to recognize and more amenable to therapeutic approaches. Patients with acute pain can usually be treated for the cause of their pain, and are more likely to respond to analgesics and other modalities. In chronic pain, the persistent pain has usually failed to respond to treatments directed at the etiology of the pain. In general, these patients respond poorly to the use of analgesics, and have developed significant changes in personality, lifestyle, and functional ability. Such patients need a management approach which encompasses both the cause of their pain and the complications which have ensued in their functional ability, their social lives, and their personalities. It is this particular group of patients that challenges physicians in the management of pain.

Within this group of patients with chronic pain, three types of patients emerge. The first type is the patient with chronic medical illness in whom pain is an intimate part of the disease process, i.e., pain with metastatic disease, rheumatoid arthritis, sickle cell anemia, or hemophilia. In these patients, the severity of pain may fluctuate. They may have pain-free intervals or may have continuous mild pain with acute severe exacerbations superimposed. This group often responds well to a series of modalities including analgesics. The second group of patients are those with chronic pain in whom the pain which began as a definable pain syndrome has evolved into a disease unto itself. Although the site may vary and commonly involves the face or lower back, the pain often consumes the patient's daily life and limits activity. This group have been referred to as the chronic intractable pain syndrome. The third type is the patient with chronic pain without a definable cause. These patients characteristically complain of diffuse myalgias and arthralgias, have had multiple diagnostic studies, and often multiple surgical procedures without any clear evolution of a definable pain syndrome.

Patients with chronic pain have often failed treatment directed at the cause of their pain and therefore are forced to live with their "pain problem." For this group of patients, the use of drug therapy is complicated because tolerance to the narcotic type analgesics, and perhaps to some of the adjuvant analgesic drugs, limits their long-term efficacy. Similarly, the long-term use of non-narcotic analgesics is associated with hepatic, gastrointestinal, and renal complications. In some patients, the component of suffering is significant with anxiety and depression, providing an added burden and confounding the assessment of the pain complaint. The role of narcotic-type analgesics in the management of pain in this population of patients is very controversial. Yet, there are no long-term data to support the thesis that chronic use of narcotic-type analgesics alone causes psychological dependence. In certain patients with chronic pain, such as the cancer patient, narcotic-type analgesics have been used successfully for both acute and chronic pain.

The purpose of this chapter is to discuss the pharmacological principles and properties that form the basis for the clinical use of the narcotic-type analgesics in the management of pain. Particular emphasis is placed on using these principles and properties to develop guidelines (practical considerations) for the therapeutic use of these drugs.

THE PHARMACOLOGICAL BASIS FOR THE CLINICAL USE OF NARCOTIC-TYPE ANALGESICS

Morphine is the prototype and standard of comparison for narcotic-type analgesics to be used for the relief of moderate to severe pain. Since the isolation of morphine from opium in 1803, there has been a proliferation of semisynthetic and synthetic derivatives of morphine and related opioids that provide the physician with a wide choice of analgesic drugs. As is discussed in chapters 2, 3, and 4, the analgesic effects of morphine and chemically-related opioids result from interactions with stereospecific and saturable binding sites, or receptors in the CNS. These opiate receptors are the site of action for several endogenous morphine-like peptides (endorphins). At present, β-endorphin, one of the naturally-occurring endorphins, and metkephamid, a synthetic enkephalin derivative, are under clinical evaluation as analgesics (10,21,63).

Available Narcotic-Type Analgesics

Although not completely satisfactory, a convenient classification for the narcotic-type analgesics is based on the belief that, in most situations, the intensity of pain rather than its specific etiology should determine which analgesic is suitable for a particular patient.

Table 1 lists the properties of those narcotic-type analgesics commonly used for severe pain. Table 2 contains those narcotic-type analgesics commonly used by the oral route for mild to moderate pain. Much of the information summarized in Tables 1 and 2 is derived from controlled clinical trials employing single-dose comparisons of a narcotic to morphine (34,35,36). Unfortunately, as will be indicated below, there are still gaps in our knowledge of analgesic pharmacology so that individualization of treatment is the rule rather than the exception.

The Clinical Pharmacology of Morphine

The consideration of narcotic-type analgesics begins with a definition of the clinical pharmacology of morphine. Table 3 lists the desirable and undesirable properties of morphine when used as an analgesic. Of the desirable properties, morphine is capable of producing effective analgesia over a wide range of doses. Morphine's analgesic action is relatively selective in that pain may be relieved

TABLE 1. *Narcotic-type analgesics commonly used for severe pain*

Name	Route	Equianalgesic dose[a] (mg)	Peak[b] (1 hr)	Duration[b] (hr)	Comments	Precautions
a. Morphine-like agonists						
Morphine	i.m.	10	½–1	4–6	Standard of comparison for narcotic type analgesics	Impaired ventilation, bronchial asthma, increased intracranial pressure, liver failure
	p.o.	60	1½–2	4–7		
Meperidine (Demerol)	i.m.	75	½–1	4–5	Slightly shorter acting; moderate to poor oral potency; biotransformed to normeperidine, a toxic metabolite	Normeperidine accumulates with repetitive dosing causing CNS excitation; not for patients with impaired renal function or receiving MAO inhibitors
	p.o.	300	1–2	4–6		
Methadone (Dolophine)	i.m.	10	Like i.m. morphine	Like i.m. morphine	Good oral potency, long plasma half-life	Like morphine, may accumulate with repetitive dosing causing excessive sedation
	p.o.	20	Like p.o. morphine	Like p.o. morphine		
Levorphanol (Levo-Dromoran)	i.m.	2	Like i.m. morphine	Like i.m. morphine	Like methadone	Like methadone
	p.o.	4	Like p.o. morphine	Like p.o. morphine		
Oxycodone	p.o.	30	1	4–6	Available only (5-mg doses) in combination with acetaminophen (Percocet) or aspirin (Percodan) which limits dose escalation	Like morphine
Heroin	i.m.	5	½–1	4–5	Slightly shorter acting; biotransformed to active metabolites (e.g., morphine); not available U.S.	Like morphine
	p.o.	(60)	Like p.o. morphine			

Drug	Route	Dose (mg)	Onset and duration[b]	Comments	Comments
Hydromorphone (Dilaudid)	i.m.	1.5	Like i.m. heroin	Like heroin	Like morphine
	p.o.	7.5	Like p.o. morphine		Like morphine
Oxymorphone (Numorphan)	i.m.	1	Like i.m. morphine	Like morphine	Like morphine
Codeine	i.m.	130	Like i.m. morphine	Like morphine	Like morphine
	p.o.	200		Excellent oral potency (see Table 2)	
b. Mixed agonist-antagonists					
Pentazocine (Talwin)	i.m.	60	Like i.m. morphine	Mixed agonist-antagonist; less abuse liability than morphine; included in schedule IV of controlled substances act	May cause psychotomimetic effects; may precipitate withdrawal in narcotic-dependent patients, not for myocardial infarction
	p.o.	180	Like p.o. morphine		
Nalbuphine (Nubain)	i.m.	10	Like i.m. morphine	Like pentazocine but not scheduled	Incidence of psychotomimetic effects lower than with pentazocine
Butorphanol (Stadol)	i.m.	2	Like i.m. morphine	Like nalbuphine	Like pentazocine
c. Partial agonists					
Buprenorphine (Temgesic)	i.m.	0.4	Like i.m. morphine 2–3	Partial agonist of the morphine type, less abuse liability than morphine, does not produce psychotomimetic effects, not yet available in U.S.	May precipitate withdrawal in narcotic-dependent patients
	s.l.	0.8	5–6		
d. Endorphins					
-Endorphin	e.d.	ND	ND	Investigational drug	
	i.t.	ND			
	i.m.	ND			
metkephamid	i.m.	ND	Like i.m. merperidine	Investigational drug	

[a] These doses are recommended starting doses from which the optimal dose for each patient is determined by titration and the maximal dose limited by adverse effects.

[b] Peak time and duration of analgesia are based on mean values and refer to the stated equianalgesic doses.

Abbreviations: i.m., intramuscular; p.o., oral; s.l., sublingual; e.d., epidural; i.t., intrathecal; ND, not determined.

Modified from Table 1, Inturrisi, (42).

TABLE 2. Narcotic-type analgesics commonly used orally for mild to moderate pain compared to aspirin (650 mg).

Name	Equianalgesic dose (mg)	Peak (hr)	Duration (hr)	Comments	Precautions
a. Morphine-like agonists					
Codeine	32–65	1½–2	4–6	"Weak" morphine, often used in combination with non-narcotic analgesics; biotransformed, in part, to morphine	Impaired ventilation, bronchial asthma, increased intracranial pressure
Oxycodone (Percodan demi)	2.5	1	3–4	Available only in combination with aspirin	Like codeine
Meperidine (Demerol)	50	1–1½	4–5	Biotransformed to normeperidine, a toxic metabolite	Normeperidine accumulates with repetitive dosing causing CNS excitation, not for patients with impaired renal function or receiving MAO inhibitors
Propoxyphene HCl (Darvon)	65–130	Like codeine	Like codeine	"Weak" narcotic; often used in combination with non-narcotic analgesics; long half-life, biotransformed to potentially toxic metabolite (norpropoxyphene)	Propoxyphene and metabolite accumulate with repetitive dosing; overdose complicated by convulsions
Propoxyphene Napsylate (Darvon-N)	100–200	Like codeine	Like codeine		
b. Mixed agonist-antagonists					
Pentazocine (Talwin®)	30	Like codeine	Like codeine	Mixed agonist-antagonist	May cause psychotomimetic effects, may precipitate withdrawal in narcotic-dependent patients

Modified from Table 2, Inturrisi, (42).

TABLE 3. *The desirable and undesirable properties of morphine as an analgesic*

Desirable	Undesirable
Analgesia	Respiratory depression
Mood effects	Mental clouding
Sedation	Sedation
	Mood effects
	Dizziness
	Nausea and vomiting
	Suppression of cough reflex
	Psychological dependence
	Physical dependence
	Tolerance
	Spasmogenic
	Constipation
	Poor oral potency

without the loss of other sensory modalities, although fully effective doses may produce some alteration in consciousness or behavior. Clinically, morphine-induced analgesia does not appear to have a "ceiling effect." That is, as the dose is increased on a logarithmic scale, the increment in analgesic effect appears to be linear, virtually to the point of loss of consciousness. However, before that level is reached, undesirable effects that can be seen after a single dose, notably, sedation, mental clouding, nausea and vomiting, and/or respiratory depression may impose a practical limit on the dose useful for any particular patient.

The ability of morphine to alter mood can be manifest as the relief of anxiety and/or induction of a sense of euphoria or well being. Certainly, in the patient suffering from advanced cancer, these mood effects, when they occur, can be considered a desirable property. Sedation, while desirable when morphine is used as a preanesthetic medication, is not useful as a general accompaniment of analgesia in the management of acute or chronic pain.

On the undesirable side, the properties of morphine that are most likely to lead to its being misused, or the patient mistreated, are effects mediated in the CNS and seen after chronic administration, including psychological dependence, physical dependence, and tolerance. Although it is recognized that the mood-altering effects of morphine in some individuals may lead to the compulsive drug-seeking behavior exhibited by the narcotic addict, the number of patients who become addicted in this sense is extremely small relative to those receiving narcotics chronically in the course of the legitimate practice of medicine (37,47).

Physical dependence is manifest by the appearance of withdrawal symptoms and signs characteristic of the well-known abstinence syndrome when the drug is abruptly discontinued or if a narcotic antagonist is administered. The severity of withdrawal is a function of the dose and duration of administration of the narcotic just discontinued (i.e., the patient's prior narcotic experience). The administration of a narcotic antagonist to a physically dependent individual produces an immediate precipitation of the withdrawal syndrome.

Tolerance develops when a given dose of a drug produces a decreasing effect, or when a larger dose is required to maintain the original effect. Tolerance and physical dependence to these drugs seem to develop with a parallel time course, so that a patient who requires an increase in the dose to maintain analgesia (tolerance) should not be abruptly withdrawn from a narcotic-type analgesic even if, for whatever reason, the patient's pain is suddenly alleviated. Fortunately, tolerance develops at comparable rates to the analgesic and some of the dose-limiting adverse effects, including sedation and respiratory depression, thus permitting the required increase in dosage. However, tolerance develops more slowly to the smooth muscle effects of narcotics.

A patient tolerant to one narcotic will also exhibit tolerance to another. However, Houde et al. (33,37) have observed that, in patients with chronic pain due to cancer, cross-tolerance tends not to be complete.

Viewed from the perspective of what might be considered the properties of an ideal, strong analgesic, morphine certainly falls short. Thus, for nearly 100 years there has been a continuing search for the better morphine--a drug with the analgesic effectiveness of morphine but without one or more of its undesirable properties. Because of the narcotic abuse in this country, a large part of this effort has been directed to the development of strong analgesics that might possess less abuse liability than morphine. Although it may be reasonably argued that this approach is likely to have little impact on the availability or use of heroin by "street addicts," it has had an important influence on drug development.

How Do Available Narcotic-Type Analgesics Differ from Morphine?

The decision on whether to use one of the narcotic drugs given in Table 1 in preference to morphine requires a consideration of how the substitute may differ from morphine, and whether this difference offers any clinical advantage. At least nine characteristics can be identified that distinguish the narcotic-type analgesics from morphine and in some cases from one another.

Source

The earliest classification of narcotics was based on the source from which they were obtained. Morphine and codeine are naturally-occurring substances derived from opium. Semisynthetic derivatives are made by modification of the morphine molecule (heroin and hydromorphone) or alteration of the opium alkaloid thebaine (oxymorphone, oxycodone, nalbuphine, and buprenorphine). Meperidine, methadone, levorphanol, pentazocine, and butorphanol are produced by completely synthetic procedures. Although β-endorphin is found in the pituitary and brain, it is produced by synthetic procedures for clinical (research) use. Metkephamid is a synthetic peptide. The source of the narcotic is ordinarily of little consequence to the practicing physician, unless world events or government policy were to severely limit the availability of opium for legitimate medical use and restrict or eliminate the supplies of morphine, codeine, and the semisynthetics.

Balance of Agonist and Antagonist Activity

In addition to their chemical diversity, the narcotic drugs are also characterized by important pharmacological differences, which are believed to be derived from the complex interactions of these drugs with multiple CNS opiate receptors (38,46,62,70). Operationally, we may consider that, as a result of chemical modifications, narcotic drugs have been produced with properties that vary along a continuous spectrum of pharmacological activity. At one end is morphine and the pure morphine-like agonist drugs, and at the other end of the spectrum are the antagonists such as naloxone. In between we can place drugs with pharmacological properties that require their classification as partial agonists or mixed agonist-antagonists.

The morphine-like agonist drugs identified in Tables 1 and 2 may differ from morphine in quantitative characteristics such as relative analgesic potency, peak, and duration of analgesia or oral potency (see below). Qualitatively, they can be considered to mimic the pharmacological profile of morphine, including both desirable and undesirable effects as given in Table 3.

The mixed agonist-antagonists include pentazocine, butorphanol, and nalbuphine. When administered to patients in pain who have limited prior narcotic experience, they produce analgesia and other narcotic effects characteristic of morphine. However, there is a ceiling on the capacity of mixed agonist-antagonists to produce respiratory depression, and they are considered to have a significantly lower abuse-liability than the morphine-like drugs. They are not, however, devoid of abuse liability, and pentazocine has recently been placed in schedule IV as a controlled substance. In therapeutic doses, they may produce certain self-limiting psychotomimetic effects in some patients. Pentazocine seems to be the worst offender, and nalbuphine the least likely to produce these effects (6,38). It has been suggested that the rate of development of tolerance to their analgesic effect is slower than that seen with the morphine-like drugs (6,38). If this observation is confirmed, it would provide the agonist-antagonists with a significant advantage over the morphine-like drugs.

Patients who have received repeated doses of a morphine-like drug to the point where they are physically dependent may experience a narcotic withdrawal reaction when given a mixed agonist-antagonist. Prior exposure to a morphine-like drug can be shown to greatly increase a patient's sensitivity to the antagonist component of a mixed agonist-antagonist (37,38). Therefore, when used for chronic pain, they should be tried before initiating prolonged administration of a morphine-like drug.

Like the mixed agonist-antagonists, the partial agonist buprenorphine has less abuse liability than the morphine-like drugs and may precipitate narcotic withdrawal in dependent patients. However, buprenorphine does not produce psychotomimetic effects. It is currently marketed in the United Kingdom and soon should be available for use in this country (49,77).

Relative Analgesic Potency

When compared by the intramuscular route, the narcotic-type analgesics listed in Table 1 differ in analgesic potency by a factor of nearly 200 (0.4 mg of buprenorphine is approximately equianalgesic to 75 mg of meperidine). Nevertheless, increased potency alone has not provided any selective advantage, because the more potent drugs also exhibit a parallel increase in their ability to produce undesirable effects. An important distinction must be made between the terms relative analgesic potency and analgesic efficacy. Relative analgesic potency is the ratio of the doses of two analgesics required to produce the same analgesic effect. Analgesic efficacy refers to the level or degree of analgesia that can be achieved by increasing the dose of the drug to the point of limiting side effects. Figure 1 provides an illustration of the determination of relative potency from a study carried out in cancer patients by Beaver et al. (5). The treatment included, in random order, two doses of morphine, two doses of oxymorphone, and a placebo. Analgesia, expressed as a change in pain intensity, is plotted as a function of the logarithm of

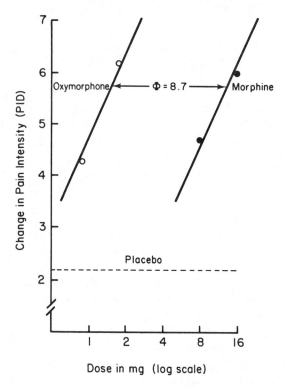

FIG. 1. Dose-response curves for i.m. oxymorphone (○) and morphine (●). Change in pain intensity (pain intensity difference) on the ordinate is plotted against dose in milligrams (mg) on the abscissa. Each point represents the mean effect for a mean dose of morphine or oxymorphone. The lines represent the common slopes plotted through the mean effects for each drug. The dotted line represents the mean placebo score (5).

the dose of each drug. The arrows connect the equieffective doses and phi (ϕ) represents the relative potency estimate. In this study, oxymorphone was found to be nine times more potent than morphine. However, as far as we can tell, oxymorphone is not capable of producing a superior analgesic effect to that of morphine. Based on a body of information gathered from dose-response studies, such as the one shown in Fig. 1, we may conclude that each of the drugs in Table 1 for which relative potency estimates are available, appear to be equally capable of relieving pain in the nontolerant patient, i.e., they are equal in their analgesic effectiveness or efficacy. If we were to compare the ability of morphine and aspirin to relieve severe pain, we would conclude that morphine is not only more potent than aspirin, but that it possesses the potential for exerting a much greater maximum analgesic effect (i.e., has greater analgesic efficacy) than aspirin.

Relative potency estimates provide a rational basis for selecting the appropriate dose when changing the route of administration or the drug. Tables 1 and 2 list the best estimates of the equianalgesic doses for the narcotic-type analgesics. The equianalgesic dose is the recommended starting dose; the optimal dose for each patient being determined by adjustment of the dose. The values in Table 1 are compared to morphine so that it can be used as a common reference when selecting an equieffective dose for any drug listed in the table.

Time-Action of Analgesia

The time-action curve of a narcotic analgesic is the result of many factors, including the dose, the intensity of pain, the criteria for analgesia, individual pharmacokinetic variation (i.e., the patient's ability to absorb, distribute, biotransform, and eliminate the drug), and the patient's prior narcotic experience (37). Therefore, rather than an absolute expression for time-action, the appropriate comparison, as given in Table 1, is the relative duration of action for each analgesic at the dose that produces a peak equivalent to that of morphine. Figure 2 shows the mean data for a comparison of morphine and meperidine after intramuscular administration. Pain relief is plotted as a function of time after drug administration. In this study, drugs produced equivalent peak analgesia at 1 hr, with the duration of action of morphine exceeding that of meperidine. When compared in this manner, no parenteral analgesic has a longer duration of action than morphine, but meperidine, heroin, and hydromorphone appear, on the average, to be slightly shorter acting. It is not always possible to extrapolate these data and predict the duration of action with chronic drug administration. At present, we lack well-controlled comparisons of the influence of pharmacokinetic factors on time-action characteristics of the narcotics when they are given repeatedly, which is the way they are administered for chronic pain (30) (*see* below).

Oral Potency

In the management of chronic pain, the oral route of drug administration avoids the discomfort and potential complications of repeated injections, is more conve-

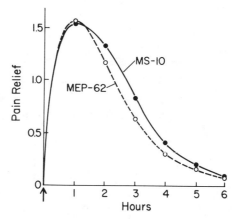

FIG. 2. Time-action curves for intramuscular (I.M.) morphine (MS), and meperidine (MEP). Pain relief scores (ordinate) are plotted against time in hours (abscissa). Each point represents the mean effect for the mean dose of 10 mg of MS (●) or 62 mg of MEP (○). (Houde, R. W., and Wallenstein, S. L. (1958): Proceedings of the 19th meeting of the National Academy of Sciences, National Research Council Committee on Drug Addiction and Narcotics, p. 1794.)

nient, and can provide a smooth curve of action. However, the narcotic drugs differ substantially in the degree to which they are inactivated as they are absorbed from the gastrointestinal tract, and pass through the liver into the systemic circulation (presystemic elimination). Furthermore, not all of the narcotic-type analgesics are biotransformed to inactive metabolites (*see* below). As indicated in Table 1, morphine, hydromorphone, and oxymorphone have oral to intramuscular (po/i.m.) potency ratios of 1/5 to 1/6. The po/i.m. potency ratio is the inverse of the equieffective po/i.m. dose ratio. Methadone, levorphanol, and oxycodone are subject to less presystemic elimination resulting in a po/im potency ratio of at least 1/ 2. Meperidine and pentazocine have intermediate ratios. The failure to recognize these differences often results in a substantial reduction in analgesia when the change from parenteral to oral administration is attempted without upward adjustment of the dose. Consideration of the po/i.m. potency ratio obtained from the equieffective i.m. and po doses, as given in Table 1, provides the starting point for dose titration.

Adverse Effects

Although the narcotic-type analgesics listed in Tables 1 and 2 may vary in chemical structure and in their affinity for the several opioid receptor types, they share the ability to produce a number of adverse effects similar to those described for morphine (Table 3). These include respiratory depression, sedation, and drowsiness, nausea and vomiting, constipation, and spasm of the biliary and urinary tracts. In this section, we will discuss the clinical significance of each of these adverse effects, and point out those drugs where clinical studies support qualitative or quantitative differences from morphine in the occurrence of adverse effects.

Respiratory depression is the most serious adverse effect of these drugs. The morphine-like agonists act on brainstem respiratory centers to produce, as a function of dose, increasing respiratory depression to the point of apnea. In man, death because of an overdose of a morphine-like agonist is nearly always owing to respiratory arrest. Therapeutic doses of morphine may initially depress all phases of respiratory activity (rate, minute volume, and tidal exchange). However, as CO_2 accumulates, it stimulates the respiratory center, resulting in a compensatory increase in respiratory rate, which masks the degree of respiratory depression. At equianalgesic doses, the morphine-like agonists produce an equivalent degree of respiratory depression. For these reasons, individuals with impaired respiratory function or bronchial asthma are at greatest risk of experiencing clinically significant respiratory depression in response to usual doses of these drugs. Respiratory depression and CO_2 retention result in cerebral vasodilation and an increase in cerebrospinal fluid pressure unless PCO_2 is maintained at normal levels by artificial ventilation (*see* Precautions, Table 1). The treatment of narcotic induced respiratory depression is discussed below. The mixed agonist-antagonists (pentazocine, nalbuphine, and butorphanol) and the partial agonist (buprenorphine) appear to differ in the dose-response characteristics of their respiratory depression curves from that of the morphine-like drugs. Therefore, although therapeutic doses of pentazocine produce respiratory depression equivalent to that of morphine, increasing the dose does not ordinarily produce a proportional increase in respiratory depression. Whether this apparent ceiling to respiratory depression offers any clinical advantage remains to be determined. Also, the clinical symptoms of a large overdose of these drugs with particular respect to respiratory depression has not been well defined (48).

The narcotic-type analgesics produce sedation and drowsiness. Although these effects may be useful in certain clinical situations (e.g., preanesthesia), they are not usually desirable concomitants of analgesia, particularly in ambulatory patients. The CNS depressant actions of these drugs can be expected to be at least additive with the sedative and respiratory depressant effects of sedative-hypnotics such as alcohol and the barbiturates. Although it has been suggested that methadone produces more sedation than morphine, this has not been supported by single-dose controlled trials (4) or surveys in hospitalized patients (65). However, the half-life of methadone is substantially longer than morphine, and could result in cumulative CNS depression after repeated doses for pain.

Toxic doses of meperidine and propoxyphene produce not only CNS and respiratory depression, but also CNS excitation that can be manifested as convulsions (*see* below).

The mixed agonist-antagonists, as have already been discussed, produce certain psychotomimetic effects not seen with other narcotic-type analgesics.

The concurrent administration of monoamine oxidase (MAO) inhibitors and meperidine has been reported to result in severe reactions, and even death (64).

The morphine-like drugs produce nausea and vomiting by an action on the medullary chemoreceptor trigger zone. The incidence of nausea and vomiting is markedly increased in ambulatory patients, suggesting that the morphine-like drugs also alter vestibular sensitivity.

The most common adverse effect of the morphine-like drugs is constipation (48). These drugs act at multiple sites in the gastrointestinal tract and in the spinal cord to produce a decrease in intestinal secretions and peristalsis, resulting in a dry stool and constipation. Tolerance develops slowly, so that constipation will continue when the drugs are used repeatedly over time. The morphine-like agonists increase smooth muscle tone and can cause bladder spasm and an increase in sphincter tone, leading to urinary retention. Biliary tract spasms produced by these drugs can cause a marked increase in the pressure in the biliary tract. Clinical studies suggest that apparent equianalgesic doses of meperidine produce less biliary spasms than morphine (48). Nevertheless, Gaensler et al. (26) reported that, in two of their study patients, meperidine produced spasms of the sphincter sufficiently severe to produce a typical attack of biliary colic.

The effects of the morphine-like agonists on the cardiovascular system are generally benign. Morphine causes a decrease in peripheral resistance and an increased capacity of the peripheral vascular compartment (peripheral pooling of blood). These effects may result in orthostatic hypotension and fainting. These same cardiovascular effects reduce the work load on the heart, and, together with its antianxiety action, are believed responsible for the efficacy of morphine in relieving the dyspnea of pulmonary edema secondary to acute left-sided heart failure. Furthermore, by virtue of its ability to decrease myocardial oxygen consumption, cardiac index, left ventricular end-diastolic pressure, and cardiac work morphine can relieve the severe pain of acute myocardial infarction without producing undesirable cardiovascular effects. The cardiovascular responses to pentazocine and butorphanol differ somewhat from those described above for morphine. Pentazocine increases aortic systolic pressure, left ventricular and diastolic pressure, and mean pulmonary artery pressure, and causes an increase in cardiac work. Thus, morphine is the drug of choice for use in patients who have suffered an acute myocardial infarction, except in hypotensive patients, where an increased aortic pressure is desirable.

As has already been discussed, the mixed agonist-antagonists and the partial agonist are capable of precipitating narcotic withdrawal in a patient who is physically dependent on a morphine-like agonist. These drugs also have significantly less abuse liability than morphine-like agonists. Codeine and propoxyphene, although classified with the morphine-like agonists, are considered to have significantly less abuse liability than morphine.

The endorphins have been the subject of only a few controlled clinical trials. Calimlim et al. (10) found that, in addition to morphine-like side effects (e.g., drowsiness), adverse effects unique to metkephamid include a sensation of burning at the injection site, fatigue, dry mouth, and nasal congestion. These adverse effects do not appear to be disturbing to patients (10). Additional controlled studies of the endorphins are needed to provide a more complete understanding of their spectrum of pharmacodynamic effects, so that an informed judgment can be made of the role, if any, of exogenously administered endorphins in the management of pain.

Biotransformation to Active Metabolites

The narcotic-type analgesics are primarily eliminated by hepatic biotransformation to inactive metabolites. Certain narcotic-type analgesics (Table 4) are biotransformed to active metabolites that may contribute to the therapeutic or toxic effects seen after administration of the parent drug.

Dispositional studies demonstrating the presence of morphine in the plasma and urine of individuals given codeine, and the very low affinity of codeine for the opiate receptor, support the contention that the analgesic effect of codeine may be due, in large part, to its conversion to morphine (48). In man, heroin given by intravenous injection or infusion, is rapidly biotransformed into acetylmorphine and morphine (40,41,50). Both of these active metabolites appear to make a significant contribution to the duration of the analgesic effects of heroin (40,41). Oxymorphone can be found in the urine of subjects who have received oxycodone (12). Propoxyphene is biotransformed to norpropoxyphene, a metabolite practically devoid of analgesic activity but capable of producing cardiotoxicity in animals (60). Both propoxyphene and norpropoxyphene accumulate during repeated dosing, and therefore, both may contribute to the symptoms of propoxyphene poisoning (44). Chronic administration of large parenteral doses of meperidine (e.g., 250 mg or more per day) results in the accumulation, most rapidly in patients with compromised renal function, of normeperidine, a toxic metabolite (43,51,82). Normeperidine-induced toxicity is characterized by CNS excitation, including shaky feelings, tremors, twitches, and/or convulsions (43,51). The pharmacokinetic and pharmacodynamic factors associated with CNS toxicity in patients receiving meperidine, and the prevention and treatment of this adverse reaction has been reviewed (43).

Pharmacokinetics

The narcotic-type analgesics may differ in their pharmocokinetic characteristics as represented by the plasma elimination half-life, so that methadone, levorphanol, and propoxyphene have relatively long plasma elimination half-lives compared with morphine (Table 5). When the duration of action of a single dose of parenteral

TABLE 4. *Active metabolites of narcotic-type analgesics*

Parent drug	Active metabolite
Codeine	Morphine
Heroin	Acetylmorphine and morphine
Oxycodone	Oxymorphone
Meperidine	Normeperidine
Propoxyphene	Norpropoxyphene

TABLE 5. *Plasma half-life values for narcotic-type analgesics*

Drug	Plasma half-life (hr)
Morphine	2–3.5
Meperidine	3–4
Normeperidine	14–21
Methadone	15–30
Levorphanol	12–16
Heroin[a]	.05
Hydromorphone	2–3
Pentazocine	2–3
Nalbuphine	5
Butorphanol	2.5–3.5
Codeine	3
Propoxyphene	12
Norpropoxyphene	30–40

[a]Biotransformed to acetylmorphine and morphine.
[b]From Inturrisi, (42).

methodone or levorphanol is compared with that of morphine (Table 1), it is obvious that their long half-lives are not reflected in the duration of analgesia seen after a single dose. However, the longer half-life drugs will accumulate with repetitive dosing so that some adjustment of dose and interval may be necessary with methadone or levorphanol to prevent excessive sedation. Much more information is required before definite guidelines can be drawn.

Cirrhosis

Many narcotic-type analgesics can undergo substantial biotransformation in the gastrointestinal tract or liver before reaching the systemic circulation. This presystemic elimination or first-pass effect results in the low bioavailability (30%) of oral morphine, and is reflected in the relatively poor oral analgesic potency reported for morphine in single dose analgesic assays (Table 1). In healthy individuals, virtually all the blood perfusing the areas of the GI tract, from which orally administered drugs are absorbed, passes into the portal vein and through the liver. In cirrhotic patients, a collateral circulation develops. Shunting can occur, resulting in a pronounced increase in the systemic availability, and a decrease in the systemic clearance of drugs subject to an extensive first-pass effect. Pharmacokinetic studies comparing normal and cirrhotic patients have revealed that meperidine (74), pentazocine (68), and propoxyphene (28) have increased bioavailability and half-life, and a decreased systemic clearance in cirrhotics. Thus, both absorption and elimination of these drugs is altered in cirrhotics so as to favor accumulation. Furthermore, although the cirrhosis-induced decrease in systemic clearance results in a decreased rate of formation of active metabolites (normeperidine from meperidine and norpropoxyphene from propoxyphene) cirrhotics may actually be at increased risk of metabolite-induced cumulative toxicity, owing to the slower than normal rate of metabolite elimination. In contrast, Patwardan et al. (71) found that the disposition and elimination of morphine are unchanged in cirrhotic patients. This unexpected finding suggests that morphine probably undergoes substantial extra-heptic metabolism, which is presumably unchanged by cirrhosis.

Renal disease

Renal excretion is a major route of elimination for the active metabolites, nor-porpoxyphene and normeperidine (*see* Table 4). The elimination of these metab-olites is decreased in patients with renal failure, resulting in accumulation (43,44).

Age

Berkowitz et al. (7) found that the initial serum levels of morphine were higher in patients over 50 yr of age, compared with younger surgical patients. The serum elimination half-life of morphine was not age dependent. Whether the difference in initial serum morphine levels is indicative of a decrease of morphine clearance in older patients was not explored.

Kaiko et al. (54) have reviewed the seven pharmacokinetic studies of intravenous morphine in adults. Unfortunately, no single study allows a direct comparison of the same type of patient as a function of age. The pooled data suggest that the clearance of morphine is twice as rapid in subjects with a mean age under 50, compared with subjects older than 50 yr of age.

Modification of the enzymes of biotransformation

The concurrent administration of drugs that induce the hepatic mixed function oxidase system can alter the disposition of certain narcotics. The metabolism of meperidine is increased by phenytoin (73) and that of methadone is increased by rifampin (56).

Overview

The pharmacokinetic studies cited above demonstrate that cirrhotic patients and renal failure patients are at a greater risk of accumulating pentazocine, meperidine, propoxyphene, and their active metabolites than normals, and that age or exposure to enzyme-inducing agents may modify the disposition of morphine or meperidine. Studies that have measured drug disposition and adverse effects in the same patients have demonstrated that the accumulation of normeperidine after meperidine admin-istration results in CNS toxicity (51). Cirrhotics (57), renal failure patients (18), and the aged (52) have been reported to exhibit increased CNS sensitivity to narcotic-type analgesics. Additional studies are needed to begin to define the relative contribution of pharmacokinetic factors and changes in intrinsic CNS sensitivity to responses to narcotic-type analgesics seen in these groups of patients. At present, these drugs should be used with caution in cirrhotics, renal failure patients, or the aged. Also, it would seem prudent to avoid drugs such as meperidine and propoxyphene that impose the added burden of active metabolites.

Pharmaceutical Properties

The development of tolerance to narcotic-type analgesics is manifest as a shift to the right along the log dose axis. A fixed incremental increase in dose, although initially adequate, may prove insufficient with the development of tolerance. In the tolerant patient, the availability of a suitable parenteral dosage form that can provide adequate pain relief without the necessity of injecting an unreasonably large volume of solution into a cachectic patient, may greatly restrict the drug choice. Table 6 lists the available narcotic-type analgesics, their equianalgesic dose, and the parenteral form, providing the maximum drug concentration per milliliter of solution. From this information, the maximum number of analgesic equivalents that are available per milliliter of solution has been calculated (Table 6). With the exception of morphine and codeine, the narcotic analgesics are available only as fixed dose solutions (Table 6), and therefore subject to volume limitations. While morphine and codeine are available as soluble tablets, they are less soluble than other narcotic-type analgesics (*see* below), so that solubility considerations preclude the administration of morphine concentrations greater than 65 mg/ml (6). Hydromorphone, which is approximately five times more soluble and nearly seven times more potent than morphine, could provide the flexibility required for dose titration in the tolerant patient. The recently introduced 10 mg/ml parenteral dose form is an important step in this direction. Hydromorphone's pharmacologic profile (Table 1) and pharmaceutical properties (Table 6) indicate that in the tolerant cancer patient, it could serve the same role as does heroin in the United Kingdom (59,85).

Table 7 provides information on the analgesic equivalents predicted for oral preparations of narcotic analgesics. It is worth noting, that because of the reduced potency of orally administered narcotics (Table 1), a single unit oral dosage form will provide considerably less analgesic equivalent than the parenteral form (Table 6). As with the parenteral forms, the unavailability of more concentrated dosage

TABLE 6. *Narcotic-type analgesics: dosage forms available for parenteral administration*

Drug	Equianalgesic dose (mg)	Parenteral form[a] (mg/ml)	Equivalents per ml
Morphine	10	30[b]	3.0
Meperidine	75	100	1.3
Methadone	10	10	1.0
Levorphanol	2	2	1.0
Hydromorphone	1.5	10	6.7
Oxymorphone	1	1.5	1.5
Codeine	130	60[b]	0.46
Pentazocine	60	30	0.5
Nalbuphine	10	10	1.0
Butorphanol	2	2	1.0

[a]Maximum available concentration.
[b]Soluble tablet.

TABLE 7. *Narcotic-type analgesics: dosage forms available for oral administration*

Drug	Equianalgesic dose	Dosage form	Equivalents per Tab[a] or 5 ml. OS[b]
Morphine	60	Tab—30 mg	0.50
Morphine	60	OS—20 mg/5 ml	0.33
Meperidine	300[c]	Tab—100 mg	0.33
Meperidine	300[c]	OS—50 mg/5 ml	0.17
Methadone	20	Tab—10 mg	0.50
Methadone	20	OS—5 mg/5 ml	0.25
Levorphanol	4	Tab— 2 mg	0.50
Hydromorphone	7.5	Tab— 4 mg	0.53
Pentazocine	180[c]	Tab—50 mg	0.28
Oxycodone	30	OS—5 mg/5 ml	0.17

[a]Tab, tablet.
[b]OS, oral solution.
[c]not recommended (see text).

forms may, to some degree, limit the use of the oral route in certain tolerant patients (*see* below).

CLINICAL USE OF NARCOTIC ANALGESICS: PRACTICAL CONSIDERATIONS

The major goal of effective pain therapy should be to enable the patients to tolerate the necessary diagnostic and therapeutic approaches to assess the nature of pain, or in patients for whom the treatment of the cause of pain has not been effective, to treat the pain symptom and to allow the patient to remain as functional as possible. Any practical approach must be individualized for each patient to provide optimal pain control. Some general guidelines for the rational use of narcotic-type analgesics are detailed below.

Treat the Patient Not the Symptom

The physician tries to believe the patient's report of pain. Through a careful history, physical and neurological examination, the physician can place this pain complaint in the total evaluation of the patient. Are anxiety and depression playing a major role in the patient's pain complaint? What does the patient fear? What does the pain signify? Does the complaint merely represent a cry for help in a patient with masked depression?

To date, there is no battery of psychological tests which provide more useful information than those obtained from a structured psychiatric interview of the patient with pain. It is also of particular importance to recognize that no matter how anxious or depressed the patient, how bizarre the symptomatology, the physician must carefully evaluate the symptoms, and attempt to establish or rule out the presence or absence of a physiological basis for pain. In the process of evaluating the patient with pain, analgesics represent the mainstay of therapy. However, pain treatment both during the evaluation, and when the nature of the pain is understood, does not stop with a prescription. It requires a commitment by the physician to help the patient achieve adequate pain control.

Start with a Specific Drug for a Specific Type of Pain

In patients with acute, severe pain, parenteral morphine is the drug of choice. In patients with mild to moderate pain, an oral analgesic such as codeine, oxycodone, or meperidine is the appropriate choice as listed in Table 2. The choice of a narcotic-type analgesic depends on the patient's prior narcotic experience as well as on his/her current physical and neurologic status, all of which must be fully assessed to provide adequate prescribing practices. Each patient must be given an adequate trial of one drug before switching to an alternative agent. Such a trial should include administration of the drug at regular intervals to maximum levels. The doses described in Tables 1 and 2 are those which represent recommended starting doses. The effective dose to control pain must be determined in the individual patient. The dose that produces analgesia is the dose appropriate to the individual patient. There is significant variation among patients in their response to pain medication, as this results in part from the fact that drug disposition shows marked individual variation (1,7,9,39,80). To fully assess whether a drug can produce effective analgesia in the individual patient, the doses should be escalated until limiting side effects occur.

Know the Pharmacology of the Drug Prescribed

Know the type of drug

The narcotic mixed agonist-antagonist drugs such as pentazocine produce psychotomimetic effects with increasing doses. Although pentazocine has less abuse potential than some of the commonly used narcotic agonists, these psychotomimetic effects limit its clinical usefulness.

Know the duration of the analgesic effect

The duration of the analgesic effect varies with the drug and its route of administration. Tables 1 and 2 list the time course for the commonly-used drugs. Each drug has a specific time course, for example, Percocet or Percodan (oxycodone 5 mg plus acetaminophen or aspirin) only acts for 3 to 4 hr in contrast to morphine, methadone, or levorphanol which produce analgesia for 4 to 6 hr. In general, drugs administered by mouth have a slower onset of action and a longer duration of effect, whereas drugs given parenterally have a rapid onset of action but with a shorter duration of effect. Recognition of these differences will allow for appropriate prescribing techniques.

Know the pharmacokinetics of the drug

The plasma half-life of the narcotics vary widely and do not correlate with the analgesic time course. Narcotics such as methadone (half-life 15 to 30 hr) (39) and levorphanol (half-life 12–16 hr) (15,16) produce analgesia for 4 to 6 hr, and must be given at 4 to 6 hr intervals to maintain adequate analgesia. However, with repetitive dosing, these drugs, with long plasma half-lives, may accumulate in plasma. Such accumulation may account for the untoward effects of sedation and respiratory depression (17,81). In using such drugs, adjustment of dose and dosing interval, based on the plasma half-life, may be necessary during introduction of the drug. The plasma half-life can be altered by both compromised hepatic and renal failure as previously discussed. Dose adjustment and dosing interval must be individualized to provide maximal analgesic effects. In the elderly patient, one-half the recommended starting dose should be given initially because of the effects of age on drug clearance (54).

Know the equianalgesic doses for the drug and its route of administration

When switching from one narcotic-type analgesic to another, and from one route of administration to another, knowledge of these equianalgesic doses can ensure more appropriate drug use. Lack of attention to these differences in drug dose is the most common cause of undermedication of pain patients (61). Lack of knowledge of these differences in equianalgesic doses can also lead to overmedication of patients. This occurs when the oral doses are given by the parenteral route, as in the case of the patient who, in the hospital, can no longer tolerate oral drugs. The doses are detailed in Tables 1 and 2. In patients who have been receiving one narcotic-type analgesic chronically, and are then switched to another narcotic for better analgesia, halving the equianalgesic dose of the new drug has usually provided effective analgesia. As previously discussed, cross-tolerance is not complete. From our clinical experience, this is most commonly seen when switching from drugs such as morphine, hydromorphone, and levorphanol to methadone. This clinical experience suggests that the relative potency of some of the narcotic-type analgesics may change with repetitive doses. Controlled studies to assess this are currently in progress.

Administer Analgesics Regularly

In general, medication should be administered on a regular basis which, if necessary, should include awakening the patient from sleep. This approach will help maintain the patient's pain at a tolerable level. It may also allow for the reduction in the total amount of drug taken in a 24-hr period. Studies suggest that such an approach reduces abnormal pain behavior in a hospitalized patient. When patients are given control of their analgesic regimen in the hospital, effective pain management can be achieved (14,24). The pharmacological rationale is to maintain the plasma level of the drug above the "minimal effective concentration" for pain relief (1). Before accepting that a narcotic-type analgesic is ineffective in an individual patient, the drug should be given on a regular basis with the interval between the doses based on the duration of effect of the drug. This approach will allow the patient to reach a "steady state" of plasma drug concentration. The time to reach a steady state level depends upon the half-life of a drug. For example, with morphine, steady state levels can be reached with five to six doses in a 24-hr period. Whereas, with repeated doses of methadone, it may take up to 5 to 7 days to reach "steady state." Therefore, full assessment of the analgesic efficacy of a drug regimen can not be completed in a 1- or 2-day period. Therefore, both patient and physician must recognize that adequate pain control requires time. Both patient and physician must be "patient" in developing the best analgesic dose and dosing schedule. For patients receiving methadone, it has been observed that once they reach steady state, they require a smaller amount of the drug than initially prescribed to control pain (78).

Use a Combination of Drugs

This approach is based on the fact that when a narcotic is combined with a non-narcotic and certain adjuvant analgesic drugs, additive analgesia occurs. Such an approach, then, enables the physician to enhance the patient's analgesia without escalation of the narcotic dose.

Narcotic + non-narcotic

The addition of 650 mg of aspirin or acetaminophen to the standard narcotic dose on a regular basis will produce additive analgesia (2,35).

Narcotic + an antihistamine, hydroxyzine

Studies by Beaver (3) have demonstrated that hydroxyzine (Vistaril) produces additive analgesic effects when compared with morphine. Pain relief from 100 mg of hydroxyzine i.m. combined with 8 mg morphine sulfate i.m. was statistically superior to 8 mg of morphine sulfate alone, 100 mg of hydroxyzine alone, and placebo. The sedative effect of the combination was only slightly greater than that of morphine alone. In clinical practice, hydroxyzine, 25 mg p.o., in combination with a narcotic has been used on a regular basis with the anecdotal observations that it is an effective analgesic combination. Studies to evaluate this dose in such a combination are currently not available.

Narcotic and an amphetamine

In single dose studies, 10 mg of i.m. Dexedrine combined with 10 mg i.m. morphine counteracted the sedative effects of morphine and enhanced its analgesic effects (25). Repeated dose studies are lacking. From clinical experience, amphetamine in 5-mg doses twice a day can often be effective to reduce the sedation in the patient excessively sedated, but receiving adequate analgesia.

Narcotic plus a tricyclic antidepressant, amitriptyline

In animal studies (8), amitriptyline produces additive analgesic effects with morphine. Comparable studies in man are lacking. In patients with migraine (13), and in patients with postherpetic neuralgia (84,89), doses of amitriptyline in a 25 to 75 mg range were associated with analgesic effects, and occurred independent of any significant alterations in mood, specifically depression. In the management of patients with cancer pain, amitriptyline in doses of 10 to 50 mg is used as the primary sleeping medication.

It is a potent hypnotic, and in low doses has analgesic properties. Again, anecdotally, it has been a useful additional drug to control cancer pain.

Narcotic plus a benzodiazepine, diazepam

Controlled studies in patients with postoperative pain demonstrate that diazepam does not produce additive analgesic effects with morphine but does produce additive sedative effects (79). There is some evidence to suggest that the benzodiazepines may have antianalgesic properties (31).

Narcotic plus cocaine

Studies by Mount et al. (67) and Twycross (86,87) have demonstrated that cocaine, when combined with a narcotic in the Brompton mixture, does not provide additive analgesic effects. Animal studies (69), however, suggest that cocaine does potentiate narcotic analgesia, but the appropriate clinical studies have not been done.

Narcotic and a phenothiazine, chlorpromazine

Studies of Houde and Wallenstein (32) demonstrate that chlorpromazine administered in doses of 25 mg i.m. did not enhance the analgesic activity of morphine. It did, however, enhance the sedative effects. In some instances, the sedative effects of certain drugs may act to limit the amount of narcotic analgesic used (66). This is often a disservice to a patient who is over-sedated with drugs that are not primarily analgesics. Recognition of the usefulness of certain combinations of drugs that provide analgesia can improve the success of the analgesic regimen.

Gear the Route of Administration to the Patient's Needs

Orally administered drugs have a slower onset of action than parenterally administered drugs. In the patient who requires immediate relief, parenteral administration, either i.m. or i.v., is the route of choice. The rectal route of administration should be considered for patients who cannot take oral drugs, or in patients for whom parenteral administration is contraindicated. Intravenous administration of a narcotic produces the most rapid onset of action, with analgesia occurring within 10 to 15 min of injection; however, the duration of analgesia is also markedly reduced, requiring frequent dosing at 1 or 2 hr intervals. Continuous infusions of narcotic drugs play an important role in the management of patients with certain chronic states, specifically, children with acute or chronic pain, and adults and children with terminal illness. Such infusions maintain smooth analgesic control, obviating the difficulties of erratic absorption by the oral or parenteral route, particularly in patients with either significant GI disturbances or limited muscle mass. Several types of infusions by various routes are currently in use: intravenous, subcutaneous, epidural, and intrathecal (11,53,63,83). With intravenous infusions, the starting dose varies with the drug, and is approximately one-half the parenteral dose, calculated according to the patient's prior narcotic experience, and adjusted to the individual needs. Subcutaneous infusions, using 25 gauge butterfly needles attached to the currently available insulin infusion pumps, can be used to provide analgesia in patients who require parenteral drug administration, but in whom repetitive injections are traumatic (children) or contraindicated. Epidural and intrathecal infusions are currently experimental approaches, and their role in the management of patients with chronic pain remains controversial (53,63).

Treat the Side Effects Appropriately

Since the side effects of the narcotic-type analgesics often limit their effective use, careful attention to managing them is essential. The most common side effects include sedation, respiratory depression, nausea, vomiting, and constipation.

Sedation

This effect varies with the drug and dose, but occurs most commonly with repeated administration of drugs with long plasma half-lives, such as levorphanol and methadone. Switching to a drug with a short plasma half-life, or reducing the individual drug's dose, while giving it more frequently, are the approaches that may obviate this side effect. For example, in a patient receiving 20 mg of morphine i.m. every 4 hr, the use of 10 mg of morphine i.m. every 2 hr may obviate this effect. Amphetamines, in combination with a narcotic, have been reported to counteract the sedative effects of the narcotic-type analgesics (25). It is also important to discontinue all other drugs which might exacerbate the sedative effects of the narcotic-type analgesics. These include a wide variety of medications, such as cimetidine, barbiturates, and other anxiolytic medications.

Respiratory depression

This effect occurs most commonly in patients following acute administration of the narcotic, and is associated with other signs of CNS depression, including sedation and mental clouding. Tolerance develops rapidly to this effect with repeated drug administration, allowing the narcotic-type analgesics to be used chronically in the management of certain pain states without significant risk of respiratory depression. If respiratory depression occurs, it can be reversed by administering the specific narcotic antagonist, naloxone. The dose suggested is 0.4 mg per cc of naloxone. Naloxone is a short-acting drug, and repeated administration, including an i.v. drip, may be necessary to prevent respiratory arrest in such patients. In patients chronically receiving narcotics who develop respiratory depression, diluted doses of naloxone (0.4 mg in 10 cc of saline) should be titrated carefully to prevent the precipitation of severe withdrawal symptoms, while reversing the respiratory depression. In certain patients, the use of naloxone to reverse drug-induced respiratory depression can be dangerous. An endotracheal tube should be placed in the comatose patient before administering naloxone. This is done to prevent aspiration associated with respiratory compromise with excessive salivation and bronchial spasm. In patients receiving meperidine chronically, naloxone may precipitate seizures by lowering the seizure threshold, allowing the convulsant activity of the active metabolite normeperidine, to become evident (43,51). In this instance, special attention to this potential seizure effect must be taken. If naloxone is to be used, diluted doses slowly titrated with appropriate seizure precautions are advised. There is insufficient clinical experience to make specific recommendations. If respiratory support can be effected by other means, e.g. continuous stimulation to maintain the patient's wakefulness, such approaches may place the patient at less risk.

Nausea and vomiting

Tolerance develops to these side effects with repeated administration. Nausea with one drug does not mean that all narcotic-type analgesics will produce similar symptoms, because the ability of the narcotic-type analgesic to produce nausea and vomiting varies from drug to drug and patient to patient. Switching to alternative narcotic-type analgesics, or using an antiemetic in combination with the narcotic-type analgesic, are methods to obviate this side effect.

Constipation

At the same time that narcotic-type analgesics are started, provisions for a regular bowel regimen, including cathartics and stool softeners should be instituted to prevent this inevitable side effect. Certain bowel regimens have been suggested because of their specific effects to counteract the narcotic drugs, but none of these have been studied in any carefully controlled way (45,88). The anecdotal surveys suggest that doses far above those used for routine bowel management are necessary to counteract the constipatory effects of the narcotics. Careful attention to dietary factors along with the use of a bowel regimen can dramatically reduce patients complaints. Similarly, tolerance develops to this effect over time.

Watch for the Development of Tolerance

In all patients taking narcotic drugs chronically, tolerance will occur within days of starting drug therapy. The earliest sign of development of tolerance is the patient's complaint that the duration of effective analgesia has decreased. In such cases, increasing the frequency of drug administration, or increasing the amount of drug at each dose are necessary to overcome tolerance. There is no limit to tolerance, but escalation of drug dosage often requires almost doubling the dose to produce a better analgesic effect. From our clinical experience, patients can and do continue to obtain analgesia. The dose of the drug should not be the major concern of the prescribing physician. This phenomenon is seen most often in the terminally ill cancer patient who may require and "tolerate" huge doses of narcotics, up to 200 mg of i.v. morphine per hr. In our clinical experience, i.v. administration of narcotics produces rapid development of tolerance with patients requiring escalation of the drug dose every 12 to 24 hr to maintain adequate analgesia. This phenomenon is not well understood, but it has led us to use intravenous narcotics as a second line approach while attempting to maximize oral use of the drugs. In Table 7, the dosage forms available for oral administration are listed. When either the number of tablets or the volume of the oral solution is poorly tolerated by the patient, we usually crush the drugs into powder form and mix it in a fruit mixture, or take the parenteral preparation and give it orally mixed with a palatable syrup. These practical methods can allow for prolonged oral dosing. Since cross-tolerance among the narcotic-type analgesics is not complete, switching from one narcotic drug to another, often improves the analgesic effect, and in an individual patient can provide more adequate pain control. This is best done by switching to an alternative narcotic drug using a dose of one-half the equianalgesic dose. Escalation or reduction of the dose then follows according to the drug's analgesic efficacy. Another alternative to consider in treating the patient who is tolerant is to add a non-narcotic analgesic to the narcotic regimen. Such an approach may provide additive analgesia without escalating the dose of the narcotic drug. A third alternative is to use a phenothiazine analgesic such as methotrimeprazine to produce analgesia. This drug works through a nonopiate receptor system, and therefore produces analgesia in patients tolerant to the narcotic-type analgesics. Methotrimeprazine, 15 mg, i.m., is equivalent to 15 mg of morphine i.m. (58). This drug may produce excessive sedation and postural hypotension, and should therefore be used with caution in the management of the tolerant patient. Finally, in patients with localized pain in the buttocks or lower extremities, the use of continuous epidural infusions of a local anesthetic can produce significant analgesia to allow the narcotic analgesics to be reduced. This provides a method to reverse tolerance in the cancer patient who is chronically receiving narcotics.

Withdraw the Medication Slowly

Abrupt withdrawal of medication in a patient receiving narcotic-type analgesics chronically will produce signs and symptoms of withdrawal characterized by agitation, tremors, insomnia, fever, and marked autonomic nervous system hyperexcitability. Slowly tapering the dose of the narcotic-type analgesic will prevent such symptomatology. The appearance of abstinence symptoms from the time of drug withdrawal is related to the elimination curve of the particular drug. The nature of the abstinence symptoms similarly varies with the individual drug; for example, with morphine, withdrawal symptoms will occur within 6 to 12 hr after cessation of the drug. Reinstituting the drug in doses of approximately 25% of the previous daily dose will suppress these symptoms.

Respect Individual Differences Among Patients

The disposition of narcotic drugs is so variable that individual variations in analgesia and side effects commonly have a pharmacologic basis and are not caused by the psychological state of the patients. All attempts should be made to optimize therapy for the individual patient.

Do Not Use Placebos to Assess the Nature of the Pain

The placebo response is a potent phenomenon in clinical medicine, although its appropriate use is not widely recognized (29). In a patient with pain, a positive analgesic effect from i.m. saline suggests that the patient is a placebo responder. It does not suggest that the pain is unreal or less severe than is reported by the patient. Such misuse of placebos tends to allow the development of distrust between the patient and the physician. This can interfere with adequate pain control.

Complications

Major complications of narcotic-type analgesics are considered briefly. These include overdose, tolerance and physical dependence, psychological dependence or addiction, and multifocal myoclonous and seizures. Overdose with the narcotic-type analgesics occurs in two forms: intentional, when the patient takes an excessive amount of a drug in a suicide attempt, street abuse of narcotics, or unintentionally, when the recommended doses accidentally produce excessive sedation and respiratory depression. In both instances, this complication can be effectively treated with the use of a narcotic antagonist as outlined previously. Overdose in patients previously stabilized on a narcotic regimen for pain is rarely caused by drug intake alone. More commonly it is the medical deterioration of the patient with a superimposed metabolic encephalopathy. This occurs most commonly in cancer patients. Reduction of the narcotic drug dosage, and careful assessment of the patient's metabolic status will usually provide the differential diagnosis. Psychological dependence or addiction is characterized by a concomitant behavioral pattern of drug abuse, characterized by craving a drug for other than pain relief, and becoming overwhelmingly involved in the use and procurement of the drug. This is a distinct state from tolerance and physical dependence, which are responses to the pharmacologic effects of chronic narcotic administration. Fear of addiction limits the use of narcotic analgesics in clinical practice (20,61). In fact, there is little available published data to determine the degree of tolerance, physical dependence, substance abuse, or addiction in patients receiving narcotic analgesics for chronic illness and pain. Many of the published studies do not adhere to strict definitions for drug use and abuse, making any review of such data practically impossible; however, studies by Pescor (72) and Rayport (76) suggested that there was a high incidence of drug addiction in patients with chronic medical illness. Their studies, however, present a biased view of the subject, because narcotic addicts admitted to treatment facilities were used as subjects of the studies. In more recent prospective studies by Porter and Jick (75), 39,946 hospitalized medical patients were monitored for the incidence of narcotic addiction. Of 11,882 who received at least one narcotic preparation, there were only 4 cases of reasonably well-documented addiction in patients who had no history of addiction. These data, taken from a survey of a general population, suggest that medical use of narcotics is rarely, if ever, associated with the development of addiction. The dearth of clinical studies, therefore, offer limited support to the belief that chronic narcotic use for analgesia is associated with the high risk of addiction. Analysis of the patterns of drug intake in our series of cancer paitents (55) suggests that drug abuse and drug addiction should not be the primary concern of the prescribing physician. Our data suggest that drug use alone is not the major factor in the development of addiction, but other medical, social, and economic conditions seem to play an important role. This phenomenon has been well supported by studies of U.S. military personnel addicted to opiates in Vietnam.

Signs and symptoms of central nervous hyperirritability can occur with toxic doses of all the narcotic-type analgesics. Multifocal myoclonous and seizures have been reported in patients receiving multiple doses of meperidine. In these patients, accumulation of the active metabolite, normeperidine, produces CNS hyperirritability (43,51,82), as discussed above.

SUMMARY

Narcotic analgesics represent the mainstay of therapy in the management of patients with acute and chronic pain. There is no question that chronic painful medical illness represents a difficult clinical problem for both the patient and physician. A careful attempt to evaluate the usefulness, the appropriate role, and long-term effects of narcotic analgesics in this population may allow us to adequately treat patients with both acute and chronic pain on a more scientific and less anecdotal and fearful basis.

ACKNOWLEDGMENTS

This work was supported in part by the Patricia Drake Hemingway Fund and USPHS grants DA-01707, DA-01457, and CA-32897. Dr. Foley is a Rita Allen Scholar.

REFERENCES

1. Aherne, G. W., Pial, E. M., and Twycross, R. G. (1979): Serum morphine concentrations after oral administration of diamorphine hydrochloride and morphine sulfate. *Br. J. Pharmacol.*, 8:577–850.
2. Beaver, W. T. (1965): Mild analgesics: A review of their clinical pharmacology. *Am. J. Med. Sci.*, 251:576–599.
3. Beaver, W. T. (1967): Comparison of analgesic effects of morphine sulfate, hydroxyzine and their combination in patients with postoperative pain. In: *Advances in Pain Research and Therapy, Vol. 2*, edited by J. J. Bonica and V. Ventafridda, pp. 553–557. Raven Press, New York.
4. Beaver, W. T., Wallenstein, S. L., Houde, R. W., and Rogers, A. (1967): A clinical comparison

of the analgesic effects of methadone and morphine administered intramuscularly, and of orally and parenterally administered methadone. *Clin. Pharmacol. Ther.*, 8:415–426.

5. Beaver, W. T., Wallenstein, S. L., Houde, R. W., and Rogers, A. (1977): Comparisons of the analgesic effects of oral and intramuscular oxymorphone and of intramuscular oxymorphone and morphine in patients with cancer. *J. Clin. Pharmacol.*, 17:186–198.

6. Beaver, W. T. (1980): Management of cancer pain with parenteral medication. *J.A.M.A.*, 244:2653–2657.

7. Berkowitz, B. A., Ngai, S. H., Yang, J. C., Hempstead, J., and Spector, S. (1975): The disposition of morphine in surgical patients. *Clin. Pharmacol. Ther.*, 17:629–635.

8. Botney, M., and Fields, H. L. (1983): Amitriptyline potentiates morphine analgesia by a direct action on the central nervous system. *Ann. Neurol.*, 13:160–164.

9. Brunk, S. F., and Delle, M. (1974): Morphine metabolism in man. *Clin. Pharmacol. Ther.*, 16:51–57.

10. Calimlim, J. F., Wardell, W. M., Sriwatanakul, K., Lasagna, L., and Cox, C. (1982): Analgesic efficacy of parenteral metkephamid acetate in treatment of postoperative pain. *Lancet*, 1374–1375.

11. Campbell, C. F., Mason, J. B., and Weiler, J. M. (1983): Continuous subcutaneous infusion of morphine for the pain of terminal malignancy. *Ann. Int. Med.*, 98:51–52.

12. Cone, E. J. (1982): Personal communication.

13. Couch, J. R., Ziergler, D. R. T., and Hassanein, R. (1976): Amitriptyline on the prophylaxis of migraine. *Neurology*, 26:121–127.

14. Coyle, N. (1979): Analgesics at the bedside. *Am. J. Nurs.*, 112:1154–1157.

15. Dixon, R., Crews, T., Mohacsi, E., Inturrisi, C., and Foley, K. (1981): Levorphanol: A simplified radioimmunoassay for clinical use. *Res. Commun. Chem. Pathol. Pharmacol.*, 32:545–548.

16. Dixon, R., Crews, T., Mohacsi, E., Inturrisi, C., and Foley, K. (1980): Levorphanol: radioimmunoassay and plasma concentration profiles in dog and man. *Res. Commun. Chem. Pathol. Pharmacol.*, 29:535–547.

17. Ettinger, D. S., Vitale, P. J., and Trump, D. C. (1979): Important clinical pharmacologic considerations in the use of methadone in cancer patients. *Cancer Treat. Rev.*, 63:457–459.

18. Fabre, J., and Balont, L. (1976): Renal failure, drug pharmacokinetics and drug action. *Clin. Pharmacokinet.*, 1:99–120.

19. Foley, K. M., and Posner, J. B. (1976): Pain. In: *American Academy of Neurology Review Book*, pp. 199–217. American Academy of Neurology, Minneapolis.

20. Foley, K. M. (1979): The management of pain of malignant origin. In: *Current Neurology, Vol. 2*, edited by H. R. Tyler and D. M. Dawson, pp. 279–302. Houghton Mifflin, Boston.

21. Foley, K. M., Kourides, I. A., Inturrisi, C. E., Kaiko, R. F., Zaroulis, C. G., Posner, J. B., Houde, R. W., and Li, C. H. (1979): B-Endorphin: Analgesic and hormonal effects in humans. *Proc. Natl. Acad. Sci. U.S.A.*, 76:5377–5381.

22. Foley, K. M. (1981): Current controversies in the management of cancer pain. In: *New Approaches to Treatment of Chronic Pain. National Institute of Drug Abuse Research Series*, edited by K. Y. Ng, #36, pp. 169–181. Rockville, Maryland.

23. Foley, K. M. (1982): The practical use of narcotic analgesics. In: *The Medical Clinics of North America*, edited by M. M. Reidenberg, pp. 1091–1104. W. B. Saunders Co., Philadelphia.

24. Fordyce, W. E., Fowles, R. S., Lehmann, J., et al. (1973): Operant conditioning in the treatment of chronic pain. *Arch. Phys. Med. Rehab.*, 54:399–408.

25. Forrest, W. H., et al. (1977): Dextroamphetamine with morphine for the treatment of postoperative pain. *N. Engl. J. Med.*, 296:712–715.

26. Gaensler, E. A., McGowan, J. M., and Henderoen, F. F. (1948): A comparative study of the action of demerol and opium alkaloids in relation to biliary spasm. *Surgery*, 23:211–220.

27. Gerbershagen, H. U. (1979): Non-narcotic analgesics. In: *Advances in Pain Research and Therapy, Vol. 2*, edited by J. J. Bonica, V. Ventafridda. Raven Press, New York.

28. Giacomini, K. M., Giacomini, J. C., Gibson, T. P., and Levy, G. (1980): Propoxyphene and norpropoxyphene plasma concentrations after oral propoxyphene in cirrhotic patients with and without surgically constructed portacaval shunt. *Clin. Pharmacol. Ther.*, 28:417–423.

29. Goodman, J. S., Goodman, J. M., and Vogel, A. V. (1979): Knowledge and use of placebos by house officers and nurses. *Ann. Int. Med.*, 91:106–110.

30. Grabinski, P., Kaiko, R., Walsh, T., Foley, K., and Houde, R. (1983): Morphine radioimmu-

noassay specificity before and after extraction of plasma and cerebrospinal fluid. *J. Pharm. Sci.*, 72:27–30.

31. Halpern, L. W. (1979): Psychotropics, ataractics and related drugs. In: *Advances in Pain Research and Therapy, Vol. 2*, edited by J. J. Bonica and V. Ventafridda. Raven Press, New York.

32. Houde, R. W., and Wallenstein, S. L. (1955): Analgesic power of chlorpromazine alone and in combination with morphine. *Fed. Proc. (Abstr.)*, 14:353.

33. Houde, R. W., Wallenstein, S. L., and Beaver, W. T. (1965): Clinical management of pain. In: *Analgetics*, edited by G. De Stevens, pp. 75–122. *Academic Press, Inc.*, New York.

34. Houde, R. W., Wallenstein, S. L., and Beaver, W. T. (1966): Evaluation of analgesics in patients with cancer pain. In: *International Encyclopedia of Pharmacology and Therapeutics, Section 6, Clinical Pharmacology*, edited by L. Lasagna, pp. 59–99. Pergamon Press, New York.

35. Houde, R. W. (1966): On assaying analgesics in man. In: *Pain, 1st ed.*, edited by R. S. Knighton and P. R. Dumke, pp. 183–196. Little, Brown and Company, Boston.

36. Houde, R. W. (1979): Systemic analgesics and related drugs: Narcotic analgesics. In: *Advances in Pain Research and Therapy, Vol. 2*, edited by J. J. Bonica and V. Ventafridda. Raven Press, New York.

37. Houde, R. W. (1974): The use and misuse of narcotics in the treatment of chronic pain. *Adv. Neurol.*, 4:527–536.

38. Houde, R. W. (1979): Analgesic effectiveness of the narcotic agonist-antagonists. *Br. J. Clin. Pharmacol.*, 7:297s–308s.

39. Inturrisi, C. E., Foley, K. M., Kaiko, R. F., and Houde, R. W. (1981): Disposition and effects of intravenous (iv) methadone (met) in cancer patients. *Pain* (Suppl. 1) 99.

40. Inturrisi, C. E., Max, M., Umans, J., Schultz, M., Shin, S., Foley, K. M., and Houde, R. (1982): Heroin: Disposition in cancer patients. *Clin. Pharmacol. Ther.*, 31:235.

41. Inturrisi, C. E., Max, M., Foley, K., and Houde, R. (1984): Heroin: Oral and parenteral pharmacokinetics in cancer patients. *Proceedings II World Conf on Clin Pharmacol Ther*, *(in press)*.

42. Inturrisi, C. E. (1982): Narcotic Drugs. *Med. Clin. North Am.*, 66:1061–1071.

43. Inturrisi, C. E., and Umans, J. G. (1983): Pethidine and its active metabolite, norpethidine. *Clin. Anesthesiol.*, 1:123–138.

44. Inturrisi, C. E., Colburn, W. A., Verebey, K., Dayton, H. E., Wood, G. E., and O'Brien, C. P. (1982): Propoxyphene and norpropoxyphene kinetics after single and repeated doses of propoxyphene. *Clin. Pharmacol. Ther.*, 31:157–167.

45. Izard, M. W., and Ellison, F. S. (1962): Treatment of drug-induced constipation with a purified senna derivative. *Conn. Med.*, 26:589–592.

46. Iwamoto, E. T., and Martin, W. M. (1981): Multiple opiate receptors. *Med. Res. Rev.*, 1,4:411–440.

47. Jaffe, J. H. (1968): Narcotics in the treatment of pain. *Med. Clin. North. Am.*, 52:33–45.

48. Jaffe, J. H., and Martin, W. R. (1980): Opioid analgesics and antagonists. In: *The Pharmacological Basis of Therapeutics, 6th ed.*, edited by A. G. Gilman, A. S. Goodman, and A. Gilman, pp. 494–534. MacMillan Publishing Co., New York.

49. Jasinksi, D., Pernich, J. S., and Griffith, J. D. (1978): Human pharmacology and abuse potential of the analgesic buprenorphine. *Arch. Gen. Psychiatry*, 35:501–516.

50. Kaiko, R. F., Wallenstein, S. L., Rogers, A. G., Grabinski, P. Y., and Houde, R. W. (1981): Analgesic and mood effects of heroin and morphine in cancer patients with post-operative pain. *N. Engl. J. Med.*, 304:1501–1505.

51. Kaiko, R. F., Foley, K. M., Grabinski, P. Y., Heidrich, G., Rogers, A. G., Inturrisi, C. E., and Reidenberg, M. M. (1983): Central nervous system excitatory effects of meperidine in cancer patients. *Ann. Neurol.*, 13:180–185.

52. Kaiko, R. F. (1980): Age and morphine analgesia in cancer patients with postoperative pain. *Clin. Pharmacol. Ther.*, 28:823–826.

53. Kaiko, R. F., Foley, K. M., Houde, R. W., and Inturrisi, C. E. (1978): Narcotic levels in cerebrospinal fluid and plasma in man. In: *Charcteristics and Function of Opioids*, edited by J. M. Van Ree and L. Terenius, pp. 221–222. Elsevier/North-Holland Biomedical Press, Amsterdam.

54. Kaiko, R. F., Wallenstein, S. L., Rogers, A. G., Grabinski, P. V., and Houde, R. W. (1983): Narcotics in the elderly. *Med. Clin. North Am.*, 66:1079–1089.

55. Kanner, R. M., and Foley, K. M. (1981): Patterns of narcotic drug use in a cancer pain clinic. *Ann. N.Y. Acad. Sci.*, 362:161–172.

56. Kreek, M. J., Garfield, J. W., Gutjahr, C. L., and Guisti, L. M. (1976): Rifampin-induced methadone withdrawal. *N. Engl. J. Med.*, 294:1104–1106.
57. Laidlaw, J., Read, A. E., and Sherlock, S. (1961): Morphine tolerance in hepatic cirrhosis. *Gastroenterology*, 40:389–396.
58. Lasagna, L., and DeKornfeld, J. J. (1961): Methotrimeprazine: A new phenothiazine derivative with analgetic properties. *J.A.M.A.*, 178:887–890.
59. Lasagna, L. (1981): Heroin: A medical "Me Too." *New Engl. J. Med.*, 304:1539–1540.
60. Lund-Jacobson, H. (1978): Cardio-respiratory toxicity of propoxyphene and norpropoxyphene in conscious rabbits. *Acta. Pharmacol. Toxicol.*, 42:171–178.
61. Marks, R. M., and Sachar, E. J. (1973): Undertreatment of medical inpatients with narcotic analgesics. *Ann. Int. Med.*, 78:173–181.
62. Martin, W. R. (1967): Opioid antagonists. *Pharmacol. Rev.*, 10:463–521.
63. Max, M. B., Foley, K. M., Inturrisi, C. E., and Kaiko, R. F., et al. (1983): Epidural and intrathecal opiates: Distribution in CSF and plasma and analgesic effects in patients with cancer (submitted for publication).
64. Meyer, D., and Halfin, V. (1981): Toxicity secondary to meperidine in patients on monoamine oxidase inhibitators: A case report and critical review. *J. Clin. Psychopharmacol.*, 1:319–321.
65. Miller, R. R. (1980): Clinical effects of parenteral narcotics in hospitalized medical patients. *J. Clin. Pharmacol.*, 20:165–171.
66. Moore, J., and Dundee, J. W. (1961): Alterations in response to somatic pain associated with anesthesia VII. The effect of nine phenothiazine derivatives. *Br. J. Anaesth.*, 33:422–431.
67. Mount, B. M., Ajemian, I., and Scott, J. F. (1976): Use of Brompton mixture in treating the chronic pain of malignant disease. *Can. Med. Assoc. J.*, 115:122–124.
68. Neal, E. A., Meffin, P. J., Gregory, P. B., and Blaschke, T. F. (1979): Enhanced bioavailability and decreased clearance of analgesics in patients with cirrhosis. *Gastroenterology*, 77:96–102.
69. Nott, M. W. (1968): Potentiation of morphine analgesia by cocaine in mice. *Eur. J. Pharmacol.*, 5:93–99.
70. Pasternak, G. W., Childers, S. R., Snyder, S. H. (1980): Opiate analgesia: Evidence for mediation by a subpopulation of opiate receptors. *Science*, 208:514–516.
71. Patwardan, R. V., Johnson, R. F., Hoyumpa, A., Jr., Shiehan, J. J., Desmond, P. V., Wilkinson, G., Branch, R. A., and Schenker, S. (1981): Normal metabolism of morphine in cirrhosis. *Gastroenterology*, 81:1006–1011.
72. Pescor, M. J. (1939): The Kolb classification of drug addicts. In: *Public Health Rep (Suppl.)*, 155:1–10.
73. Pond, S. M., and Kretschzmar, K. M. (1981): Effect of phenytoin on meperidine clearance and normeperidine formation. *J. Clin. Pharmacol. Ther.*, 30:680–686.
74. Pond, S. M., Tang, T., Benowitz, N. L., Jacob, P., and Kigod, J. (1981): Presystemic metabolism of meperidine to normeperidine in normal and cirrhotic subjects. *Clin. Pharmacol. Ther.*, 30:183–188.
75. Porter, J., and Jick, H. (1980): Addiction rare in patients treated with narcotics. *N. Engl. J. Med.*, 302:123.
76. Rayport, M. (1954): Experience in the management of patients medically addicted to narcotics. *J.A.M.A.*, 156:684–691.
77. Robbie, D. S. (1979): A trial of sublingual buprenorphine in cancer pain. *Br. J. Clin. Pharmacol.*, 7:3155–3185.
78. Sawe, J., Hansen, J. Ginman, C., Hartvig, P., Jakobsson, P. A., Milsson, M.-I., Rane, A., and Anggard, E. (1981): Patient-controlled dose regimen of methadone for chronic cancer pain. *Br. Med. J.*, 282:771–773.
79. Singh, P. N., Sharma, P., Gupta, S., et al. (1981): Clinical evaluation of diazepam for relief of postoperative pain. *Br. J. Anaesth.*, 53:831–835.
80. Stanski, D. R., Greenblatt, D. J., and Lowenstein, E. (1978): Kinetics of intravenous and intramuscular morphine. *Clin. Pharmacol. Ther.*, 24:52–59.
81. Symonds, P. (1977): Methadone and the elderly. *Br. Med. J.*, 1:512.
82. Szeto, H. H., Inturrisi, C. E., Houde, R., Saal, S., Cheigh, J., and Reidenberg, M. M. (1977): Accumulation of normeperidine, an active metabolite of meperidine, in patients with renal failure or cancer. *Ann. Int. Med.*, 86:738–741.
83. Tamsen, A., Harlvig, P., Dahlstrom, B., Landstrom, B., and Holmdahl, M. H. (1979): Patient

controlled analgesic therapy in the early postoperative period. *Acta Anesthesiol. Scand.*, 23:462–470.

84. Taub, A. (1973): Relief of post-herpetic neuralgia with psychotropic drugs. *J. Neurosurg.*, 39:235–241.
85. Twycross, R. G. (1974): Clinical experience with diamorphine in advanced malignant disease. *Int. J. Clin. Pharmacol.*, 9:184–198.
86. Twycross, R. (1977): Value of cocaine in opiate containing elixirs. *Br. Med. J.*, 2:1348.
87. Twycross, R. G. (1977): A comparison of diamorphine with cocaine and methadone. *Br. J. Clin. Pharmacol.*, 4:691–693.
88. Twycross, R. G., and Ventafridda, V. (1980): *The Continuing Care of Terminal Cancer Patients*, pp. 3–279. Pergamon Press, New York.
89. Watson, C. P., Evans, R. J., Reid, K., Merskey, H., Goldsmith, L., and Warsh, J. (1982): Amitriptyline versus placebo in postherpetic neuralgia. *Neurology*, 32:671–673.

Analgesics: Neurochemical, Behavioral, and Clinical Perspectives, edited by M. Kuhar and G. Pasternak. Raven Press, New York © 1984.

Peripherally-Acting Analgesics

T. G. Kantor

New York University Medical Center, Department of Medicine, New York, New York 10016

The pharmacological relief of pain was conveniently divided into two drug categories by the studies of Lim and associates (48). In cross-profusion experiments in dogs, he demonstrated that the narcotic analgesic opiates and opioids worked exclusively in the central nervous system, as opposed to nonsteroidal anti-inflammatory drugs (NSAID) and acetaminophen, which worked exclusively in the periphery where the pain was engendered. The identification of specific narcotic receptor sites has confirmed these observations (69), and now analgesic drugs may be categorized as to whether or not they bind with strong affinity to such sites. The finding of narcotic receptor sites in the gut, salivary glands, adrenal glands, and spinal cord has modified Lim's original conception, but operationally, the peripheral action of non-narcotic drugs has been established.

Although it is known that the endings in the periphery of the relatively unmyelinated A-delta and C fibers are responsible for picking up the pain signal, the exact events leading to production of the signal are as yet obscure.

Most human pain seems to be associated with an inflammatory process. Our understanding of the mediation of inflammation is growing. The histological events associated with the initiation of inflammation have been well described (17a).

After an appropriate stimulus, capillaries in the immediate area begin to dilate, probably as the result of histamine excretion by local mast cells. Very quickly, the capillary wall becomes leaky, and plasma exudes into the inflamed area. White cells then marginate along the interior capillary wall and diapedese out through openings between the endothelial cells. The polymorphonuclear leukocytes, now in the interstitial area, begin to ingest the offending stimulus or other detritus, and, in doing so, "regurgitate while feeding" various enzymes which would ordinarily attack ingested material interiorized into phagosomes (79). The enzymes released into the interstitium include proteases and lipases.

Mediating substances which can perform or amplify any of these events include bradykinin, a nonopeptide digested from alpha globulin by the proteases noted above, prostaglandin products digested from membrane bilayers, other lipids by the lipases, and complement split products which are digested by still other proteases (Table 1). In addition, degradation products of some of these mediators call forth a further white cell response, and opsonize material to be ingested. Mononuclear

TABLE 1. *Summary of the most important
endogenous mediators of inflammation*

Increased vascular permeability
  Vasoactive amines (histamine)
  Kinins (bradykinin)
  Prostaglandins
Leukocyte infiltration (chemotaxis)
  Neutrophils (leukotrienes)
  Complement system by-products (C5 fragments)
  Mononuclear phagocytes (leukotrienes)
  Neutrophil lysosomal cationic protein
  Eosinophils
  Complement system by-products (C5 fragments)
  Eosinophil chemotactic factor of anaphylaxis
Tissue damage
  Neutrophil lysosomal products (neutral proteases)
    Oxygen radicals

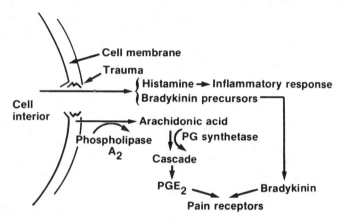

FIG. 1. Proposed peripheral mechanisms of pain. Schema for activation of peripheral pain receptors which in turn trigger A-δ and C nerve fibers carrying pain impulses to the spinal cord.

cells brought into the area can trigger immune events and produce products which further amplify the histological events (58).

It has been shown by Lim and ourselves, that bradykinin can cause immediate pain when injected intra-arterially and into serosal lined body cavities, but not when injected intradermally or intramuscularly (35). Later, Ferreira showed that subcutaneous tissues primed with prostaglandins and then injected with bradykinin gave an immediate pain response (19). Prostaglandins injected alone also gave pain, but only after a prolonged latent period. It is assumed therefore that bradykinin is not only an inflammation mediator, but a direct stimulant of the pain sensation, either alone in some locations or in congress with prostaglandins in others (Fig. 1). The exact interaction of prostaglandin and bradykinin is unknown.

The recent development of nonsteroidal anti-inflammatory agents has been characterized by many different chemical classes, all of which antagonize the enzyme cyclo-oxygenase (Fig. 2). Indeed, the search for effective anti-inflammatory drugs has hinged almost entirely on tests for prostaglandin inhibition. Potential developments through interference with other inflammation mediators have been hampered by difficult and often unreproducible methodology. Such difficulties have beset all of the theories of NSAID action listed in Table 2. Drugs specifically developed to interfere with inflammation mediating pathways other than prostaglandins are very much in the minority.

Obviously, drugs that completely suppress inflammation owing to all mediators, would represent a disservice to the total organism. Corticosteroids come close to doing just that, and are therefore more dangerous to use because of reduction of resistance to infection and interference with wound healing. Part of the effect of corticosteroids is to stabilize membranes in such a way that the in-facing membrane lipid components of the bilayer are not perturbed, and phospholipase digestion to arachidonic acid does not occur (26). Thus, all components of the prostaglandin cascade are blocked (Fig. 3).

Development of anti-inflammatory and analgesic drugs was at first quite empirical. Inflammation models, such as the granuloma pouch and irritants injected into footpaws, are affected by all NSAIDs including the original standard aspirin. The

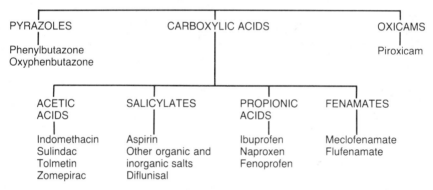

FIG. 2. Chemical classes of nonsteroidal anti-inflammatory and analgesic drugs.

TABLE 2. *Mechanism of action of non-steroidal anti-inflammatory drugs (NAIDs)*

1. Interference with prostaglandin synthesis
2. Uncoupling oxidative phosphorylation
3. Endogenous NSAID
4. Membrane stabilization
5. Interference with superoxide production
6. Antichemical mediation of pain
7. Inhibition of other inflammation mediators
8. Adrenal mechanism
9. Leukocyte migration and function

Mechanisms theorized to explain the analgesic and anti-inflammatory effects of NSAIDs.

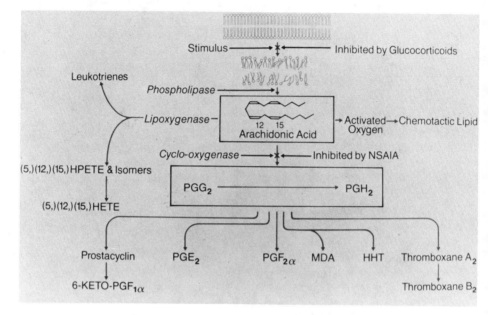

FIG. 3. The arachidonic acid cascade. Arrow labeled "Inhibited by NSAID" shows point where nonsteroidal anti-inflammatory drugs inhibit prostaglandin synthesis. Arrow labeled "Inhibited by glucocorticoids" shows point where corticosteroids inhibit prostaglandin synthesis.

hot-plate and tail flick tests, using heat as a stimulus and time as a measurement parameter as tests for analgesia, pick up all the opioids except some agonist-antagonists, but are also responded to by most NSAIDs, though relatively weakly. More recently, binding to narcotic receptor models and *in vitro* antagonism to the enzyme cyclo-oxygenase have been used. Test systems to show blocking of the production or biological effects of kinins, complement, or oxygen radicals are not so well developed.

Perhaps because of the test systems used in pharmacological experiments, clear-cut distinctions are made in the United States between drugs with analgesic effects and those with anti-inflammatory ones. Such a distinction can clearly be made for the opioids, but clinically, the NSAIDs as a group are both analgesic and anti-inflammatory. There may well be a relationship between the two effects for NSAIDs (37). However, acetaminophen, which is a peripherally-acting analgesic, has very little anti-inflammatory action, whereas there is a probable disproportion favoring analgesia between the two effects for zomepirac (*see* below).

The remainder of this chapter will be devoted to a description of those NSAIDs which have analgetic effects, and some peripherally-acting drugs which may not affect inflammation to a significant degree. As far as possible, these agents will be described in historical progression.

These medications are indicated for mild to moderate pain of any type, although some are potent enough to supplant morphine in acute pain. Almost all are in oral form, a few have parenteral versions, and one or two can be used as suppositories.

GENERAL CONSIDERATIONS OF NSAIDs AS ANALGESICS

The choice of which NSAID to use is often empiric because it is impossible to predict to which one an individual patient will respond or tolerate (32). This puzzling difference in response is apparently not because of differences in drug kinetics, and may be instead owing to genetic differences in the mediating pathways by which an inflammatory response is mounted, or to differences in the mediators utilized at varying stages of the disease to be treated. For example, one individual may primarily use products of the cyclo-oxygenase pathway in response to a given stimulus, whereas another may primarily use the lipoxygenase pathway. The former individual may respond well to many of the NSAIDs, although the latter will not. Similarly, in rheumatoid arthritis, early stages may be characterized by prostaglandin-mediated inflammation, and later stages by complement mediation. In this case, all the NSAIDs might act better at an earlier stage.

An interesting study illustrating this point selected patients with rheumatoid arthritis who responded well to indomethacin, and compared them with similar patients who never responded to indomethacin. There were no kinetic differences in the way the two groups handled the drug. However, some of the nonresponders had less inhibition of the platelet prostaglandin end-product than responders (2). A study by Scott et al. has shown an augmentation of the lipoxygenase pathway at the expense of the cyclo-oxygenase pathway in human microphages treated with indomethacin (64). If this type of response is under genetic control, it may explain nonresponse in that the leukotrienes produced by the lipoxygenase prostaglandin pathway may be at least as powerful mediators of inflammation as those produced by the cyclo-oxygenase pathway.

It seems obvious that all drugs which inhibit cyclo-oxygenase are both analgesic and anti-inflammatory. The fact that "dolor" is one of the cardinal signs of inflammation should make this no surprise. There may be some dose discrepancy between their analgesic effects and anti-inflammatory effects, but this may be owing to the sensitivity by which we measure these phenomena. I believe that there is a continuum between the two pharmacologic effects. Anaglesia is easier to produce and measure (39). Whether or not prostaglandin synthesis inhibition is solely responsible for both effects, the common adverse reactions of all these diverse chemical entities can certainly be explained by this one feature.

As noted in the section on aspirin, there is a target population, very small, in whom prostaglandin synthesis inhibition can cause severe adverse effects. Subjects who from early life have been subjected to bronchial asthma and nasal polyps may develop hives and severe breathing restriction from all NSAIDs. It is interesting that such individuals are often also sensitive to certain tetrazine dyes used in tablet manufacture.

None of these drugs should be given to patients with active peptic ulcers, hiatus hernias, or peptic esophagitis. Patients with a history of these conditions may be cautiously treated with a concurrent full anti-ulcer regimen. When possible, doses should not be taken on an empty stomach.

Patients with renal defects should be treated cautiously. Many drugs are associated with interstitial nephritis as an adverse effect. The NSAIDs are no exception. Possibly related to their usual long-term use in arthritis, there seems to be a somewhat higher incidence of this complication than for other types of drugs. In short-term analgetic use, this adverse effect is almost nonexistent. In long-term use, the incidence is still quite low.

Salt and water retention is a significant feature of all of these drugs, the fenamates possibly excepted. Caution should be exercised in cases of borderline congestive heart failure and hypertension.

Since uterine contractility is partially under prostaglandin control, use of these drugs in pregnant women may prolong labor and their platelet effects increase bleeding.

Stopping and restarting the NSAIDs has been reported to produce a low incidence of anaphylactoid reactions.

With the possible exception of the fenamates, teratogenicity is not a problem with NSAIDs.

Patients with drug induced or disease related aberrancies in the coagulation cascade should also be treated with caution, particularly with aspirin which irreversibly inhibits platelet function throughout their lifetime in the platelet (4 to 8 days). Many surgeons feel that all of these drugs should be stopped 1 week or more before elective surgery. A few are grateful for the anti-thrombotic effect. NSAIDs other than aspirin all have minor effects on platelet function which is quickly reversible.

Of all NSAIDs, only phenylbutazone and oxyphenbutazone self-induce their own metabolism to any significant degree, and even these pyrazoles are limited in this respect. It can therefore be safely assumed that NSAIDs never change either their analgesic or anti-inflammatory effects over long-term administration unless the condition treated waxes or wanes.

Since all the above described drugs are acid in function and thereby bound to serum albumin to a greater or lesser degree depending on their affinity, they may displace or be displaced from albumin binding. Unbound drug is generally more pharmacologically active. From a practical standpoint, only hypoglycemic drugs and coumarin derivatives are clinically affected by NSAIDs, both being slightly displaced from albumin and therefore more active. The acidic function of NSAIDs may allow more ready penetration into the acid milieu of inflammation.

Ceiling Effect

For reasons which are unclear, all of the NSAIDs used as analgetics seem to have a ceiling analgesic effect beyond which no increment in dose increases the analgetic effect. This ceiling has not been accurately determined for each drug, but toxicity will probably modify individual experimentation. In some instances, such as piroxicam, there is a known upper limit dictated by toxicity.

Fever

Since the central nervous system fever center is apparently triggered by prostaglandins, one might expect that all NSAIDs would reduce fever. This is indeed so but access to the central nervous system is necessary and there are some variations among these drugs in this regard.

Other Drugs

Other drugs such as acetaminophen and compounds which are antihistaminic or derived from antihistaminics have analgesic properties. Except that these drugs do not bind significantly to central nervous system narcotic binding sites or affect prostaglandin synthesis, little is known about the mode by which they cause analgesia.

ACETAMINOPHEN

Pharmacology

This phenacetin derivative has milligram for milligram analgesic potency compared to aspirin (4) with very limited anti-inflammatory effect. It is said to be a superoxide dismutase (41). Since it only slightly inhibits cyclo-oxygenase and hardly affects prostaglandin synthesis in any significant way, this drug has none of the gastrointestinal or renal adverse effects of the NSAIDs. It enters the central nervous system and reduces fever (20). It is extensively metabolized in the liver with a limiting step being chemical reduction.

Toxicity

Although acetaminophen is a relatively safe analgetic, in high doses over a prolonged period, its metabolism may exhaust the enzyme systems responsible for its reduction. This in turn may paralyze the capacity of the liver to reduce other toxic substances in addition to the drug itself. This can lead to death, with earlier symptoms of hepatic failure. Therapy for this kind of toxicity consists of the replenishment of sulfhydryl radicals necessary to the activity of the depleted enzyme. Methionine glutathiase or acetylcysteine are satisfactory for this purpose and may be lifesaving (34). O_2 radicals produced during metabolism may also be responsible for hepatotoxicity. Cimetidine, which interferes with hydroxylation by the liver, has also been suggested as a treatment for overdose (1).

Use

Acetaminophen may be given in doses up to 975 mg every 4 hr for analgesia. It is not known if the ceiling effect exists. The drug may be preferential as a mild to moderate analgetic in patients with active upper gastrointestinal peptic disease.

Other drugs in this class, such as phenacetin and aminopyrine, are no longer used because of renal and bone marrow toxicity, respectively.

ASPIRIN AND THE SALICYLATES

Aspirin, as such, was first commercially produced at the Bayer Laboratories by Felix Hofmann in 1893, although Von Gerhardt had first synthesized it 50 years previously. The analgetic effects of salicylates in general had been noted by Hippocrates. Botanical preparations of willow bark to reduce fever were described by Stone in 1763 and Leroux isolated the active ingredient, salicin, in 1829 (73).

Ironically, Hofmann's father, who probably had rheumatoid arthritis, was the first patient treated with the drug, and its anti-inflammatory properties were quickly realized by his physician who then promoted aspirin's use. The antipyretic and analgesic properties of crude salicylate preparations had been previously noted.

Early in the 20th century, the use of high-dose salicylate therapy for rheumatic fever was championed by Coburn (11) and others. A controversy raged among rheumatologists as to whether aspirin's salutory effects on rheumatic fever and other forms of arthritis were due simply to its analgesic effect, or to anti-inflammatory properties. These two effects were considered to be separate, and other salicylate preparations such as sodium salicylate were used as well.

However, the studies of Boardman and Hart (7), and Fremont-Smith and Bayles (25) clearly demonstrated the anti-inflammatory effect of high dose aspirin in patients with rheumatoid arthritis. Most authorities now agree that this is the primary effect of aspirin in inflammatory arthritis. However, many believe that in lower doses, aspirin produces only an analgesic effect where no anti-inflammatory effect can be demonstrated. In latter day clinical trials, these lower doses are understood to be analgetic for a variety of pain models including headache, post-fracture, postoperative, postpartum, and postdental extraction (4). Aspirin is also analgetic in cancer pain (53,54). With the predominance of aspirin as a commercially nonprescription salicylate analgesic, the use of other salicylates has faded, although such entities as sodium salicylate are available. Many others, such as salsalate, magnesium salicylate, and choline salicylate, are available by prescription, but none are as potent milligram for milligram as aspirin for either analgesia or anti-inflammatory effect.

The analgesia of salicylates is an old clinical story. The pharmacological effect responsible for this was suggested by Vane's experiments which showed that salicylates *in vivo* suppressed protaglandin synthesis, whereas only aspirin did so in *in vitro* experiments (76). Further studies demonstrated the irrevocable destruction of the enzyme cyclo-oxygenase associated with the donation of aspirin's acetyl group to this enzyme (62). Cyclo-oxygenase is central to one of the three pathways known to stem from the formation of arachidonic acid by phospholipases. Of course, this still does not explain why nonacetylated salicylates work *in vivo*. There is no evidence that salicylate as a chemical moiety acts simply as a "dump truck" moving acetyl groups from one tissue location to another, nor evidence that they interfere with other enzymatic derivatives of arachidonic acid.

Pharmacology

Aspirin is somewhat unique in that it does not follow first order pharmacokinetics. Instead, the higher the dose, the longer the elimination half-life (45). For all doses, total plasma residence time of acetylsalicylate per se is a mere 90 min. Powerful esterases, which are higher in concentration in males than in females (51), quickly convert the parent compound into salicylate which is then the major component to be metabolized and excreted. There are five known metabolic products of salicylate but only conjugation with glycine to form salicyluric acid and production of a glucoronide are quantitatively important (46). Both of these, particularly the former, are overloaded at total daily doses of more than 4 grams a day, so that higher doses will greatly increase the plasma salicylate level. However, the early acetylsalicylate peak is unaffected.

This latter feature is crucial to our understanding of the primary biologic effects of aspirin. Since the destruction of the enzyme cyclo-oxygenase is irrevocable and further enzyme activity is dependent on its own remanufacture, salicylate kinetics may not be too important if one believes in the necessity of the acetyl group and its effect on prostaglandin synthesis. However, the time-effect curves for aspirin analgesia are incompatible with the half-life of acetylsalicylate. The clinically demonstrable analgesic effect of nonacetylated salicylates cannot be explained. In fact, the time-effect curves for analgesia are compatible with the half-life of nonacetylated salicylate (4).

In chronic doses, a steady state of salicylate plasma level is achieved after 3 days of dosage using a variety of schedules (47). So-called long-acting salicylates have, therefore, no advantage over plain aspirin tablets in therapy lasting longer than 3 continuous days.

Special Pharmacologic Considerations

Aspirin, but not nonacetylated salicylates, has a direct mucosal destructive effect on the stomach with back diffusion of acid adding to the damage (3). This can be avoided by buffering or by the use of enteric-coated preparations. Adequate buffering, such as the Ascriptin formulation, leads to more rapid absorption. However, increased alkalinization of urine can lead to facilitation of excretion (16). Until relatively recently, absorption of enteric-coated preparations was irregular at best. Better pharmaceutical finishing has improved the situation so that recent studies have shown no difference between the absorption of ordinary aspirin tablets and enteric-coated preparations, such as Lilly's Enseals or Ecotrin (59).

Aspirin is unique in that it is the only NSAID with proven direct mucosal destructive effects. In addition, aspirin shares with other NSAIDs the pharmacologic gastric effects associated with prostaglandin inhibition in gastric mucosa. Prostaglandins present in the gastric mucosa increase mucus production, decrease acid production, and increase mucosal blood supply. Body wide reduction of prostaglandin synthesis, including the stomach, leads to less gastric mucus, more acid and less mucosal blood supply, and, thus, more gastric irritation and potential ulcer formation (10,61). Similarly, prostaglandins modulate salt and water metabolism and free-water excretion by the kidney. Reduction of prostaglandin synthesis produces salt and free-water retention which can lead to hypervolemia and its consequences (44).

Apparently also related to the prostaglandin effect is a true hypersensitivity in patients with a history of nasal polyps and asthma (63). This is very rare.

Therapy

Single doses of 650 mg aspirin can be shown to confer analgesia in a variety of pain models when compared double-blind to placebo (4). Doses as low as 325 mg can occasionally be shown to do so. Twelve hundred milligrams is significantly more analgetic than 650 mg. However, there is controversy as to whether or not a ceiling effect for analgesia exists above 1,200 mg. In any case, the dose-effect positive slope is on the average more shallow than opioids. Maintenance of dosage maintains reduction of inflammation causing pain. This is an important point to be related to the patient about all NSAIDs, if used for anti-inflammatory effect.

Toxicity

Doses of aspirin up to 1,200 mg at a time rarely cause toxic effects when used for acute pain. In these cases, the assumption is made that the necessity for analgesic doses in acutely painful conditions will rarely extend for more than 4 to 5 days. Toxicity is certainly related to salicylate plasma level, although plasma levels bear only an uncertain relation to the desired pharmacologic effect.

At about 30 mg% salicylate plasma level, ototoxicity is almost universal with reversible tinnitus and/or reduction in hearing being noted. Above 30 mg%, metabolic changes take place. By central stimulation of the respiratory center, a respiratory alkalosis may occur, and at levels over 50 mg%, metabolic acidosis may occur, owing to the acidity of salicylate itself and its metabolic products (16). In addition, nonspecific central nervous system effects may be noted leading to psychosis and coma.

After several days of high-dose therapy, the direct mucosal irritating effect and the secondary reduction of prostaglandins in the gastric mucosa may cause pyrosis, nausea, and vomiting. Constipation is not infrequent in chronic therapy. Comcomitant antacid therapy with a magnesium hydroxide product may overcome both of these problems and a good enteric-coated product can deal with some of the gastric toxicity. A suppository form is available but may be irritating to the rectal mucosa.

The acetylation of the cyclo-oxygenase present in platelets reduces their ability to aggregate, and thereby initiates the clotting process (55). This effect lasts throughout the lifetime of the platelet (4 to 8 days), since platelets are unable to manufacture new proteins, and the effect on the enzyme is, therefore, permanent.

Large doses over several days interfere with prothrombin production by the liver and produce an added hazard. Therefore, use of aspirin in patients with bleeding diathesis, whether endogenous or produced by coumarin products, is hazardous.

In doses under 3.6 grams daily, aspirin interferes with uric acid tubular excretion, and may elevate serum uric acid levels and overcome the effects of uricosuric agents or allopurinol (83).

Large doses of aspirin in children or patients with systemic lupus erythematosus may lead to hepatic toxicity (65), but other patients seem at little risk for this adverse effect.

Alkaline diuresis rapidly reduces acute toxic symptoms owing to overdose, and salicylate is eminently dialyzable (75).

Salsalate in doses of 3,000 mg daily (50), and magnesium choline salicylate preparations in doses of 2,500 mg daily (12) are also analgetic. Perhaps because they are nonacetylated, they do not interfere with platelet aggregation or cause as much gastrointestinal problems as aspirin. They are, however, prescription drugs, cost a good deal more than aspirin preparations, and have a weaker analgetic effect. Choline salicylate is available in a liquid formulation. Magnesium choline salicylate in tablet form (12) and a long-acting fluorinated salicylate preparation, diflunisal, are also available.

Diflunisal has recently been marketed. It is a fluorinated derivative of salicylate. Although it is not metabolized as a salicylate, it performs more or less like other nonacetylated salicylates. It has an elimination half-life of about 10 hr, and at a dose of 250 to 500 mg every 12 hr, produces effective analgesia as documented in a variety of pain models (21,31).

PYRAZOLES

The pyrazoles are characterized by a five-membered ring structure containing two nitrogens. There are only two drugs in common use from this class, phenylbutazone and oxyphenbutazone.

Phenylbutazone was introduced as an anti-inflammatory agent in 1955. There have been no adequate trials of the drug as a pure analgesic, but the potency of its anti-inflammatory effect reduces pain rapidly in acute musculoskeletal conditions such as gout, tendonitis, and sprains (68).

Pharmacology

Oxyphenbutazone is a metabolic product of phenylbutazone and has similar potency to the parent compound. Both interfere with prostaglandin synthesis by inhibition of the enzyme cyclo-oxygenase although, unlike aspirin, the effect is reversible after metabolism or excretion of the drug. There seems, in addition, a preferential effect inhibiting production of the endoperoxide PGG_2 while allowing production of PGH_2 (40). This may confer special properties on these drugs, and account for their potency.

Kinetics

Both drugs have prolonged half-lives of 40 to 90 hr. However, they both are capable of self-induction of their own metabolism which makes the effective half-life in chronic therapy somewhat lower (15). Metabolism takes place extensively in the liver.

Toxicity

As are all drugs which reduce prostaglandin synthesis, the two drugs are potentially ulcerogenic and are capable of producing pyrosis, nausea, and vomiting.

There are additional hazards peculiar to this group of drugs. They are the most potent salt-retaining compounds of the NSAIDs (18). In addition, direct renal and hepatic toxic effects can occur. Bone marrow toxicity, particularly thrombocytopenia, has been noted and seems both dose related and, more rarely, idiosyncratic. Psychotomimetic effects have also been noted (8).

Careful monitoring of blood counts, urine, and blood pressure should be undertaken when these drugs are used in chronic therapy.

Use

These drugs should be given only with great caution in patients with known heart disease, hypertension, liver, or renal disease, or those with a history of peptic ulcer, esophagitis, or hiatus hernia.

In doses of 4 to 600 mg daily for over a week, they are relatively safe. In certain inflammatory arthritides with a spinal component, such as ankylosing spondylitis, Reiter's syndrome, or juvenile rheumatoid arthritis, these drugs have a seeming specificity. A chronic dosage of 200 mg daily is often beneficial and safe for long periods of time. Higher doses should be used much more cautiously.

In effect, there is no advantage of oxyphenbutzone over phenylbutazone, although the latter has more uricosuric effect but each is as toxic as the other and the addition of small amounts of antacid in a combination preparation is essentially useless as a GI mucoprotectant.

PYROLES

Drugs in this chemical class contain five membered rings containing one nitrogen, occasionally with a phenyl group attached which resembles the configuration seen in serotonin. They are all powerful inhibitors of cyclo-oxygenase in a time-dependent fashion, and the effect is almost completely reversible. They include the drugs indomethacin, tolmetin, sulindac, and zomepirac.

Indomethacin

Pharmacology and Kinetics

This drug has a half-life of some 3 hr and requires dosage on a three or four times a day basis. It is extensively metabolized in the liver. Metabolites and parent drug are excreted by the kidney. It can be used in a suppository form. A formal trial of indomethacin as an analgetic has been performed in postoperative patients, and 50 mg was essentially the equivalent of 650 mg of aspirin in this population (71). Its dosage as an anti-inflammatory is between 75 and 200 mg daily in divided doses and it has been used in a single nighttime dose to suppress early morning stiffness in arthritis.

Toxicity

As a prostaglandin synthesis inhibitor, and a very potent one, the drug is ulcerogenic and causes pyrosis, nausea, and vomiting in a high incidence. Advantage is taken of its renal effect in the management of Bartter's syndrome (28), and it can also be used in the treatment of patent ductus arteriosus (30), the patency of which is under the control of prostaglandins. The renal effect in patients with otherwise normal kidneys can cause significant retention of salt and water, although not as severe as phenylbutazone.

A peculiar kind of migraine headache, for which there is no ready explanation, can occur, especially after the earliest morning dose (33). Other central nervous system effects include psychotomimetic problems. A patient with a history of a psychotic break should not receive this drug. This may be related to the serotonin-like chemical configuration.

Use

Indomethacin's use as an analgetic seems to be more prevalent in Europe than in the United States. There, it is used in both capsule and suppository form in essentially the anti-inflammatory doses noted above. The suppository form is nonexistent in the United States but can be made up as a 100 mg dose in a simple cocoa butter suppository.

There is some evidence that bony metastases are surrounded by a cloud of prostaglandins, presumably involved in leaching away the bony matrix and allowing further tumor growth (66). In doses of 25 mg four times daily, I have seen an occasional patient become pain free and sometimes normocalcemic after 2 or 3 days. The effect is spectacular enough to warrant trial in every such case before potent opioids are used.

A recently introduced sustained release preparation may allow once a day dosage.

Tolmetin

Pharmacology and Kinetics

This drug has not been extensively tested as an analgetic but is closely enough related to zomepirac to warrant its use. It has a short half-life of 90 min, but high doses often seem to extend its effect for far longer, at least for its anti-inflammatory effect (27). It is rapidly metabolized by the liver.

Toxicity

The toxic effects of tolmetin are, in general, those of indomethacin. However, central nervous system effects, including headaches, seem to be in lower incidence, perhaps associated with the drugs shorter elimination half-life.

Use

Since tolmetin is still under trial as a pure analgetic, its dose is uncertain for this effect. A four times daily dose schedule would theoretically be optimum at 400 mg per dose. The drug is one of the few NSAIDs cleared for use in children, and might be useful as an analgetic in pediatrics.

Sulindac

Pharmacology and Kinetics

This drug is of pharmacologic interest because it is a prodrug; the parent drug is not biologically active. It must be converted into a sulfide after oral absorption to produce anti-inflammatory effects. The sulfide has a 13- to 18- hr half-life (17). The drug has a few clinical trials suggesting moderate analgesic effect, and as with all of these compounds, potent cyclo-oxygenase inhibition of the reversible type occurs. A sulfone is also a metabolite which undergoes an enterohepatic circulation.

Toxicity

In addition to the usual cyclo-oxygenase inhibition-associated symptoms of gastric irritation and fluid retention, the sulfone may cause severe diarrhea.

Use

The literature on sulindac as an analgesic is sparse but suggestive enough to warrant its use. The long half-life of the active metabolite suggests a dose of 150 to 200 mg every 12 hr and perhaps a dosage of once a day in patients with renal disease. The only dose form is oral. As with all NSAIDs, taking the medication after a meal is most acceptable to the gastrointestinal tract.

Zomepirac[1]

Pharmacology and Kinetics

Laboratory testing of zomepirac suggested analgesia but most investigators were surprised at the potency of this effect in humans. The drug itself is active and extensively metabolized in the liver. Its half-life is about 4 to 9 hr (57). Trials for analgetic potency are commonly done in single dose double-blind protocols. Several excellent studies suggest that 100 mg of oral zomepirac is equivalent to 8 to 16 mg of injected morphine (24,78).

Toxicity

Zomepirac shares the toxic effects of its group having potent cyclo-oxygenase inhibiting effects. Despite its lipophilicity, it seems to have little in the way of CNS adverse effects or long-lasting adverse effects. Adrenal tumors have been reported after long-term use in high dose in animals.

THIAZINES

This category of drugs has been associated with hepatic toxicity to an extent which delayed their introduction for human use. As of this writing, only one is marketed in the United States, piroxicam.

Piroxicam

Pharmacology

This drug seems to have a similar effect on cyclo-oxygenase as other NSAIDs. However, it has a much longer half-life, 30 to 40 hr, and greater lipophilicity than the others. The long half-life allows once a day dosage as an anti-inflammatory drug (81). Conventional trials for analgesic effects are not as yet completed. Its lipophilicity allows greater penetrations into the central nervous system which may confer separate pharmacologic properties.

Toxicity and Use

Although the adverse effects of piroxicam are essentially those of the other NSAIDs, its longer half-life is associated with a narrow dose range. At dose levels of 40 mg and higher, it has an unacceptably high incidence of gastrointestinal toxicity and peptic ulcer formation. At doses less than 20 mg daily, it is sharply reduced in effect. A dose of 20 to 30 mg daily is as safe and effective as other NSAIDs for anti-inflammation (74). Its short-term analgesic dose schedule is yet

---

[1]The drug has been voluntarily removed from the market by the McNeil Company because of analphylactic reactions mostly occurring on second presentations which resulted in a few deaths.

to be determined. It seems to have little hepatotoxicity and about the same range of renal toxicity as other NSAIDs.

PROPIONIC ACIDS

After an exploration of various alkanoic acids for medicinal purposes, it was discovered that some propionic acid derivatives have anti-inflammatory properties. As of this writing, three are available to American physicians (ibuprofen, fenoprofen, and naproxen), but many others are in daily use in other countries. With the realization that all three were inhibitors of prostaglandin synthesis, clinical trials have established their effects as mild to moderate oral analgetics.

Ibuprofen

The first one introduced in America was ibuprofen. This drug had already been noted to have at least analgetic properties if not anti-inflammatory action in the doses used in Europe. On its introduction in the United Kingdom, the suggested daily dose was 600 mg daily. When marketed in America 7 years later, the suggested dose was 1,200 to 1,600 mg daily. In present usage, starting doses of over 4,000 mg daily have been reported (67).

Trials in various analgetic models have suggested that 600 to 800 mg may form a ceiling for acute analgetic effects (6,13,38,52,60). Poor models available for chronic clinical pain evaluation make higher doses over long periods difficult to evaluate except in trials for arthritic pain. This shortcoming is true for all the peripherally-acting analgetic drugs.

Dysmenorrhea has been shown to be related to production of prostaglandins within the uterine cavity. All of the propionic drugs appear to be more effective than aspirin for this type of pain (60,70).

Pharmacology

Ibuprofen has an elimination half-life of approximately 3 hr, and this requires dosing on a three or four times a day schedule. Attempts to use higher individual doses, up to 1,200 mg, to produce effective analgesia on a twice a day schedule have been equivocal.

The drug is extensively metabolized in the liver with a minimal amount of the parent drug excreted in the urine unchanged. Prostaglandin synthesis reduction is accomplished by reversible inhibition of the enzyme cyclo-oxygenase as with other NSAIDs. For ibuprofen, there is also some evidence of lipoxygenase inhibition (14).

Toxicity

All drugs that inhibit prostaglandin synthesis cause upper gastrointestinal irritation to the extent of occasional peptic ulcer production, but ibuprofen seems less ulcerogenic than others. There are rare reports of diarrhea production.

Perhaps also on the basis of prostaglandin inhibition, renal toxicity in the form of an interstitial nephritis has been reported for ibuprofen. Although the exact incidences are unknown, ibuprofen is probably safer in this regard than the other propionic acids.

Ibuprofen does cause significant blurring of vision in a few patients, but original fears of retinal toxicity do not seem to be well founded. As with other drugs, rare instances of bone marrow and skin toxicity have been reported. Transient elevations of liver transaminases are occasionally noted, but cessation of the drug seems to almost universally reverse this trend. Effect on inhibition of platelet function seems to be minimal but should be considered (39).

Use

Doses of 300 to 600 mg every 4 to 6 hr produce satisfactory analgesia in mild to moderate pain. Higher dose schedules to 1,200 mg every 6 to 8 hr are occasionally used for anti-inflammatory effect in arthritis but are attended by a higher incidence of gastrointestinal intolerance. However, ibuprofen is characterized by the wide range of potential dose schedules which seem to be tolerated by most patients.

Blood counts, urine determinations, and liver profiles can be used to monitor toxicity in chronic use.

Fenoprofen

Pharmacology

While it is a different propionic acid derivative than ibuprofen, fenoprofen has a very similar pharmacologic profile. It has a 2- to 3-hr half-life and inhibits cyclooxygenase reversibly. Doses above 200 mg have been shown to be analgetic in a wide variety of pain models with a ceiling of about 1,200 mg for mild to moderate pain (43).

Toxicity

There have been more reports of renal toxicity with fenoprofen than with ibuprofen (49). Otherwise, the same spectrum of adverse effects holds for fenoprofen as for ibuprofen.

Use

Doses of 50 to 200 mg every 4 to 6 hr are useful for mild to moderate pain. The ceiling for anti-inflammatory effect in arthritis has probably not been adequately explored but would be limited by toxicity as with other drugs in this group. A 300 mg and 600 mg capsule are available.

Naproxen

Pharmacology

This drug has essentially the same overall pharmacologic profile as ibuprofen and fenoprofen, but it has a half-life of 11 to 13 hr, which allows greater spacing of doses. The sodium salt of naproxen has recently been introduced as the analgetic form of the drug, but there is little reason to believe that it is superior in this respect to the original compound. Both forms are potent, but reversible cyclo-oxygenase inhibitors.

Toxicity

Despite its longer half-life, neither naproxen nor its sodium salt seem to have any greater incidence of increased toxicity over the other propionic acids. With very few exceptions, all drugs which inhibit cyclo-oxygenase have similar adverse effects. While it is uncertain that their desired pharmacologic effects are related to this inhibition, it is certain that their adverse effects are.

Use

Twice daily (250 mg) is a satisfactory dose schedule for the parent drug, both as an analgetic and antiarthritic drug. The sodium salt may do slightly better as an analgesic drug in a three times a day dose schedule. 375- and 500-mg tablets have recently been introduced. Anaproxen is available in 275-mg tablets. Both drugs can be utilized in children.

Benoxaprofen

This drug is not strictly a propionic acid derivative, and also has chemical relationships to the pyroles. It is pharmacologically unique in its half-life of some 31 hr which will allow once a day dosing. The drug has recently been removed from the market because of renal and hepatic toxicity resulting in the death of elderly patients. This feature was predicted by noted changes in the pharmacokinetics of benoxaprofen in the elderly when compared to younger subjects (29). Claims are made that it interferes with the lipoxygenase prostaglandin pathway more than cyclo-oxygenase, and that it modulates immune and inflammatory events by an effect on monocytes (14).

There are other reservations about its toxicity. There is a tendency to onycholysis in an incidence which is as yet unknown. In general, it seems to have a high incidence of adverse skin reactions, especially on skin surfaces exposed to sunlight. The drug should be analgetic but there are no trials reported. It is fairly well tolerated by the gastrointestinal tract.

FENAMIC ACIDS

Mefenamic and meclofenamic acids are the two examples available to American physicians. The former was originally introduced as an anti-inflammatory drug but restricted to use for 7 days only because of long-term bone marrow and renal toxicity. It has been more recently reintroduced for a dysmenorrhea indication and has general short-term mild to moderate analgesic effect.

Pharmacology and Toxicity

Both drugs inhibit cyclo-oxygenase and therefore have all of the adverse effects of other such NSAIDs. They also competitively inhibit the peripheral actions of prostaglandins, a unique property. Their half-lives are 2 to 4 hr and a three or four times daily dosage is required. Meclofenamate is associated with a greater incidence of diarrhea than other NSAIDs. Mefenamic acid has been shown to increase blood urea nitrogen and is occasionally associated with serious bone marrow toxicity and hepatic toxicity, both on long-term administration.

Use

Mefenamic acid comes in 250-mg capsules. A dose schedule of one capsule three times daily or four times daily beginning several days before an expected period is an excellent schedule for dysmenorrhea and perhaps other pains as well after they occur. Because of its potential toxicity, use for beyond 1 week is not recommended.

Meclofenamic acid is available in a 100-mg capsule. The suggested antiarthritic dose is 100 mg three times daily (77); at this dose schedule, it should be analgetic, although clinical data are lacking.

ANTIHISTAMINES AND RELATED DRUGS

Methotrimeperazine

This drug might more properly be considered among the thiazines but it has very special properties.

The only preparation available is parenteral, although an oral preparation is pending. In a dosage of 10 to 20 mg, methotrimeperazine confers fairly potent analgesia in humans (42). Its short half-life requires dosing at 3- to 4-hr intervals. It causes a high incidence of postural hypotension and sedation (9) so that it cannot be recommended for patients other than those who are recumbent. It is not recommended for use in those on antihypertension drugs. It is, however, useful in those in whom NSAID, opioids, and opiates are totally contraindicated.

Hydroxyzine

This drug was originally introduced as a sedative/tranquilizer and antihistaminic. It achieved some prominence as a preanesthetic medication and during the course of this use was found to have analgesic properties.

Pharmacology and Toxicity

Hydroxyzine does not significantly bind to narcotic receptor sites, either in the central nervous system or the gut (56). It may have an inhibiting effect on prostaglandin synthesis (82).

Use

As an analgetic, the drug was originally tested as an adjunct to meperidine but in factorial experiments was found to have analgesic properties on its own. In doses of 50 to 100 mg parenterally, it is a moderately potent analgetic (22). However, oral 100-mg doses show no analgetic effect (36), although its sedative and antihistamininc properties can still be demonstrated. This suggests that metabolites are responsible for the latter two effects and that first-pass effects destroy an analgetic component.

Other drugs which are derived from antihistaminics, such as nefopam, have been shown to have analgetic properties (72), but have not been marketed.

COMBINATIONS AND ADDITIVES

One can now understand the rationales for combining certain drugs to induce additive analgesia. Drugs that work peripherally can be combined with those that work centrally. Many such oral preparations are available. The potency of the available combinations is ordinarily based on the dose and type of the centrally-acting agent.

For example, 30 mg codeine plus 650 mg aspirin or 30 mg acetaminophen are each at the lowest measurable analgesic dose for both, but in combination, are more analgetic than either (5). The low doses reduce the possibility of side effects. Preparations containing higher doses of codeine may confer more analgesia but one runs the risk of increased adverse effects owing to the narcotic component. Similar statements can be made of available meperidine/aspirin or meperidine/acetaminophen combinations, pentazocine/aspirin or pentazocine/acetaminophen combinations, propoxyphen/aspirin or propoxyphene/acetaminophen combinations, and oxycodone/aspirin or oxycodone/acetaminophen. The latter combinations are by far the most potent but there is a risk of tolerance and habituation if more than three doses daily are given over a 1 week to 10 day period.

Combinations of two or more narcotics are irrational because the same receptor site is involved. Combinations of two or more peripherally-acting drugs may not be irrational since the receptor sites are really unknown. Aspirin and acetaminophen as a combination seem rational to this observer. Ibuprofen and fenoprofen may not be because of their chemical similarity.

Most of the package inserts for NSAIDs admonish the user not to use aspirin along with them because of a potential increase in gastrointestinal toxicity and reduction in peak plasma levels of the NSAID. The latter consideration has been shown experimentally for several NSAIDs, but there seems to be little evidence that this phenomenon, for which there is no good explanation, has any clinical importance. At least one study suggests that the clinical effect of aspirin and naproxen are additive (80). Since the side effects of all these drugs are related to reduction in prostaglandin synthesis, the side effects of two of them (aspirin plus X) will be entirely because of aspirin because of its added mucosal destructive effect. Either one of such a combination will have maximally turned off prostaglandin synthesis everywhere. The author is not so certain about the safety of aspirin and indomethacin, a combination which seems to cause more gastrointestinal toxicity than either.

Such additives as caffeine or amphetamine have seemed, in clinical trials, to confer additive analgesia, both to aspirin or to narcotics (23). However, there is little information on either of these xanthines being analgesic on their own. The mechanism for the augmenting effect is unknown. Most over-the-counter preparations which contain caffeine do so at levels up to 60 mg, which is about the caffeine content of a strong cup of coffee.

Combinations of analgesics with drugs other than analgesics are not recommended.

SUMMARY

One can be impressed with the advances made in the past 20 years to develop peripherally-acting, non-narcotic analgetics. Selection can be made from a wide variety of different chemical entities. Active research is going on to exploit derivatives of each one. The nonsteroidal group of anti-inflammatory drugs is particularly interesting because their effects, as a group, may be related to interference with a particular enzyme system. However, there are no ready explanations for the activity of other peripherally-acting non-narcotic drugs.

When we are better able to explain the exact molecular biology of the initiation of pain at the periphery, there is no doubt that other chemical entities, more powerful as analgetics and less likely to produce adverse effects, will be developed. This will require further understanding of the relationship of inflammation to pain and the biochemical trigger activating the specific nerve ending which initiates the pain signal.

REFERENCES

1. Abernethy, D. R., Greenblatt, D. J., and Divoll, M. (1982): Differential effects of cimetidine on drug oxidation versus conjugation. Potential mode of therapy for acetaminophen hepatotoxicity. *Clin. Pharm. Therap.*, 31:198 (Abstr.)
2. Baber, N., Halliday, D. C., and Van Den Heuvel, W. J. A. (1979): Indomethacin in rheumatoid arthritis. Clinical effects, pharmacokinetics and platelet studies in responders and non-responders. *Ann. Rheum. Dis.*, 38:128–137.
3. Baskin, W. N., Ivey, K. J., and Krause, W. J. (1976): Aspirin induced ultra-structural changes in human gastric mucosa. Correlation with potential difference. *Ann. Intern. Med.*, 5:299–303.
4. Beaver, W. T. (1965): Mild analgesics. A review of their clinical pharmacology. *Am. J. Med. Sci.*, 251:577–604.
5. Beaver, W. T. (1966): Mild analgesics. A review of their clinical pharmacology. *Am. J. Med. Sci.*, 251:576–599.

6. Bloomfield, S. S., Barden, T. P., and Mitchell, J. (1974): Comparative efficacy of ibuprofen and aspirin in episiotomy pain. *Clin. Pharmacol. Ther.*, 16:565–570.
7. Boardman, P. I., and Hart, F. D. (1967): Clinical management of the anti-inflammatory effects of salicylate in rheumatoid arthritis. *Br. Med. J.*, 4:264–268.
8. Butazolidine. Package insert.
9. Callaghan, P. E., and Zelenik, J. S. (1966): Methotrimeperazine for obstetric analgesia. *Am. J. Obstet. Gynecol.*, 95:636–639.
10. Chaudbury, T. K., and Jacobson, E. D. (1978): Prostaglandin cytoprotection of gastric mucosa. *Gastroenterology*, 74:59–63.
11. Coburn, A. F. (1943): Salicylate therapy in rheumatic fever. *Bull. Johns Hopkins Hospital*, 73:435–464.
12. Cohen, A., Thomas, G. B., and Cohen, E. E. (1978): Serum concentration, safety and tolerance of oral doses of choline magnesium trisalicylate. *Curr. Ther. Res.*, 23:358–364.
13. Cooper, S. A., Needle, S. E., and Kruger, G. O. (1977): Comparative analgesic potency of aspirin and ibuprofen. *J. Oral Surg.*, 35:898–903.
14. Dawson, W. (1980): The componative pharmacology of benoxaprofen. *J. Rheumatol. (Suppl.)*, 6:5–11.
15. Domenjos, R. (1960): The pharmacology of phenylbutazone. Annals N.Y. *Acad. Sci.*, 86:263–291.
16. Dromgoole, S. H., Furst, D. E., and Paulus, H. E. (1981): Rational approaches to the use of salicylates in the treatment of rheumatoid arthritis. *Semin. Arthritis Rheum.*, 11:257–283.
17. Duggan, D. E., Hare, L. E., and Ditzler, C. A. (1977): The disposition of sulindac. *Clin. Pharmacol. Ther.*, 21:326–335.
17a. Ebert, R. H. (1965): The experimental approach to inflammation. In: *The Inflammatory Process*, edited by B. W. Zweifuch, L. Grunt, and R. T. McCluskey. Academic Press, Inc., New York.
18. Feldman, D., and Couropmitree, C. (1976): Intrinsic mineralocorticoid agonist activity of some non-steroidal anti-inflammatory drugs. *J. Clin. Invest.*, 57:1–7.
19. Ferreira, S. H. (1972): Prostaglandins, aspirin-like drugs and analgesia. *Nature*, 240:200–203.
20. Flower, R. J., and Vane, J. R. (1972): Inhibition of prostaglandin synthesis in brain explains the anti-pyretic activity of paracetamol (4-acetaminophenal). *Nature*, 240:410–411.
21. Forbes, J. A., Calderazzo, J. P., and Fowser, M. W. (1982): A 12 hour evaluation of the analgesic efficacy of diflunisal, aspirin and placebo in postoperative dental pain. *J. Clin. Pharmacol.*, 22:89–96.
22. Forrest, W. H. Jr., and Beaver, W. T. (1976): Hydroxyzine added to narcotics for analgesia. *Hosp. Pract.*, (Special Report) 11:20–29.
23. Forrest, W. H. Jr., Brown, B. W., and Brown, C. R. (1977): Dextroamphetamine with morphine for the treatment of post-operative pain. *N. Engl. J. Med.*, 296:712–715.
24. Forrest, W. H. Jr. (1980): Orally administered zomepirac and parenterally administered morphine. *J.A.M.A.*, 244:2298–2302.
25. Freemont-Smith, K., and Bayles, T. B. (1965): Salicylate therapy in rheumatoid arthritis. *J.A.M.A.*, 192:103–106.
26. Goldstein, I. M., Roos, D., and Weissmann, G. (1976): Influence of corticosteroids on human polymorphonuclear leukocyte function in vitro. Reduction of lysosomal enzyme release and superoxide production. *Inflammation*, 1:305–315.
27. Grindel, J. M., Migdalof, B. H., and Plostnieks, J. (1979): Absorption and excretion of tolmetin in arthritic patients. *Clin. Pharmacol. Ther.*, 26:122–128.
28. Halushka, P. V., Wohltman, H., and Privitera, P. J. (1977): Bartter's syndrome: Urinary prostaglandins E-like material and kallekrein. Indomethacin effects. *Ann. Int. Med.*, 87:281–286.
29. Hamdy, R. C., Murnane, B., and Perera, V. (1982): The pharmacokinetics of benoxaprofen in elderly subjects. *Eur. J. Rheum. Inflamm.*, 5:69–75.
30. Heymann, M. A., Rudolph, A. M., and Silverman, N. H. (1976): Closure of the ductus arteriosus in premature infants by inhibiting of prostaglandin synthesis. *N. Engl. J. Med.*, 295:530–533.
31. Honig, W. J., Cremer, C. W., and Manni, J. C. (1978): A single dose study comparing the analgesic effects of diflunisal, acetylsalicylic acid and placebo in pain following meniscectomy. *J. Int. Med. Res.*, 6:172–179.
32. Huskisson, E. C., Woolf, D. L., and Baume, H. (1976): Four new anti-inflammatory drugs: Responses and variations. *Br. Med. J.*, 1:1048–1049.
33. Indocin. Package insert.

34. James, O., Roberts, S. H., and Douglas, A. (1975): Liver damage after paracetamol overdosage. *Lancet*, 2:578–579.
35. Kantor, T. G., Jarvik, M., and Wolff, B. B. (1967): Bradykinin as a mediator of human pain. *Proc. Soc. Exp. Biol. Med.*, 126:505–506.
36. Kantor, T. G., and Steinberg, F. P. (1976): Studies of tranquilizing agents and meperidine in clinical pain. Hydroxyzine and meprobamate. In: *Advances in Pain Research and Therapy, Vol. I*, edited by J. J. Bonica and D. AlbeFessard, pp. 567–572. Raven Press, New York.
37. Kantor, T. G., Streem, A. and Laska, E. (1977): Estimates of doses of anti-inflammatory drugs in man by testing for analgesic potency. *Arthritis Rheum.*, 20:1381–1387.
38. Kantor, T. G. (1979): *Ibuprofen. Ann. Int. Med.*, 91:877–882.
39. Kantor, T. G. (1982): Antiinflammatory drug therapy for back pain. In: *Chronic Low Back Pain*, edited by M. Stanton-Hicks and R. Boas, pp. 157–169. Raven Press, New York.
40. Kuehl, F. A., Jr., Humes, J. L., and Egan, R. W. (1977): Role of prostaglandin endoperoxide PGG_2 in anti-inflammatory processes. *Nature*, 265:170–173.
41. Kuehl, F. A. Jr. (personal communication).
42. Lasagna, L., and DeKornfeld, T. J. (1961): Methotrimeperazine: A new phenothiazine derivative with analgesic properties. *J.A.M.A.*, 178:887–890.
43. Laska, E. M., and Sunshine, A. (1981): Fenoprofen and codeine analgesia. *Clin. Pharmacol. Ther.*, 29:606–616.
44. Levy, G., and Leonards, J. R. (1971): Urine pH and salicylate therapy. *J.A.M.A.*, 217:81.
45. Levy, G., and Tsuchiya, T. (1972): Salicylate accumulation kinetics in man. *N. Engl. J. Med.*, 287:430–432.
46. Levy, G., Tsuchiya, T., and Amsel, L. P. (1972): Limited capacity for salicyl phenolic glucuronide formation and its effect on the kinetics of salicylate elimination in man. *Clin. Pharmacol. Ther.*, 13:258–268.
47. Levy, G., and Giacomini, K. M. (1978): Rational aspirin dosage regimens. *Clin. Pharmacol. Ther.*, 23:247–252.
48. Lim, R. K. S. (1968): Neuropharmacology of pain and analgesia. In: *Pharmacology of Pain*, edited by R. K. S. Lim, D. Armstong, and E. G. Pardo. Pergamon Press, Oxford.
49. Linton, A. L., Clark, W. F., and Driedger, A. A. (1980): Acute interstitial nephritis due to drugs. *Ann. Int. Med.*, 93:735–741.
50. Liyanage, S. P., and Tambar, P. K. (1978): Comparative study of salsalate and aspirin in osteoarthrosis of the hip or knee. *Curr. Med. Res. Opin.*, 5:450–453.
51. Menguy, R., Desbaillets, L., and Masters, Y. (1972): Evidence for a sex-linked difference in aspirin metabolism. *Nature*, 239:102–103.
52. Miller, R. R. (1981): Evaluation of the analgesic effecacy of ibuprofen. *Pharmacotherapy*, 1:21–27.
53. Moertel, C. G., Ahmann, D. L., and Taylor, W. F. (1971): Aspirin and pancreatic cancer pain. *Castroenterology*, 60:552–553.
54. Moertel, C. G. (1980): Treatment of cancer pain with orally administered medications. *J.A.M.A.*, 244:2448–2450.
55. Moncada, S., and Vane, J. R. (1979): Arachidonic acid metabolites and the interaction between platelets and blood vessel walls. *N. Engl. J. Med.*, 300:1142–1147.
56. Musacchio, J. (personal communication).
57. Muschek, L. D., and Grindel, J. M. (1980): Review of the pharmacokinetics and metabolism of zomepirac in man and animals. *J. Clin. Pharmacol.*, 20:223–229.
58. Nathan, C. F., Murray, H. W., and Cohen, Z. A. (1980): The macrophage as an effector cell. *N. Engl. J. Med.*, 303:622–626.
59. Orozco-Alcala, J. J., and Baum, J. (1979): Regular and enteric coated aspirin. A re-evaluation. *Arthritis Rheum.*, 22:1034–1037.
60. Pulkkinen, M. O., and Csapo, A. I. (1978): The effect of ibuprofen on the intrauterine pressure and menstrual pain of dysmenorrhea patients. *Prostaglandins*, 15:1055–1062.
61. Robert, A. (1974): Effects of prostaglandins on the stomach and the intestine. *Prostaglandins*, 6:523–532.
62. Roth, G. J., Standord, N., and Majerus, P. W. (1975): Acetylation of prostaglandin synthetase by aspirin. *Proc. Natl. Acad. Sci. U.S.A.*, 72:3073–3076.
63. Samter, M. (1973): Intolerance to aspirin. *Hosp. Pract.*, 8:85–90.

64. Scott, W. A., Pawlowski, W. A., and Andreach, M. (1982): Resting macrophages produce distinct metabolites from exogenous arachidonic acid. *J. Exp. Med.*, 155:535–547.
65. Seaman, W. E., and Plotz, P. H. (1976): Effect of aspirin on liver tests in patients with rheumatoid arthritis or systemic lupus erythematosus and in normal volunteers. *Arthritis Rheum.*, 19:155–160.
66. Seyberth, H. W., Raisz, L. G., and Oates, J. A. (1978): Prostaglandins and hypercalcemic states. *Annu. Rev. Med.*, 29:23–29.
67. Smith, D. C., and Regan, M. G. (1980): Ibuprofen in psoriatic arthritis. *Arthritis Rheum.*, 23:961–962.
68. Smyth, C. J., and Percy, J. S. (1973): Comparison of indomethacin and phenylbutazone in acute gout. *Ann. Rheum. Dis.*, 32:351–353.
69. Snyder, S. H. (1979): Receptors, neurotransmitters and drug responses. *N. Engl. J. Med.*, 300:465–472.
70. Sorbie, J. (1982): Prostaglandin inhibitors—Rational therapy for dysmenorrhea. *Canad. Fam. Phys.*, 28:91–95.
71. Sunshine, A., Laska, E., and Meisner, M. (1964): Analgesic studies of indomethacin as analyzed by computer techniques. *Clin. Pharmacol. Ther.*, 5:699–707.
72. Sunshine, A., Laska, E., and Slafta, J. (1978): Oral nefopam and aspirin. *Clin. Pharmacol. Ther.*, 24:555–559.
73. Tainter, M. L., and Ferris, A. J. (1969): History. In: *Aspirin in Modern Therapy*, p. 1–3. Bayer Co. Div. of Sterling Drug, Inc., New York.
74. Tausch, G. (1982): Placebo controlled study of piroxicam in the treatment of rheumatoid arthritis. *Am. J. Med. (Suppl.)*, 72:18–22.
75. Temple, A. R., George, D. J., and Dore, A. K. (1976): Salicylate poisoning complicated by fluid retention. *Clin. Toxicol.*, 9:61–68.
76. Vane, J. R. (1972): Prostaglandins and the aspirin-like drugs. *Hosp. Pract.*, 7:61–71.
77. Vreede, P. D., and Parrino, G. R. (1982): Double-blind comparison of meclofenamate (Meclomen) with placebo in the treatment of rheumatoid arthritis. *Curr. Ther. Res.*, 32:288–294.
78. Wallenstein, S. L., Rogers, A., and Kaiko, R. F. (1980): Relative analgesic potency of oral zomepirac and intramuscular morphine in cancer patients with postoperative pain. *J. Clin. Pharmacol.*, 20:250–258.
79. Weissman, G., Smolen, J. E., and Korchak, H. M. (1980): Release of inflammatory mediators from stimulated neutrophils. *N. Engl. J. Med.*, 303:27–34.
80. Willkens, R. F., and Segre, E. J. (1976): Combination therapy with naproxen and aspirin in rheumatoid arthritis. *Arthritis Rheum.*, 19:677–681.
81. Wiseman, E. H., and Hobbs, D. C. (1982): Review of pharmacokinetic studies with piroxicam. *Am. J. Med. (Suppl.)*, 72:9–17.
82. Wiseman, E. (personal communication).
83. Yu, T. F., Dayton, G., and Gutman, A. B. (1963): Mutual suppression of the uricosuric effects of sulfinpyrazone and salicylate. *J. Clin. Invest.*, 42:1330–1339.

Analgesics: Neurochemical, Behavioral, and Clinical Perspectives, edited by M. Kuhar and G. Pasternak. Raven Press, New York © 1984.

Future Vistas

E. Leong Way

Department of Pharmacology, University of California at San Francisco, San Francisco, California 94143

Crystal ball gazing may not be legitimate science, but it may still have some validity for guiding future investigative approaches. In looking forward, it is always advantageous first to look back so that past errors will not be repeated and the building can start from imaginative concepts that have withstood the test of time.

The present volume tells of the amazing progress that has been made in the anatomy, physiology, biochemistry, and pharmacology of pain. The authors have summarized most of the recent developments and hence, for my task, I need only to give emphasis to some of their commentaries and fill in some crevices with my biases. Although some of the notions may not be entirely my own, I shall not make too many citations, since an extensive bibliography is already provided in each chapter.

Some more significant basic discoveries made within the past decade deserve special emphasis, because in addition to augmenting the understanding of the etiology of pain, they provided the stimulus and impetus for initiating so many other basic and clinical studies. For example, the finding that aspirin-like compounds act by inhibiting prostaglandin synthesis was a major breakthrough. Of similar significance were the identification of opioid recognition or binding sites and the isolation of native peptide ligands with morphine-like activity.

With respect to the opioid receptor and ligand studies, I should like to insert a personal note about a prophesy. At the embryonic stage of the work, I had the privilege of hearing the most terse yet foretelling statement of the current state of the art in this area, and I have never forgotten the words. When Vincent Dole was asked in 1974 to keynote a symposium on "The Opiate Receptor," he rose and said, "I object to all three words."

With time, the statement has revealed Dole's deep insight and perspective. It has become increasingly apparent that "binding sites" and "receptors" are not synonymous, and furthermore, multiple opioid recognition or binding sites have been demonstrated. Also, more than one native ligand with opiate-like properties have been discovered, but all are peptides instead of alkaloids. In projecting to the future, therefore, it is necessary for me to borrow from the wisdom provided by the words of an admired friend and colleague.

313

LESSONS FROM HISTORY

Looking at new vistas dictates the necessity of repeating the cliché about maintaining an open mind. Outmoded beliefs must be quickly abandoned in the face of new facts that are well derived and difficult to refute. History has taught that entrenchment in dogma can be a major hindrance to the development of innovative conceptual approaches. Lasagna's overview (chapter 1) has placed the subject in proper perspective. Long-held beliefs are difficult to discard even when the facts are straightforward and obvious.

A good example to illustrate this point can be learned from the notions concerning the mode of the action of aspirin. It had been long assumed that aspirin produces pain relief by a central effect, despite the fact that pharmacologists were unable to demonstrate an antinociceptive action for the compound by either the conventional tail flick or hot-plate procedures, which give excellent predictions of opiate agonist analgetic potency and efficacy. In fairness, there was some basis for the misconception. After all, aspirin and other antipyretic analgetics had been shown to lower body temperature, apparently by promoting heat loss via an effect on the hypothalamus. It appeared only reasonable to conclude, therefore, that aspirin afforded pain relief by action in the brain, even if the site and effect could not be demonstrated convincingly in the laboratory. Of course, we know now that injections of prostaglandins will cause both pain and fever but this was not known in 1962 when Lim showed, by his elegant cross-perfusion experiments in dogs, that aspirin and other antipyretic analgetics elicit their effects by a local action (*see* chapter 11). Although the data were most convincing, acceptance of the fact was still extremely slow and grudging. Even a decade after this study was published, aspirin was classified usually in pharmacologic texts as a centrally-acting analgetic, and Lim's findings were hardly mentioned.

As documented by Brune (chapter 6), it was not until 1971, when two British laboratories independently demonstrated that aspirin-like drugs inhibit prostaglandin biosynthesis, was there general dawning that the compounds might indeed be producing analgesia by a local action. It appeared only reasonable that compounds with dissimilar structures, but sharing the same therapeutic and side effects, should also share an effect on a common biochemical pathway. The studies finally convinced the skeptics. Subsequent studies by Vane and his associates rekindled interest in the aspirin-like compounds (7). The renaissance resulted not only in the recent marketing of several potent nonsteroidal analgetics with an efficacy approaching that of the opiates, but also promoted the study of other clinical applications of aspirin such as in stroke and myocardial infarction.

The discovery of the prostaglandin synthetase inhibitory properties of aspirin opened vistas not only with respect to new clinical applications, but also to more careful application of the compound. While it had been long-recognized that prolonged high dosage of aspirin can result in gastrointestinal bleeding, because its platelet antiaggregation properties were not known, it was not readily appreciated that aspirin might promote generalized bleeding. Neurosurgeons, in particular, are now alerted to the possibility that aspirin can be a contributory cause of cerebro-vascular accidents and be a complicating factor when surgery is required.

METHODOLOGY

Progress in any given area of scientific research is governed principally by the tools that can be applied. In the case of brain peptides with opioid-like activity, although the discovery of the first one was announced only as recently as late 1975, the number of publications on these substances since then likely exceed the total on all other neuropeptides combined. The frenetic activity on the opioid peptides, of course, does not mean that they have greater biologic significance than the other peptides, but only that investigators have followed the path of least resistance, and are carrying out research on the substances easiest to study. Earlier workers in narcotic research have provided those enticed freshly from related disciplines with simple *in vitro* and *in vivo* tools for studying peptides with mor-phine-like activity.

We have learned from both Michne and Wood (chapters 5 and 7) of the wide assortment of experimental procedures available for assessing analgetic compounds. The battery of tests include, in addition to the usual *in vivo* ones, some valuable *in vitro* techniques. Of particular interest is the ability of certain *in vitro* methods to provide highly predictive data with respect to analgetic potency and efficacy. In the guinea pig ileum, for example, the correlation between the ability of μ agonists to inhibit electrically-induced contractions and clinical potency is extremely good. Even with chemical binding tests, affinity and rank order of pharmacologic potency correlate surprisingly well. The use of Na^+ to antagonize or enhance opiate binding provides further insight into agonist or antagonist activity. However, even with the plethora of excellent procedures at hand, it needs to be emphasized that they measure essentially the activity of known prototypic compounds and can not be expected to reveal new classes of agents. A substance that yields a positive anti-nociceptive response by either the rodent tail flick or hot-paw technique is also liable to produce respiratory depression, tolerance, and physical dependence, and, on the other hand, a novel innovative compound might well be missed in the screen. However, for the mixed antagonist-agonist analgetics, the tail flick and hot-plate procedures can be used for reverse screening. When a compound indicated analgetic activity by the writing test, Harris then used a positive tail flick or hot-plate response to discard the compound because of its likelihood of producing addiction liability similar to morphine.

The main need in methodology is better animal procedures for evaluating chronic pain. The present models for acute pain often miss the mark because they do not always provide valid information concerning chronic pain. They are essentially based on anatomic and physiologic aspects of pain, and do not yield information on the reactive components, because emotional and psychologic factors are difficult to assess. Nonetheless, in chronic headaches, back disorders, causalgia, postherpetic neuralgia, cancer, etc., these factors are major considerations that can not be ignored. Perhaps, those demands are too much for an inarticulate animal but at least approaches can be made.

Some inroads have been made in producing animal models for chronic pain by deafferentation of select sites such as the spinal cord, brainstem, thalamus, and cortex. Several models for autoimmune disease are also available. One example for rheumatoid arthritis and perhaps other connective tissue disease is the use of type II collagen to induce chronic peripheral polyarthritis by immunization in the rat. Validity and applicability of the model is suggested by the fact that the arthritis developed may result from an "autoimmune response." Also, difference in the susceptibility to this procedure by various strains of rats indicate that the disease has a genetic basis.

Clinical assessment of analgetic drugs have come a long way, and the battery of available techniques have been thoroughly documented (Wallenstein, chapter 9). Although double-blind testing with a placebo originated from clinical assessment of analgetic drugs (Lasagna, chapter 1), I have reservations about the necessity for the use of placebos. I recognize that there is a relatively high incidence of placebo reactors when drugs are tested for alleviation of symptoms, but this does not mean that a clinical study has to be performed double-blind with a placebo. I object to the use of placebo for philosophic and pharmacologic reasons. Ethically, it does not seem right to deny medication to a person suffering from pain, especially if it may not be at all necessary. We teach the beginning medical student the simple dictum that drugs exhibit a dose-response relationship, and an increasing effect may be expected with increasing dosage until a ceiling is reached. Thus, any new compounds introduced today should have sufficient analgetic potency and efficacy to yield a good dose-response curve. Hence, after preliminary dose-ranging studies on a test substance, dose-response studies can be carried out on a double-blind basis without a placebo. In most instances, the lowest dose of the compound would serve as the placebo, but such studies would be justified morally and scientifically because the investigator wishes to find the lowest effective dose that causes minimal side effects. It will be argued on practical grounds that such a study would be too expensive. However, many clinical assessments are now made comparing a placebo with two doses of a test compound. I would argue that a satisfactory dose-response curve could be obtained with three doses and such experiments would yield more valid data without much more effort in time and money.

LIGANDS AND MORE LIGANDS

The number of peptides with opiate-like activity now approximate at least a dozen, and it appears that only the tip of the iceberg has been exposed. The announcement of many other active peptides can be expected. The formidable task lies ahead to map their neuronal pathways and elucidate their function.

It has become increasingly clear that there are at least three types of peptides in the brain with opioid-like activity. They are distinct, with respect to their receptors, neuronal distribution, and biosynthetic pathways (Frederickson, chapter 2). The

systems may be conveniently named enkephalingeric, endorphinergic, and dynorphinergic. Although endorphin was originally proposed as the generic name for
opioid-like peptides, the term has not been generally accepted. Often endorphins
have been loosely associated with systems identified with β-endorphin. Perhaps it
should be reserved only for this purpose, in which case, the family name for all
peptides might well be termed opiopeptins.

Many of the active peptides that have been identified may be fragments of larger
precursor molecules, and the true identity of each native ligand needs to be established. The answer lies in part on ascertaining the biosynthetic pathways of these
substances with more refined technology that will allow determination of closely
related peptides with greater precision and specificity than current immunoreactive
procedures.

Greater specificity in peptide analysis will almost certainly be achieved by the
use of hybridomal cell lines to make monocloncal antibodies against the various
opiopeptins. Also, changes in immunoreactivity can be followed by the use of
enzymatic digestion with various peptide fragments before incubation with antibodies. Moreover, the binding properties of these antibodies with opioid agonists
and antagonists likely can mimic those of the drug receptor and thus provide clues
with respect to its structure, configuration, and conformation.

The presence of relatively large amounts of enkephalin-like material in the adrenal
medulla raises a number of questions concerning the active species of the enkephalins, since only a small proportion of the total enkephalin-like immunoreactivity
is in the form of free methionine- or leucine-enkephalin. In particular, the precursor
molecule with a molecular weight of about 50,000 daltons which, after digestion
gives rise to approximately six molecules of Met-enkephalin to one of Leu-enkephalin, appears to contain repeating sequences of the two enkephalins. It now
appears that this enkephalin precursor is also present in the brain, because potent
biologically active low molecular weight Met-enkephalin and Leu-enkephalin peptides have recently been identified there. The fact that gene cloning experiments
provide evidence that the amino acid sequence of the Pro-enkephalin macromolecule
from human pheochromocytomas is similar to that from the bovine adrenal medulla
gives added meaning to this 50 K dalton protein. Also of interest is the active
heptapeptide (Met-enkephalin Arg[6]-Phe[7]) that has been isolated from the striatum
as well as the adrenal medulla. These studies raise important questions concerning
the role of Met-enkephalin and Leu-enkephalin. It can be argued that they may not
be true native neuromodulators or transmitters, but merely end-product fragments
that retain some of the biologic activity of a more active common precursor. The
next decade will almost surely provide the answers.

The fact that the enkephalins and the catecholamines are stored in the same
chromaffin vesicle and are coreleased from the adrenal gland on stimulation is most
intriguing. The task remains to determine which of the opioid-like peptides are
released into the bloodstream. Since the native enkephalins appear to have very
short half-lives, it is possible that they may act locally in the adrenal gland and/or
that larger precursor peptides are transported via the circulatory system to their

peripheral site of action. Independent of the function of these medullary peptides, it appears that the adrenal medulla is a highly useful model for studying the biosynthesis of the enkephalins. Whether enkephalins in the brain are derived from a common precursor or are processed by similar enzymes as in the adrenal gland are important points that need to be clarified. Although exogenously administered enkephalins have very short half-lives in the body, and can be cleaved by a variety of ubiquitous peptidases, the two enkephalinases which have been purified from the brain hold perhaps greater relevance should further studies reveal that their distribution parallel that of the enkephalins and their receptors.

A large variety of peptides have been examined, but the attempts to develop specific enkephalinase inhibitors have been rather disappointing. However, more recent studies look promising. Inhibitors that can potentiate the central actions of the enkephalins have been recently reported. In particular, the finding that thiorphan, not only blocks the *in vitro* degradation of the enkephalins at micromolar concentrations, but also produces analgesia that is naloxone reversible, offers new hope that new agents can be developed by inhibiting enkephalin degradation. Other enkephalin analogs, relatively resistant to enzymatic degradation and exhibiting strong analgetic properties after minor chemical modification, also display interesting pharmacologic characteristics. They more closely resemble morphine or β-endorphin in central action.

RECEPTOROLOGY

With so many active ligands being isolated with varying degrees of morphine-like properties, it is difficult indeed to keep pace with studies that can identify the receptor corresponding with the ligand, even though it appears that the different receptors may have subtypes (Goodman and Pasternak, chapter 3). It seems rather unlikely that the number of receptor subtypes can equal the number of active peptides, because many of the latter may be active fragments of a common precursor. Another complication is the fact that one ligand may bind to several receptor subtypes. Having irreversible antagonists that selectively bind to specific receptors would facilitate their identification.

It should be emphasized that the opiate receptor is still a figment of the imagination of pharmacologists. Although opiate binding or recognition sites have been identified, the receptor remains to be isolated. The state of the art is such that receptor isolation and characterization studies are being carried out without regard to whether there are actually, in fact, the different opioid subtypes suggested by pharmacologic and binding studies. For the present, the solubilization and purification of any membrane material capable of binding endogenous or exgenous opioid ligands would represent a major technologic advance.

The concept of having multiple opioid receptors simplifies and complicates the thinking concerning opiate action. For explaining mixed antagonist-agonist effects, it is convenient to classify a compound such as nalorphine as a μ-antagonist and a κ-agonist, were it not for the fact that not all antagonist-agonists fit this mold.

Invoking the δ receptor to explain selective effects of the enkephalins on the mouse vas deferens would have more significance if binding studies on this preparation yielded more definitive data. If δ receptors in the brain are not involved in analgetic action, what does agonist affinity at specific brain sites translate into in terms of a behavioral effect that can be applied for correlative studies? Will it be necessary to invoke more and more subsets of distinct receptors, or will it be possible to establish different conformations of a parent type?

The concept of multiple receptors provides a reasonable explanation for some of the inconsistencies in the action of the enkephalins. One of the disappointments after the discovery of the enkephalins was the fact that they exhibited little or no analgetic activity. To explain this failure it was proposed initially that the effects of the enkephalins were dissipated by rapid metabolism. This argument was made in the face of evidence that the enkephalins failed to produce analgetic effects at a reasonably high dose, even after their injection at sensitive sites, that behavioral effects other than analgesia could be elicited after systemic administration, that fairly long-lasting effects could be obtained with isolated tissue preparations, and that the binding properties of the enkephalins different from those of the opiate alkaloids. Fortunately, it was not too long before Martin's theory of opiate receptors dualism, which he first proposed in 1967 and substantiated in 1976, was invoked to provide a more plausible explanation.

A conceptual approach that might serve to reduce the number of subsets of opiate receptors is encompassed in the model proposed by Lee and her associates for the β-endorphin receptor (9). Based on both pharmacologic and binding data, β-endorphin has been visualized to interact at a receptor containing both a μ and a δ site. It is argued that since β-endorphin is as potent as morphine in the ileum and as potent as enkephalin in the mouse vas deferens, and since β-endorphin displaces either type of ligand equally well and vice versa (that is, radioactive β-endorphin is displaced to about the same degree by opiate alkaloids and the enkephalins), β-endorphin must interact concomitantly with at least two sites. To bolster further the case, structure-activity relationship studies were cited to indicate that the intact β-endorphin molecule is required for expressing full biological as well as binding activity. Thus, shortening of the β-endorphin chain by removal of the middle peptide sequences decreases biologic activity and binding. Moreover, modifications of the five N-terminal amino acids having the Met-enkephalin sequence decreases both binding to brain tissue and biological potency, and although less critical, sequential removal of C-terminal amino acids also gradually results in reduction in binding and biological activity.

The above results are interpreted to indicate that the active site of β-endorphin resides at its N-terminus and at another site, 14 to 24 carbons removed from the N-terminus, the first site being the δ-site where enkephalin binds and the latter one the μ-site where morphine interacts. Although each of these two types of ligands can initiate activity by binding to their receptive receptor, β-endorphin must bind simultaneously at both loci. Thus, the β-endorphin receptor is viewed as a complex containing both μ and δ binding sites. Based on other evidence, it is further proposed that the enkephalin site may be contained in a protein and the morphine site may be lipid associated. This concept has the advantage of unifying a great deal of information hitherto explained in terms of multiple opiate receptors, but like all other operational postulates, good and bad, it needs to be verified by the isolation of the receptor.

Studies on the chemical nature of the opiate receptor do suggest it to consist of lipids as well as protein. Cerebroside sulfate (CS), in particular, holds particular interest. The case for CS has been summarized (Goodman and Pasternak, chapter 3). Although, the widespread occurrence of CS appears to conflict with the specific pattern of opiate receptor distribution, it can be argued that only the CS strategically localized at membrane sites is critical (10). Thus, CS or other glycolipids in association with certain unknown proteins may well represent a functional opiate receptor, which would not only permit specific opiate-receptor binding, but would also allow opiate-Ca^{2+}-lipid (CS) interactions.

With respect to the protein moiety involved in opiate receptor activity, solubilization of brain membranes using nonionic mild detergents have been disappointing in that a reduction in stereospecific binding invariably results. It becomes increasingly apparent that the procedures amenable for the isolation of the acetylcholine receptor are not entirely applicable for the opiate receptor. Perhaps solubilization of the opiate receptor by ultrasonication offers a new approach, since it circumvents the presence of solubilization agents which interfere with opiate binding (4).

MECHANISM OF ACTION

A number of hypotheses have been advanced to explain the mode of action of the opiate drugs. In the past, the postulates have been directed toward implicating one of several putative neurotransmitters found in the brain. Acetylcholine, 5-hydroxy-tryptamine, norepinephrine, dopamine, δ-aminobutyric acid, and substance P have been among those investigated (Basbaum, chapter 4, Haubrich et al., chapter 8). Experimental evidence can be cited to argue a role for any one of the substances in opiate action. It is likely that they are all involved in the expression of opiate effects. In view of this, it appears more probable that the primary mechanism should involve an action common to all these native brain ligands. One of the links might be concerned with a second messenger such as Ca^{2+} or cAMP, and indeed, both agents have been postulated to be responsible for opiate action. Although a role can be argued for both substances, the evidence supporting a case for Ca^{2+} is rather extensive and includes *in vitro* as well as *in vivo* findings, whereas the data for cAMP are derived mainly from experiments on cultured hybrid cells. The arguments implicating Ca^{2+} in opioid action are summarized below from recent reviews which cite the original studies (2,3).

There is considerable electrophysiologic data to support an opioid action on Ca^{2+} flux. Opiates appear to act primarily as inhibitors of sensitive neurons to prevent firing. In instances where the effects of opiates are found to be excitatory, they have been found to occur from disinhibition. The electrophysiologic data argue for a presynaptic site for opiate action, but do not preclude a postsynaptic mechanism. The opioid-induced presynaptic inhibition appears to be related to the inhibition of neurotransmitter release that is coupled with Ca^{2+} disposition. An enkephalin analog D-Ala$_2$-enkephalinamide not only inhibits depolarized Ca^{2+}-dependent release of substance P from sensory neurons grown in dispersed cell culture, but also decreases the duration of the Ca^{2+} action potential recorded from the cell body. A similar effect on Ca^{2+} channels located at nerve endings would explain the action of opiates on neurotransmitter release. Also Ca^{2+} antagonizes the inhibitory effects of opioids on excitatory junction potentials of the stimulated mouse vas deferens as well as the firing of neurons in the myenteric plexus. Based on intracellular recordings made from neurons in the myenteric ganglia of the guinea pig ileum and ciliary ganglion of the cat, it seems that opiates may act by impairing K^+ conductance; the consequence would be altered Ca^{2+} disposition, hyperpolarization, and inhibition of neuronal firing.

There is also pharmacologic evidence indicating that Ca^{2+} can inhibit a wide variety of acute effects of opiates both *in vivo* and *in vitro*. In addition, opiates produce a rapid fall in neuronal Ca^{2+} levels after acute treatment, and an adaptive gradual increase in Ca^{2+} levels occurs as tolerance develops after prolonged opiate treatment. These two opposing effects on Ca^{2+} disposition have been used to formulate an hypothesis which provides an explanation for the classic effects of opiates. Thus, analgesia, tolerance, and physical dependence are considered to depend on the functional state of the neuron as regulated by its Ca^{2+} levels.

When acute opiate treatment causes decreasing Ca^{2+} binding and/or fluxes at nerve endings, this results in reduced neurotransmitter release, since the latter effect is dependent on Ca^{2+} influx. In support of this postulate, it has been shown that Ca^{2+} antagonists such as the Ca^{2+} chelator, ethylene glycol-bis(β-amino ethyl ether)-N,N' tētre acetic acid (EGTA), and La^{3+}, which blocks Ca^{2+} entry, can enhance opiate analgesia and can themselves produce analgesia. These agents are less potent than opiates, possibly because they act generally, whereas opiates appear to act at specific Ca^{2+} pools associated with synaptic plasma membranes (SPM) and synaptic vesicles. Conversely, Ca^{2+} not only can antagonize opiate-induced analgesia, but can also produce hyperalgesia. Furthermore, the ionophores X537A and A23187, which facilitate Ca^{2+} influx, enhance Ca^{2+} antagonism of opiate action.

With prolonged opiate administration, a counteradaptive mechanism increasingly takes over to retain Ca^{2+}. This results in increased Ca^{2+} and/or uptake at synaptic vesicles and SPM sites. The elevated Ca^{2+} tends to oppose acute opiate effects and as a result more opiate is required to again reduce intracellular Ca^{2+} accumulation. As a consequence, one might expect that the augmented Ca^{2+} should antagonize the analgetic effects of La^{3+} and EGTA; the cross-tolerance to these two agents noted in the morphine tolerant state is consistent with this notion.

The increase in Ca^{2+} cumulation requires the continual presence of the opiate and this may explain physical dependence development. Thus, when opiate discontinuance or antagonist treatment removes the agonist, the high synaptosomal Ca^{2+}

content in the absence of the agonist produces greatly increased neurotransmitter release. This neuronal hyperexcitability then gives rise to withdrawal signs and symptoms. Hyperalgesia, for example, may occur after dissipation of morphine at receptor sites below a critical level. Indeed, the hyperalgesia can be further enhanced by intracerebroventricular injection of Ca^{2+}. Also according to this model, the abstinence syndrome can be attenuated by reducing intracellular Ca^{2+}. Compatible with this notion, La^{3+} administration reduces abrupt or naloxone-induced withdrawal jumping in mice.

This model further suggests that Ca^{2+} administration, by opposing opiate effects on intracellular binding, should reduce tolerance development, whereas EGTA, by decreasing Ca^{2+} availability to the same site during opiate administration, should enhance tolerance development. Thus, the hypothesis suggests the Ca^{2+} site for mediating acute pharmacologic effects is distinct from that for producing tolerance and physical dependence.

If our views concerning two opposing acute effects of opiate are correct, the possibility for developing analgetics of the opiate type without the liabilities of tolerance and physical development has some theoretic basis. Supposing, for example, if acute opiate effects concerned with acute pharmacologic action are mediated somehow via the Ca^{2+} channel, whereas those associated with tolerance and physical dependence are limited to an intracellular compartment such as the inner SPM or synaptic vesicles, it can then be expected that the affinity constants of the two sites for different agonists are likely to be different, in which case, the acute and delayed effects can indeed be separated quantitatively if not qualitatively. There is already some evidence to suggest such a possibility. In terms of analgetic potency and efficacy, morphine and methadone are nearly equal. However, it is well-established in the experimental laboratory, and the findings appear to be supported clinically, that the rate and degree of tolerance development to and dependency on methadone are less than for morphine. Furthermore, there are several studies indicating that the development of morphine tolerance and physical dependence can be blocked by inhibitors of protein synthesis at doses which do not alter acute pharmacologic action. This could be interpreted to mean that the macromolecule(s) associated with either tolerance or physical dependence development are turning over at a more rapid rate than the one associated with mediating acute effects. Such an explanation may provide the clue for why agonist or antagonist displacement binding experiments do not reveal differences between the naive and the tolerant-dependent animal.

Another explanation that is compatible with the Ca^{2+} hypothesis has been proposed to account for acute and chronic opiate effects based on changes in lipid metabolism (10). Acute opiate effects are considered to arise from alterations in membrane lipid structure owing to agonist receptor binding. Since phospholipids are known to stimulate gene expression, it is further argued that prolonged drug treatment and the consequent changes in lipid metabolism may alter the synthesis of protein necessary for tolerance and physical dependent development. This model is consistent with the Ca^{2+} model since the changes in lipid metabolism could well involve changes in Ca^{2+} metabolism after acute and chronic treatment. The specific Ca^{2+} pool(s) interacting with opiates have not been conclusively identified, but several possibilities have been considered.

ATPase enzymes represent possible site of opiate interference with Ca^{2+} flux because these enzymes have an important function in active ion transport. A number of investigators have reported positive effects of opiates on ATPase activity after *in vitro*, acute, and chronic treatment, but no clear pattern emerges from these studies that can adequately explain tolerance development. The data obtained with Mg^{2+}-dependent ATPase in synaptic vesicles perhaps have some relevance because the activity of this enzyme in synaptic vesicles was significantly increased after tolerance development, whereas the activities of the Mg^{2+}-dependent ATPase and Na^+, K^+ activated ATPase from SPM fractions were not altered. Since synaptic vesicles are known to contain neurotransmitters and Ca^{2+} is important for neurotransmitter release, the changes in synaptic vesicles Ca^{2+} content after opiate treatment may represent an interference with release mechanisms on Mg^{2+}-dependent ATPase of synaptic vesicles, in as much as this enzyme has been implicated in the regulation of neurotransmitter release and Ca^{2+} accumulation.

Another possible binding site for opioids may be calmodulin. Calmodulin regulates the activity of many enzymes including phosphodiesterase and adenylate cyclase via the formation of complexes in response to Ca^{2+} fluxes. Calmodulin appears, therefore, to be a Ca^{2+} receptor site and represents a link between different types of cell messengers, namely, Ca^{2+} and cAMP, and may thus represent an important site for Ca^{2+} opiate interactions.

Another possible form of Ca^{2+} opiate interaction is drug-induced inhibition of Ca^{2+} binding at synaptic membrane sites, but the evidence for such an effect needs considerable reinforcement. Opiates might displace Ca^{2+} from anionic binding sites on phospholipid molecules in neuronal membranes. The displacement of Ca^{2+} from these phospholipid opiate receptors would thus result in changes in membrane permeability to other ions and produce changes in neuronal excitability. Based on data that the phospholipid base-exchange reaction in nervous tissue is stimulated by Ca^{2+}, perhaps morphine alters the turnover and/or composition of membrane phospholipids by a direct effect on the Ca^{2+}-dependent base-exchange reaction. Marked alterations in exchange observed after chronic treatment possibly reflect a homeostatic adaptative change to overcome acute effects.

Attempts have been made also to relate opiate effects to adenylate cyclase and guanylate cyclase since it has been noted that Ca^{2+} must be present before opiates can induce changes in activity. Adenylate cyclase activity in neuroblastoma x glioma cell lines is inhibited by opioids, whereas prolonged treatment induces increased activity once the restraint imposed by the drug has been removed. This system has also been proposed as a model for studying opiate effects related to tolerance/dependence production.

Synaptic membrane-bound protein kinase activity is regulated by both cAMP and Ca^{2+}, and the possibility that opiates might alter protein kinase activity by reducing Ca^{2+} availability has been considered. Williams has shown that acute treatment of rats with a number of narcotics and opiate peptides results in an initial increase, followed by a subsequent decrease in striatal SPM phosphorylation *in vitro* (5). This pattern resembled that owing to Ca^{2+} changes. It was postulated that the opiates, by reducing intrasynaptosomal Ca^{2+} levels, first gave rise to optimal Ca^{2+} levels (and hence increased phosphorylation), while further reduction of Ca^{2+} levels resulted in reduced phosphorylation.

PAIN PATHWAYS AND CLINICAL ASPECTS

Much information has been generated on the pain pathways, and yet the gaps in the knowledge are tremendous. Most of the studies, particularly, have been concerned with the enkephalinergic system. Some progress has been made in defining the role of bulbospinal neurons, but the major achievements have been in delineating the involvement of the dorsal horn. As mentioned by Basbaum (chapter 4) and Haubrich (chapter 8), there is considerable data indicating that nociceptive input in the dorsal horn can be altered by peripheral, spinal, and supraspinal descending control systems. This supports the Melzack and Wall hypothesis (12) that peripheral specificity in perception can be modified peripherally and centrally, and points to the substantia gelatinosa in the spinal horn as the gate which modifies peripheral sensory input.

Long before the identification of opiate receptors, it had been established that there is a spinal component to the action of morphine and its surrogates. In patients with transected spinal cords, clinicians have used morphine to reduce the intensity of noxious stimuli below the level of the lesion. Moreover, in a spinalized animal, although an antinociceptive effect of morphine can be demonstrated, a higher dose than that in the intact animal is required. More recent validation that the spinal cord is an important site of opiate action is supported by the fact that long-lasting analgesia in the rat was produced in a dose-dependent fashion by opiates without loss of motor function by microinjection of morphine into the subarachnoid space. Thus, it appears that opioids act at both spinal and supraspinal sites. Descending tracts from supraspinal structures can modulate the effect of incoming noxious stimuli likely by effecting release of opioid peptides in the spinal cord at or near opioid receptors in the substantia gelantinosa, in which case, exogenous opioids injected at such loci should also be antinociceptive. It was only logical to expect, therefore, that there were practical benefits to be gained from using morphine and its surrogates epidurally.

The presence of opiate receptors in the spinal cord meant that opiates, when applied at these sites, should selectively elicit analgetic effects and produce minimal side effects. On a theoretic basis, the use of opiates instead of local anesthetics for the production of spinal analgesia offers several advantages. The pain relief from opiates should be achieved without impairment of motor as well as autonomic functions, and sensations other than pain should not be affected. Furthermore, the risks after accidental overdosage would be less, since, unlike local anesthetics, opiates would be less likely to cause cardiovascular collapse or convulsions and any opiate overdosage would be easily counteracted with naloxone. Since the experimental studies, a number of clinical reports demonstrating the production of long-lasting analgesia after epidural or intrathecal opiates in various types of painful conditions with relatively minimal side effects have been published. It is becoming increasingly clear that clinically these routes of administering opiates are not only feasible but under certain conditions have distinct advantages (Foley and Inturrisi, chapter 10). And in view of Martin's idea that the κ receptor is localized in the spinal cord, administration of κ-agonists at this site should be feasible and greater selectivity in action might be gained. *In vitro* data suggest that dynorphin may be an endogenous ligand for the κ-receptor in the gastrointestinal tract. Although *in vivo* findings are not entirely consistent with this notion, the rapid studies being made in mapping the dynorphinergic system should greatly enhance the knowledge concerning its role in pain mechanism.

Although much has been learned about the role of the spinal horn, and especially the substantia gelatinosa in opiate action, the vast array of other neuropeptides there raises many questions. Granted that substance P may be an excitatory component of pain mechanism in the cord, why are bombesin, cholecystokinin, vasoactive polypeptides, oxytocin, to name but a few, there, and what are they doing? Also to be considered are bulbospinal neurons where enkephalin, somatostatin, and thyrotropin-releasing hormones may coexist with biogenic amines and GABA. Do all these substances have independent pathways? Clearly, there is still much to be done in these areas.

The reticular formation has been demonstrated to be an important site for action of analgetic agents. Lesions of the reticular formation can affect reactivity to noxious stimulus. Morphine has been demonstrated to produce analgesia after local injection into various reticular sites. Thus, it appears that certain neurons in the reticular formation can be influenced by nociceptive input. However, it is well-established that this region does not relate exclusively to pain but contributes to other aspects of behavior. Since cells of the deep layer of the spinal cord are known to project to the reticular formation, intense nociceptive stimulus from this region might well have important effect on the reticular formation. Spinoreticular neurons selectively sensitive to noxious input may distribute their axons to specific groups of reticular cells, and this may be a determinant in pain behavior. Clearly, the interaction among the cells of the reticular formation is in need of greater definition and the work should be intensified in the field.

The identification of opiate receptors along the nervous pathways associated with pain certainly provides also a broader base for reinforcing the traditional viewpoint regarding pain mainly as a sensation. As several authors have noted, opiates can act both at the spinal and supraspinal levels to elevate the pain threshold by decreasing afferent input of nociceptive stimuli. However, opiates also alter reactive processes to pain, and these recent findings fortify the knowledge about the pathways that are involved. I am told that in clinical practice, pain relief can be achieved by stimulation of the spinal cord epidurally, and, likely this is owing to activation of a gating mechanism in the spinal cord. Moreover, it is well-established that aversive or similar pain-related behavior after a noxious stimulus can be modified by the limbic system and closely associated areas. The fact that opiate receptors have been localized in the medial thalamus, hypothalamus, and closely related sites lends further support for the existence of a special neural system for the modulation of pain.

Less clear is how opiates might be involved in the cognitive aspects of pain associated with the modulation of perception, evaluation, and affect that are defined by distinct physiologic and anatomic neural systems. There are in addition higher central control systems that can modulate sensory discriminative and aversive processes. Why does the amputee experience phantom pain? On the other hand, intense concentration, excitement, stress, etc. can reduce the pain experience. Also, it is recognized that patients with prefrontal lobotomy, while perceiving pain, no longer find the noxious input so bothersome and yet, sensory pathways have not been interrupted. In all likelihood, some of the effects of the opiates in affording pain relief can be associated with these phenomena. A better definition of the nervous pathways and receptor concerned with these processes remains a major goal to be attained. The increasing application of sophisticated techniques for intracellular recording and ultrastructural studies should facilitate the task.

Despite the gaps in the knowledge, the existence of at least three opiopeptin pathways is now well-accepted. There appears to be also non-endorphinergic pathways, which however, are in need of better definition (10). Their existence is based mainly on the fact that certain manipulations to produce analgesia do not yield effects that are alterable by naloxone or are only reduced in part by the antagonist. Non-neuronal pathways also contribute to modifying pain mechanism since adrenalectomy or hypophysectomy may increase sensitivity to opiates. However, the latter two manipulations do not necessarily exclude neuronal components since they do not alter foot shock induced analgesia (14).

Some of the new nonsteroidal analgetics, in addition to their anti-inflammatory properties, now approach opioids in effectiveness for relieving certain forms of pain, but there are still other types of pain that are not readily alleviated by either of these two anodyne types. My clinical colleagues inform me that it is difficult to achieve good pain relief with drugs in subjects with lesions in sensory pathways. Not always amenable to drug therapy is the paraplegic with burning pain in the leg owing to a spinal cord lesion; nor is the thalamic syndrome resulting from stroke or thrombus. Basbaum's explanation (chapter 4) that peripheral nerve damage results in significant degenerative changes of primary afferents within the spinal horn sounds plausible and provides a reasonable answer as to why treatment of peripheral neuralgia is often unsatisfactory. Progress in this area is hampered by the fact that it is extremely different to develop a suitable animal model for such conditions to assess drug affects. This remains a challenge for both basic and clinical investigators.

The fact that chronic pain is a major pressing problem that needs greater emphasis both in research and in treatment is becoming increasingly appreciated. The devastation that results from persistent recurring pain can not be minimized. Not only is there much agony and suffering for the subject and his family but the economic hardship can be severe. Bonica (1) estimates that the loss in workdays for disability headaches alone account for 124 million workdays at a cost of $1.2 billion, and when other pain states including those from musculoskeletal, orofacial, neurologic, and vascular origin, as well as from cancer are considered, the costs become staggering. Coupled with the emotional expense and impact on the subject and his family, the sociologic consequences can be overwhelming.

With respect to clinical applications of the nonsteroidal analgetics, the wide ranging effects of the prostaglandins on pain, inflammation, temperature, blood pressure, blood flow, and uterine activity indicate that different prostaglandins are involved in the regulation of these functions and that the balance between the different types is critical for normal function. The different prostaglandins may produce opposite effects and an imbalance results in abnormal regulation. Thus, it appears that therapeutic benefits with decreased adverse effects can be attained by the development of agents that selectively inhibit prostaglandin biosynthesis of pathologic but not of physiologic processes.

For the control of pain and inflammation, instead of seeking more potent inhibitors of the prostaglandin system, it appears more feasible to find agents that can selectively block the various pathways of arachadonic acid metabolism. To alleviate headaches and reduce inflammation, an agent that blocks only PGE_2 synthesis and not prostacyclin formation could eliminate the bleeding problems associated with aspirin. On the other hand, to prevent stroke or myocardial infarct, a useful compound would be one that acts specifically on thromboxane synthetase to prevent transformation of endoperoxides into thromboxane A_2, while not interfering with the ability of vascular endothelial cells to generate prostacyclin.

SERENDIPITY AND EXPLOITING ADVERSITY

Despite imaginative well-thought out approaches to provide solutions, the role of serendipity in contributing to major advances can not be ignored nor minimized. It has been an important factor in the innovation of new types of analgetic compounds and in promoting comprehension of the mechanisms involved in opiate action. How fortunate it has been that knowledgeable pharmacologists had the insight to exploit their chance observations.

To recapitulate some of the examples presented, in screening atropine congeners for antispasmodic properties, Schaumann had the perspicacity to test meperidine for analgetic properties after he noted that the compound produced the peculiar tail erection in mice similar to that of morphine (6). A well-designed study for the evaluation of a nalorphine-morphine combination by Lasagna and Beecher (8) unveiled the analgetic properties of nalorphine, and led not only to the development of potent mixed agonist-antagonist analgetics largely devoid of the respiratory depressant, tolerant and physical dependence producing properties of the morphine agonist type, but also to the discovery of an invaluable research tool, the pure antagonist, naloxone. Simple procedures for testing the dependence liability of opiate drugs and for assessing basic mechanisms in physical dependence resulted from the realization by Wikler et al. (15) that the acute explosive syndrome occurring from their attempts to antidote heroin overdosage in an addict was a precipitated abstinence-like phenomenon that could be the result of rapid displacement of the agonist from its receptors. After the discovery of a rabbit aorta contracting substance from the guinea pig lung, it was demonstrated to be on the metabolic pathway of prostaglandins. When aspirin was found to interfere with the release of both substances, the idea occurred to Vane that aspirin was interfering with the biologic generation of prostaglandin (11). Lady Luck, of course, is a perennial factor in discovery, but she will always favor the prepared mind. However, even with the dice loaded, the cast still has to be made and there can be no substitute for doing the experiment.

Although the primary purpose of this volume is to deal with basic and clinical pharmacologic perspectives in pain, we should not let our mission shut our eyes and ears to possible spin-offs. Agents that act to alleviate pain have other important effects that should not be overlooked and might be exploitable. As the role of the opiopeptins and the prostaglandins become increasingly clear, the knowledge almost surely will bring about novel and better application of pharmacologic agents that affect these systems. We have already alluded to how the understanding of the antiplatelet properties of aspirin led to its more careful application but also to its possible utility in myocardial infarction and stroke. In a similar vein, the widespread distribution of opioid receptors suggests that opiopeptins have peripheral as well as central functions.

Recent findings suggest that the opiopeptins may participate in the regulation of cardiovascular function and there is a growing number of publications implicating the opiopeptins in shock and trauma. The cardiovascular effects produced by the narcotic analgetics and the opiopeptins result from central as well as peripheral actions of these compounds. Holaday and his associates found that in experimental shock induced by endotoxin, hemorrhaging, hypoglycemia, or cervical spinal traumatization, the resulting cardiovascular collapse was alleviated by injection of naloxone (7). In addition, naloxone increased the incidence of survival of hypovolemic shock and accelerated the rate of recovery after spinal injury. Since the central injection of naloxone is highly effective in countering shock, it is likely that central as well as peripheral opiopeptinergic systems are involved.

It appears that opiopeptins are released during stress, and that the opiate antagonist must be blocking the specific opiate receptors activated. Some questions, however, remain unanswered: which of the natural opiopeptins is mobilized under these situations and where and how do they act? The involvement of the opiopeptins in the pathophysiology of shock, spinal trauma, and cerebral stroke needs clinical verification that antagonists benefit such conditions. Preliminary results to date appear encouraging.

With respect to the pathologic mental states, the role of the opiopeptins is less clear. Their discovery aroused the hope that they might find immediate application. In schizophrenia, two opposing hypotheses for its etiology evolved, one proposing hyperactivity and the other hypoactivity of the opiopeptinergic system. In both instances, despite the claims of success, the results have been disappointing. Although some of the symptoms of schizophrenia may have been alleviated by either approach, no dramatic reversal of the pathologic process was achieved.

The proponents who advocate that schizophrenia might be due to opiopeptinergic overactivity, maintain that naloxone is highly beneficial in relieving some of the symptoms of the disease but their results have been controversial. Even if the claims hold, the findings do not support a major role for opiopeptins as a causative factor in the disease and it does not appear hopeful that antagonists will have a major role in its treatment.

Investigators suggesting a deficient endorphinergic state in schizophrenia have reported beneficial effects after administering β-endorphin. Modest favorable findings have also been noted for the use of β-endorphin in endogenous depression. In view of the well-established actions of opiates on mood, such findings are hardly surprising. It would seem to us, however, that considering the prior usage of opiates for mood disorders, had opiates been truly of major benefit, prohibitive legalities notwithstanding, morphine would have been included in the physicians' armamentarium for such purposes.

Nonetheless, despite our skepticism, it may be worthwhile to remove prejudices against chronic usage of opiates because of their dependence liabilities and make more extensive assessments of opiates in schizophrenia. Even if the opiopeptins may not be directly involved in the etiology of the disease, such an approach does have some rationale, especially with the orally active longer-acting opiates such as methadone or 1-acetymethadol which have been studied fairly extensively for long-term toxicity. Opiates have been shown to have antidopaminergic effects but by a mode different from that of the phenothiazines, hence, the possible usefulness of a combination of two types of antidopaminergic agent should be examined with the modern evaluative methods that are now available. Finally, since it is now established that there are different types of opiate receptors, the question still remains as to whether opioid peptides other than β-endorphin might yield a more selective action in this condition or in other affective disorders.

COMPUTEROLOGY

The national research efforts on pain research will be greatly strengthened by national computer networks such as PROPHET which is increasingly being used for analyzing and sharing research data. To stimulate creativity and productivity, the programs are designed to provide researchers in academia, government, and industry with the opportunity to acquire the maximum available information in specific areas of interest. The cost of research is greatly reduced since the expense and effort of maintaining computer centers with programmers, statisticians, and maintenance personnel are shifted to a central facility. One of the programs of PROPHET enables pharmaceutical chemists to make correlations of molecular structure with pharmacologic activity.

By using computer graphic techniques to build visual models of compounds that have potential for application, the development of selectively acting peptides can be greatly facilitated. After creating images of molecules on a screen, the pharmaceutical chemists can then tailor drugs for specific purposes. With its memory for a vast store of facts, vivid graphics, and the ability for rapid calculation, the computer can diagram the receptor and a compound that fits to it. By looking at multidimensional data on computer screens and manipulating them to search for patterns, the complexities of drug-receptor interactions are more easily understood. This greatly facilitates further probing for agents that might have useful application, and thus, a potential drug can be designed on the screen before going into the laboratory.

As an example, an opiate analgetic might be designed without constipating properties by first visualizing the differences between the opiate receptors in the brain and intestine and then creating an agent that best fits the brain receptor and least fits the gut receptor. Such an approach may save time, energy, money, and promote greater creative interaction between chemists and pharmacologists. In addition to the computer techniques for conformational, structural, and configurational analysis of peptides, chiroptical analysis and X-ray structure studies combined with solid phase peptide synthesis should further enhance the development of tailor-made compounds. I foresee in the next decade the development of many active agonist and antagonist peptides, not only for the management of pain but also for the treatment of many other conditions.

In the final analysis, use of computer systems depends on their performance and their acceptability by researchers. Systems that rely on human mimicry are the most popular. Researchers are now programming computers with reasoning processes that mimic those of the human mind and can be explained by the computer in medical terms. But for the clinical assessment of pain, do not expect computers to do the entire job.

To remedy current deficiencies in the management of pain, proper communication is essential at all levels. This involves adequate orientation in the medical problems associated with pain in the curriculum for medical, dental, nursing, and pharmacy students and maintaining the education intensively for the practitioner on a continuing basis. In the treatment of the patient with severe pain, a holistic approach is, of course, essential but the advances from the experimental laboratory and the clinical must be appreciated. The major breakthroughs can only occur from the fundamental contribution emanating first from the experimental laboratory and this work can only flourish in an atmosphere that has economic, political, and philosophic support from an educated public at large.

REFERENCES

1. Bonica, J. (1981): Pain: Editorial. *Triangle*, 20:1–6.
2. Chapman, D. B., and Way, E. Leong (1980): Metal ion interaction with opiates. *Annu. Rev. Pharmacol. Toxicol.*, 20:553–579.
3. Chapman, D. B., and Way, E. Leong (1982): Pharmacologic consequences of calcium interactions

with opioid alkaloids and peptides. In: *Calcium Regulation and Drug Design*, ACS Symposium Series No. 201, edited by R. G. Rahivan and D. Witiak, pp. 119–142. Amer. Chem. Soc., Washington, D.C.

4. Cho, T. M., Yamato, C., and Loh, H. H. (1981): Isolation of an opiate receptor and the effect of membrane lipids on isolated receptor binding. In: *Advances in Endogenous and Exogenous Opioids*, edited by H. Takagi and E. J. Simon. Kodinsha Ltd., Tokyo.

5. Clouet, D. H., and Williams, N. (1981): In: *Advances in Endogenous and Exogenous Opioids. Proceedings of the International Narcotic Research Conference*, edited by H. Takagi and E. Simon. Kodansha Ltd., Tokyo.

6. Eisleb, O., and Schaumann, O. (1939): Dolantin ein neuratiges spasmolyticum und Analgeticum. *Dtsch. Med. Wochenschr.*, 65:967.

7. Holaday, J. W., and Faden, A. I. (1978): Naloxone reversal of endotoxin hypotension suggests role of endorphins in shock. *Nature*, 275:450.

8. Lasagna, L., and Beecher, H. K. (1954): The analgesic effectiveness of nalorphine and nalorphine-morphine combinations in man. *J. Pharmacol. Exp. Ther.*, 112:356.

9. Lee, N. M., Huidobro-Toro, J. P., Smith, A. P., and Loh, H. H. (1982): β-Endorphin receptor and its possible relationship to other opioid receptors. In: *Regulatory Peptides: From Molecular Biology to Function*, edited by E. Costa and M. Trabucchi, pp. 75–89. Raven Press, New York.

10. Loh, H. H., and Law, P. Y. (1980): The role of membrane lipids in receptor mechanism. *Annu. Rev. Pharmacol. Toxicol.*, 20:201–234.

11. Martin, W. R., Eades, C. G., Thompson, J. A., Huppler, R. E., and Gilbert, P. E. (1975): The effects of morphine and nalorphine-like drugs in the nondependent and morphine-dependent chronic spiral dog. *J. Pharmacol. Exp. Therap.*, 197:517.

12. Melzack, R., and Wall, P. D. (1965): Pain mechanisms: A new theory. *Science*, 150:971.

13. Vane, J. R. (1971): Inhibition of prostaglandin "synthesis" as a mechanism of action for aspirin-like drugs. *Nature New Biol.*, 231:235.

14. Watkins, L., and Mayer, D. J. (1982): Organization of endogenous opiate and nonopiate pain control systems. *Science*, 216:1185–1192.

15. Wikler, A., Fraser, H. F., and Isbell, H. (1953): N-allynormorphine: Effect of single doses and precipitation of acute abstinence syndromes during addiction to morphine methadine or heroin in man (post addicts). *J. Pharmacol. Exp. Ther.*, 109:8.

Subject Index

Subject Index

A

Acemetacin, 157
Acetaminophen (paracetamol),
    164,165,168,237,295–296
Acetylcholine, 216–217
Acupuncture analgesia, 112–113
Addiction risk, narcotic, 284
Adrenergic mechanisms, 214–215
Age, narcotics and, 273
D-ALA²-D-Leu-enkephalin (DADL), 75–
    76
N-Allylnorcodeine, 132–133
N-Allylnormetazocine (SKF 10,047)
    72,73,79,86–88
N-Allylnoroxymorphone, 133; *see also*
    Naloxone
Alpha-neoendorphin, 20
Amino-oxyacetic acid, 219
Aminopeptidase inhibitors, 22
Aminopeptidases, 22
4-Aminophenazone, 167
p-Aminophenol derivatives, 163
Aminopyrine, 238
Amphetamine, 237
Analgesics
    evaluation of in humans, 235–251
    exploiting adversity in, 327–329
    future vistas in, 313–330
    historical overview of, 1–8
    lessons from history of, 314
    ligands and, 316–317
    mechanisms of actions of, 320–324
    methodology for, 315–316
    novel, 187–188
    serendipity in, 327–329
    sources of variation in, 246–251
Angiotensin converting enzyme, 22–23
Animal models, 3,175–188,236–242; *see*
    also Experimental pain models
    chemical stimuli, 179–182
    chronic pain, 184
    criteria for analgesic testing, 178–179
    electrical stimulation, 183–184

hyperesthesia, 181–182
narcotic properties, 184–187
novel analgesics, 187–188
noxious heat stimuli, 182–183
pressure stimuli, 184
problem stated, 177–178
writhing assays, 179–181
Antihistamines, 307–308
Anti-inflammatory analgesics, 149–163;
    see also Nonsteroidal anti-
    inflammatory drugs
    applications of, 162–163
    characteristics of, 149–150
    duration and action of, 162
    pharmacodynamics of, 150–158
    pharmacokinetics of, 158–162
    side effects of, 156–158,160–162,163
Antipyretic analgesics, 149–163
    acidic, *see* Anti-inflammatory
        analgesics
    nonacidic, 163–168
Aryl-piperidines, 139–141
Ascending pain pathways, 108–110
Aspirin, 237–241,249,250,295–299
    pharmacokinetics of, 158
    pharmacology of, 297–298
    prostaglandins and, 314
    side effects of, 163
    toxicity of, 298–299
Aspirin asthma, 160
Autoreceptors, 217

B

Bacitracin, 22,30
Baclofen, 21,188,202,220
Beecher, Henry K., 1–8
Benorylate, 157
Benoxaprofen, 306
Benzoctadiene, 239
Benzomorphan, 84,137–139
Beta-ELI, 28
Beta-endorphin, 329
    distribution of, 11–12